TREATMENT PROCEDURES IN COMMUNICATIVE DISORDERS

TREATMENT PROCEDURES IN COMMUNICATIVE DISORDERS

Second Edition

M. N. Hegde, Ph.D.

pro·ed

8700 Shoal Creek Boulevard
Austin, Texas 78757

Printed in United States of America

Library of Congress Cataloging-in-Publication Data

Hegde, M. N. (Mahabalagiri N.), 1941–
2nd ed.
    p.   cm.
  Includes bibliographical references and indexes.
  ISBN 0–89079–563–0
1. Communicative disorders—Treatment. 2. Speech therapy.
1. Title.
  [DNLM: 1. Communicative Disorders—therapy. WL 340 H4621]
RC423.H383 1992
616.85′506—dc20
DNLM/DLC   92–3401
for Library of Congress   CIP

pro·ed

8700 Shoal Creek Boulevard
Austin, Texas 78757

2 3 4 5 6 7 8 9 10   98 97 96 95 94

To Prema and Manu

Contents

Preface

Since the first edition of *Treatment Procedures in Communicative Disorders* was published in 1985, many academic instructors and clinicians who have used the book have offered positive comments. The instructors and clinicians alike have welcomed the general approach taken in the book. They have reinforced my belief that empirically based treatment principles and procedures must continue to be explicated in our classrooms and clinics.

The book has been thoroughly revised for this second edition. The revision reflects changes in the discipline and feedback received from instructors, professionals, and students. Most chapters have been expanded with additional examples and explanations to clarify the concepts and procedures.

Chapter 8 on decreasing undesirable behaviors has been totally rewritten. It takes a different outlook on the behavioral procedures of response reduction. It reevaluates the concept of punishment, and provides a better framework for understanding and implementing response reduction procedures. The chapter includes recent research on the development of nonaversive methods of response reduction.

A new chapter (9) on working with families has been written for the second edition. This chapter summarizes a few basic concepts about counseling and focuses on problems and methods of working with persons associated with clients in their natural settings. The new chapter is consistent with the growing recognition in the field that treatment of communicative disorders involves much more than working with clients in a small treatment room. The chapter is based on the assumption that, unless clinicians work closely with people surrounding clients, the ultimate success of treatment may not be assured.

I would like to thank many instructors and professionals who have used this book and have offered constructive comments. Also, I am grateful to many students who have offered me a variety of comments. These comments have been valuable in revising the book.

Introduction

This book is written for practicing speech–language pathologists and student clinicians in training programs. The main focus of the book is the treatment principles and procedures used in treating communicative disorders. Generally, treatment of different disorders is considered separately, with the implication that each disorder is treated uniquely. The approach taken in this book, however, is that certain treatment principles and procedures can be applied to all types of communicative disorders. This is not to suggest that the uniqueness of individuals or disorders should be ignored. To the contrary, the treatment model presented in this book seeks to clarify the issue of commonality and uniqueness. It is suggested that treatment principles are based on generality and procedures on uniqueness.

This book presents an integrated model of treatment in a single source. The model has empirical bases, but it is not theoretical. A major purpose I had in writing this book is to describe techniques that clinicians can use in treating clients on a day-to-day basis. At the same time, I have made every effort to put the practical treatment procedures in the context of broader and empirically based scientific principles. I believe that speech–language pathology, which is trying to broaden its scientific bases, cannot afford to take a cookbook approach to treatment. Nor can it afford to base treatment procedures upon rational arguments and logical assumptions that are not supported empirically.

The book emphasizes clinician accountability in both legal and scientific terms. Practical methods of documenting effectiveness of treatment and improvement in client behaviors are described. Strategies for documenting treatment effectiveness in individual clients without the aid of complex statistical techniques are summarized. It is well known that clinician accountability depends upon the measurement of client behaviors. Therefore, objective and verifiable procedures of measurement are described and emphasized throughout the book.

There are common principles of selecting target behaviors for training. These principles, along with suggestions on how to select multiple target behaviors, are offered. The importance of selecting target behaviors from the standpoint of long-term maintenance is pointed out.

In the final analysis, a clinician's task is to increase certain desirable communicative behaviors in clients, while decreasing certain undesirable and interfering behaviors. Therefore, in two chapters, basic techniques of increasing a variety of communicative behaviors and of decreasing undesirable behaviors are specified. In a later chapter, a method for writing comprehensive treatment programs for clients with speech and language problems is described. In addition, the reasons for and procedures of making changes in written treatment programs are specified.

A significant clinical problem is the sequencing of treatment. A good program may be ineffective simply because of inappropriate sequencing of target behaviors. Before being taught, many target behaviors must be simplified by isolating their smaller components that may be learned somewhat easily. Subsequently, the learned components must be integrated into the final target behavior. This is shaping. Most clients need such additional procedures as modeling, instruction, prompting, and manual guidance. All of these techniques are described with examples.

A major challenge faced by clinicians today is the maintenance of clinically established behaviors. This challenge is described as "problems of generalization." It is possible, however, that the concepts and techniques associated with the term *generalization* are not appropriate for the clinical purposes of response maintenance. Some of these conceptual and methodological problems are discussed, along with several techniques designed to achieve response maintenance.

I hope that both practicing and student clinicians will find this book useful in planning and executing treatment programs for their clients. I also hope that the book will help clinicians plan treatment programs on the basis of scientific and professional principles. These principles are a basis for designing flexible treatment programs that can be modified to suit individual clients with a variety of communicative disorders. The principles and procedures described in the book seek to fulfill legal, professional, and scientific demands made on the profession.

1

A Treatment Paradigm for Communicative Disorders

- Treatment principles and procedures
- A treatment paradigm for communicative disorders
- Treatment targets versus treatment procedures
- Treatment programs and treatment variables
- A definition of treatment
- Some legal considerations

Discussions of treatment techniques in communicative disorders tend to be disorder specific. Most textbooks typically separate descriptions of the treatment of different communicative disorders. Clinicians who seek information on treatment procedures also tend to be concerned with specific disorders. Beginning clinicians believe that each disorder of communication is treated with a unique technique. Such a belief is understandable in light of the way most university curricula are organized. Students typically take separate courses on such disorders as language, articulation, or stuttering. Each academic course necessarily focuses upon the unique characteristics of a given disorder, and the treatment procedures offered in such courses tend to focus upon the unique aspects of treating a given disorder.

The belief that different disorders are treated differently may be further strengthened by the medical model that is often used in describing and assessing communicative disorders. According to this model, disorders are described under "diagnostic categories." In the assessment of communicative disorders, much emphasis is placed upon "differential diagnosis." In medicine, treatment is typically directed toward the *original* cause of physical diseases. Therefore, diagnosis, which is the detection of the causes of particular diseases, is especially important. When different causes are determined for different disorders, the disorders are treated differently.

An uncritical application of this model to the assessment and treatment of communicative disorders can create the impression that totally unique procedures are used to treat each speech and language problem. In communicative disorders, differential diagnosis often amounts to differential *descriptions* of disorders, not the detection of different causes. Furthermore, a disorder is a description of a client's behaviors. For example, a disorder of articulation may be described in terms of the production of various speech sounds, whereas stuttering may be described in terms of dysfluency forms and frequencies. Similarly, descriptions of language problems differ from those of voice problems.

Although most communicative disorders take different response forms, their treatment procedures share common features. A closer examination of treatment procedures applied to various disorders of communication reveals many common treatment elements. At the same time, the treatment of given individuals and disorders may include some unique features. Before the treatment aspects that are common across disorders and clients and those that are unique can be clarified, a distinction must be made between treatment principles and treatment procedures.

TREATMENT PRINCIPLES AND PROCEDURES

Both clinical and nonclinical behavioral research has shown that individuals with disorders share common characteristics while being unique in many other respects. Commonality exists because of similarities between disorders and people who exhibit them. Uniqueness exists because of special response characteristics of given disorders and unusual histories of individual clients.

Some unique aspects of treatment are based on the special response characteristics of particular disorders. For instance, techniques designed to evoke the correct production of /s/ are different from those evoking the preposition *on*. However, the differences are not absolute. Different response evocation techniques share common elements. For example, modeling or verbal instructions may be common across techniques.

It is generally believed that the uniqueness of treatment procedures stems from differential diagnosis of various disorders. A more important reason for some unique aspects of treatment may be that each individual is unique. Therefore, different procedures may be necessary in treating the same disorder across individuals. For example, all clients with a specific language disorder may not react positively to the same type of stimuli or consequences. Similarly, all persons who stutter may not react the same way to the same reinforcers. Thus, some unique aspects of treatment are a result of the unusual personal histories clients bring into the training situation.

Commonality and uniqueness are both real. In essence, the basic principles of treatment are common, whereas certain specifics of treatment procedures may be unique to disorders, clients, or both. **Treatment principles** are defined as empirical rules from which treatment procedures are derived. A clinician who knows a principle can derive a variety of procedures from it. Treatment principles are products of controlled experimental research.

Ideally, the principles should be based on replicated research with a certain degree of generality. This means that the data on which the principles are based are repeatedly shown to be valid and that they apply to a wide set of conditions and clients. Therefore, accepted principles should be reliable, valid, and comprehensive. When such principles are formulated, it should be possible to derive different treatment procedures from them. These procedures can then be used with different disorders and clients, and in different situations.

Treatment procedures can be defined as the technical operations the clinician performs to effect changes in the client behaviors. Treatment procedures refer to actions of clinicians. These actions induce changes in a client's communicative behaviors. In a later section, it will be shown that most clinician actions are typically performed before and after a client's attempted response.

Broad Principles and Specific Procedures

While treatment principles are broad and general, treatment procedures are specific to a given disorder or client. For example, the statement that certain consequences, when made contingent upon a behavior, increase the rate of that behavior is a principle. It is the well-known principle of positive reinforcement. There is enough empirical evidence to suggest that the principle applies to different people, different age groups, and even members of different species. Because the principle has some generality, it amounts to an empirical rule.

In applying the principle of positive reinforcement, the clinician must derive some specific procedures that suit the individual client, the disorder being treated, or both. The principle does not specify what particular thing or event will reinforce a given response in a given client; that is a matter of particular procedures that the clinician must determine. For example, a clinician might find that one client correctly produces /s/ when reinforced by verbal praise, whereas another client requires tokens backed up by 2 minutes of play activity. Each case illustrates a client-specific procedure of treatment derived from the principle of positive reinforcement.

In addition to the principle of positive reinforcement, there are such treatment principles as negative reinforcement, response reduction, punishment, discrimination, differential reinforcement, generalization, and stimulus control. Most of these principles are based on extensive laboratory research across species.

In applied behavioral analysis, these principles have been shown to be reliable and valid. In communicative disorders, many successful treatment procedures have been derived from these and other principles. In later chapters, each of these principles is described and several procedures derived from them are illustrated.

Fewer Principles, Many Procedures

Many treatment procedures may be derived from a single treatment principle. The principle of positive reinforcement, for example, has given rise to several specific reinforcement procedures, including primary reinforcers, verbal reinforcers, conditioned generalized reinforcers, and informative feedback. Similarly, the principles of punishment and extinction have generated multiple procedures to achieve reductions in response rates. Therefore, there are fewer principles and many procedures.

It is important that a clinician understands treatment principles to avoid searching for procedures every time a new client is encountered. A distinction between a professional and a technician may be made on this basis: A professional understands the principles, whereas a technician understands only the procedures that were presented to him or her.

Without an understanding of abstract treatment principles, clinicians would be baffled by new clients, disorders, and clinical settings. With an understanding of treatment principles, clinicians can design flexible treatment plans.

Procedures without principles can be rigid prescriptions that are hard to modify to suit individual clients or disorders. Such procedures are often a part of "cookbooks" of treatment. A professional discipline cannot make significant progress without underlying treatment principles that are based upon experimental evidence.

Abstract Principles, Concrete Procedures

Another distinction between treatment principles and procedures is that the former are abstract and conceptual, whereas the latter are concrete, practical, and measurable. As such, principles are the abstract conceptual bases of practical and concrete treatment techniques. Fully validated principles are summary statements of experimental evidence. The principles describe relations between events using abstract statements based on experimental evidence. For example, the principle of response reduction (punishment) is based on results of many experiments involving different kinds of stimuli, intensities of those stimuli, correlation of those stimuli with other kinds of stimuli, manner of their introduction, and so on. These various experimental observations are abstracted into the principle of response reduction, which simply states that certain stimulus events, when made contingent upon a response, can decrease the rate of that response.

An abstract principle suggests practical methods that can be applied in treatment. In deriving procedures from a principle, the clinician often has to examine the specific experimental manipulations on which the principle was based. In the example of the response reduction principle, the clinician may have to review particular kinds of stimuli that were used in the original experiments to identify tentative stimuli that may reduce behaviors.

Unlike treatment principles, the procedures are specified in operational (measurable) terms. Unless the procedures specify what the clinician should do, they cannot be used in treatment. Procedures that are not concrete cannot be replicated by other clinicians. Operationally defined procedures make it possible to measure the effectiveness of treatment, and thereby document clinician accountability.

A TREATMENT PARADIGM FOR COMMUNICATIVE DISORDERS

A **treatment paradigm** may be defined as an overall philosophy of treatment. In this book, treatment paradigm means a philosophy or view of treatment based on controlled and replicated research. The paradigm is based on certain concepts and leads to several procedures.

The Conceptual Bases of the Paradigm

The paradigm presented in this book is based on the concept that, for the most part, the behaviors with which the communicative disorders specialist deals are due to certain contingencies. A **contingency** describes an interdependent relation between certain events, often called variables or factors. In this relation, each event influences the other.

Two kinds of contingencies help create and maintain communicative behaviors. One involves genetic and neurophysiologic variables, and the other involves environmental variables. Thus, both neurophysiologic or genetic variables and environmental variables are causes of behaviors, including communicative behaviors. More importantly, the two sets of variables are interdependent, creating a complex contingency. According to the paradigm, practically all human behaviors, including communicative behaviors and disorders, are determined by this complex contingency.

Research into neurophysiologic or genetic contingencies that partially control communicative behaviors and disorders has become more sophisticated in recent years. Many genetic syndromes that are associated with communicative disorders have been described (Jung, 1989), and it is well known that an intact neurophysiologic mechanism is necessary for the normal acquisition of speech and language behaviors. Differences in the organization or functioning of neurophysiologic mechanisms can affect the way communicative behaviors are acquired or maintained. Neurophysiologic and genetic factors may restrict the rate or scope of improvement that can be obtained by treatment. They also may partly determine the amount or type of treatment needed.

Sophisticated research on how genetic or neurophysiologic mechanisms affect treatment considerations has barely begun, however. Although much of the available genetic and neurophysiologic information concerning communicative disorders may be used to counsel clients and their families, the information cannot be effectively used in the treatment process. In the near future, researchers may learn more about integrating this type of information with treatment considerations.

Manipulable Environmental Contingencies

In the treatment of communicative disorders, environmental contingencies can be manipulated more successfully than organic (neurophysiologic) contingencies. This means that clinicians can teach communicative behaviors, but they cannot change a client's genes or neurophysiology. This is also true of those communicative disorders that are described as neurologically or organically based. In dealing with either a patient with aphasia or a child with surgically repaired cleft, the task of the speech–language clinician is to modify the client's communicative behaviors using environmental manipulations. Currently, clinicians do not have direct access to those organic contingencies that create disorders of communication. For example, various genetic conditions associated with syndromes of language disorders cannot be altered directly. Similarly, brain damage that results from a cerebrovascular accident cannot be altered to eliminate aphasia.

The medical profession handles organic conditions that can be manipulated (e.g., the surgical repair of cleft palate). However, such manipulations are usually not sufficient to fully alter the communicative disorders associated with the original organic deficit. Following the organic manipulations, the speech–language clinician has to modify the communicative behaviors. The techniques available to the clinician for doing so are typically environmental. The procedures the clinician uses in treating the communicative disorders of individuals with aphasia, dysarthria, apraxia, and other neurological deficits also are environmental manipulations. Similarly, education and rehabilitation of hearing impaired individuals involves environmental manipulations.

Because the manipulable environmental contingencies are treatment procedures, clinicians need to understand the nature of such contingencies. Environmental contingencies can be defined as three sets of interdependent variables that correspond to antecedent events (stimuli), responses, and consequences. After identifying target behaviors for a client, the clinician usually arranges certain stimulus conditions for those behaviors. The clinician may select pictures, real objects, and questions that might evoke the responses. The clinician might plan on modeling the target behaviors so that the client can imitate them. Later in the training sequence, the clinician may use prompts to evoke the correct responses from the client. All of these stimulus conditions are *antecedents* of target behaviors because they are presented *before* the responses are expected.

Typically, the correct responses expected of the client are predetermined. Modeling the correct response is a way of specifying the form of an acceptable response. When the client responds to the stimuli presented (including modeling), the clinician usually judges whether the response is acceptable. If it is, the clinician responds in one manner, and if it is not, in a different manner. If the client does not respond at all, the clinician might react still differently. These clinician reactions are the consequences of the client behaviors. Some kinds of consequences create new behaviors or increase the frequency of current behaviors, whereas others make existing behaviors less probable in the future.

All of the client and the clinician behaviors form a contingency. The clinician behaviors affect what the client does, and the client behaviors determine the consequences, which are the clinician responses. In essence, the stimulus conditions, the client response characteristics, and the consequences the clinician arranges for those responses are the three interrelated variables in a contingency.

Based on the Concepts and Methods of Science

Another conceptual basis of the treatment paradigm is the philosophy of science. The paradigm dictates that all concepts and procedures used within its scope be empirically validated. There is very little room for clinical or theoretical speculation. Speculative concepts are rarely of much help to a practicing clinician. It is difficult to base effective treatment procedures on a paradigm that simply makes assumptions about the disorders that need to be treated. To be useful, the treatment paradigm should stay close to empirical evidence. Cause–effect relations must be demonstrated, not merely assumed. They should be demonstrated through experimental research in which the causal variables were actually manipulated by the researcher. This type of research is more fully described in Chapter 3.

Many of the clinical controversies and apparent treatment diversities are due to the predominance of nonexperimental research in communicative disorders. Nonexperimental research tends to encourage theoretical speculation, which in turn leads to fruitless controversies. Researchers may offer untested treatment procedures, and clinicians may vigorously advocate them. Often, treatment procedures are offered by pure theoreticians (e.g., in linguistics) who may not have an opportunity to verify their own suggestions. Although such clinical procedures or suggestions for treatment are not experimentally verified, they may stay on the books for years confusing clinicians.

The Procedural Bases of the Paradigm

The treatment paradigm offered in this book leads to procedures that can be readily applied in the treatment of communicative disorders. Ideally, treatment procedures should be objective, measurable, replicable, and empirical. Methods that help document the effectiveness of treatment should be a part of the procedures. These requirements stem from scientific, legal, and social considerations.

Response Rates as Target Behaviors

The paradigm suggests that the treatment targets should be observable rates of client responses. Client responses are also known as the dependent variables, and when they are observable behaviors, they can be verified by other clinicians. Communicative behaviors are most observable when described as response rates of speakers. The speaking behaviors can be broken down into specific responses that can be counted in real numbers. For example, clinicians can specify in actual numbers how many times a client produced a phoneme, grammatic morpheme, pragmatic language feature, or certain vocal behavior in a 10-minute conversational speech. Similarly, clinicians can measure the number of words or parts of words repeated, the duration for which a given vocal pitch was sustained, or the number of manual signs a person who is deaf produced.

Clinicians often have used measures other than the rate of responses. Rating scales are an excellent example of popular measures not based on real numbers. Disorders may be rated as *mild, moderate,* or *severe,* or assigned a number such as 3, 5, and 7. Such ratings may be considered "measurement" of communicative behaviors; however, such rating scales offer no direct and meaningful measures of specific behaviors. Based on a scale, the clinician would not know the actual number of times a given behavior was produced. Instead of saying that a person was a "severe" stutterer with a rating scale value of 7, the clinician would be more precise to say that the person exhibited dysfluencies or stutterings on 13% (or whatever) of the words spoken. The reader then can make his or her own judgments regarding the "severity" based upon the reported percentage of stuttering.

Rate of responses, measured in real numbers, can make it possible for other observers to verify treatment gains or changes in client behaviors. Other observers can count the same behaviors in the same client and see if their values agree with the clinician's values. Objectivity in clinical activity is achieved when a given clinician's measures can be verified by other clinicians.

Mere agreement among observers when no measurements are taken is no indication of objectivity. Different clinicians may hold the same opinion about a disorder and may believe in a certain treatment approach; however, if these opinions and beliefs are not supported by experimental data, such agreements do not constitute objectivity. Popular consensus should not be confused with agreement based on objective measurement and evidence.

Communicative behaviors described in terms of presumed mental, cognitive, or neurophysiologic processes are hard to measure. Such internal processes presumed to take place within individuals are theoretically based and are often not observed directly. For example, one might define a target behavior in a language training program either as linguistic competence or as production of specified grammatic morphemes, or vocabulary items (words). Linguistic competence is an inferred entity, whereas the production of grammatic morphemes or words is observable. In Chapter 3, selection and definition of target behaviors are described more fully.

Measurable Treatment Procedures

The paradigm also suggests that treatment procedures should be replicable. A treatment program is replicated when it gives similar results when used with new clients, in new settings, and by various clinicians. When such replications yield comparable and favorable results, the treatment technique is said to have generality. Techniques that have generality may be recommended for general use.

Treatment techniques described in vague and nonmeasurable terms do not lend themselves to replication. If it is not clear how a given technique was used, then it cannot be repeated.

Logical Versus Empirical Validity

Finally, the paradigm suggests that the treatment procedures should be empirical, in the sense that their effects are demonstrated, not merely supposed. When clinicians read about different treatment techniques that often conflict with each other, they may find them equally appealing, rational, and plausible. Most treatment procedures do appear logical. However, the clinician needs to distinguish between logical and empirical validity. What is logically valid may or may not be empirically valid, although empirical validity usually assures logical validity.

Statements that are mutually consistent and do not violate rules of logic have **logical validity**. However, those statements may turn out to be invalid in experience or when put to experimental test. For example, there is nothing illogical in the suggestion that lack of parental affection causes language delay in a child, or that psychosexual repressions and regressions result in stuttering. However, when parents show affection in the absence of verbal exchange, the child may not learn language, thus showing that the logical suggestion did not have empirical validity. Similarly, a treatment based exclusively on the theory of psychosexual aberrations may not reduce stuttering.

Clinicians need procedures that go beyond logical validity to **empirical validity**, which means that the procedures are experimentally demonstrated to be effective. Empirical validity refers to credibility or truthfulness of statements or procedures.

In speech–language pathology, "new" treatment programs are sometimes offered simply on the basis of logical validity. As pointed out earlier, if research clinicians refrain from offering treatment suggestions that are not experimentally verified, much controversy and confusion can be avoided.

TREATMENT TARGETS VERSUS TREATMENT PROCEDURES

In clinical literature, there is sometimes a confusion between treatment targets and treatment techniques. Although a comprehensive treatment program includes a description of both, it is necessary to distinguish treatment targets from procedures. That distinction has conceptual and technical significance.

Treatment targets are client behaviors, whereas **procedures** are mostly clinician behaviors. What the client is expected to do is the target, and what the clinician does is the treatment. This simple and rather obvious rule is sometimes violated when treatment techniques are confused with target behaviors.

In communicative disorders, examples of confusion between treatment targets and procedures abound. For example, a stuttering treatment may be described as the "airflow" technique, or a new language treatment may be described as "cognitive reorganization." Actually, however, "airflow" refers to what the stutterer is expected to do, and hence is a treatment target, not a procedure. The treatment procedure would be the actions of the clinician that are necessary to teach appropriate airflow management. Likewise, cognitive reorganization is not what the clinician does; it is what is presumed to take place within the client. The treatment would be the procedures by which cognitive reorganization is achieved, if at all. Similarly, in the area of articulation, "phonologic rules" do not refer to treatment procedures. Such rules are simply supposed to underlie observed regularities in response patterns. How such rules are taught (if they are) might constitute a treatment technique.

Perhaps not as many treatment procedures exist as may be supposed. Some descriptions of presumed treatment procedures may simply be descriptions of different target behaviors. Certain target behaviors may be more useful than others in that some may improve the overall communicative skills better than others do. It is therefore natural that clinicians keep looking for new target behaviors that are effective in improving the quality of their clients' verbal behavior. New treatment techniques are not necessarily being invented at the same time, however.

Theoretical shifts in language and articulation illustrate how target behavior changes have masqueraded as new treatment procedures. During the early days of language intervention, clinicians often focused exclusively upon vocabulary training. Subsequently, the emphasis was shifted to the training of various syntactic and morphologic aspects of language. Later, for a brief period of time, the emphasis was on training semantic notions. More recently, clinicians have been asked to train pragmatic functions or rules. In the treatment of articulation disorders, emphasis has shifted from single-phoneme training to distinctive features, and again to phonologic rules or processes.

While the answer to the question "what to train" to persons with language or articulation problems was being shifted around, new treatment procedures were rarely invented. Different methods of analysis or viewpoints did not produce new language or articulation treatment procedures. What were new at any given time were the target behaviors, or perhaps a new terminology to describe the old target behaviors. New procedures to train those new or redefined behaviors were rarely presented. Typically, the question of how to train those behaviors was not addressed at all. Therefore, such descriptions as "phonological process treatment," "distinctive feature treatment," or "pragmatic language therapy" are as inappropriate as "rate reduction treatment," "syllable prolongation treatment," or "airflow treatment."

Lack of a clear distinction between target behaviors and treatment procedures may be responsible for poor descriptions of treatment techniques in many treatment programs. Apparently, many clinicians assume that when they describe a new treatment target, they have automatically suggested a new treatment procedure. Much worse, some clinicians do not describe their treatment procedure at all; they describe only their target behaviors.

As indicated earlier, a treatment technique should specify what the clinician ought to do to achieve the treatment target. When this is done, what emerges is a description of the stimulus conditions the clinician needs to arrange, and the kinds of feedback that must be provided to the client under the differing conditions of correct, incorrect, and lack of responses. Such a description also clarifies the contingency between stimulus conditions, responses, and consequences that follow those responses. The treatment paradigm described in this book suggests that contingencies are the treatment variables in communicative disorders. Those contingencies can be placed upon any kind of empirically valid target behavior.

TREATMENT PROGRAMS AND TREATMENT VARIABLES

The term **treatment program**, as used in this book, is an overall description of target behaviors, treatment variables, measurement procedures, generalization measures, maintenance strategies, parent training and counseling, follow-up, booster treatment, and so on. As such, a program is a comprehensive plan of action that includes different kinds of clinical activities designed to achieve certain overall objectives. A treatment program describes all of the clinician and client behaviors.

Treatment variables refer only to technical operations performed by the clinician to induce, increase, reduce, or eliminate certain client behaviors. Treatment variables are also called **independent variables**, which may include certain stimulus manipulations, such as modeling. More importantly, they include consequences programmed for target behaviors. The clinician's actions that follow a client's production of a correct or incorrect response are the programmed consequences. Therefore, only a portion of a treatment program is concerned with treatment variables. In this book, such terms as *treatment variables, treatment techniques, training procedures,* and *teaching methods* refer to the manipulations of independent variables, including stimulus conditions and response consequences. These manipulations are done by the clinician or the educator. The term *treatment program*, on the other hand, is used in the broader sense to include an overall clinical or educational strategy.

A DEFINITION OF TREATMENT

The meaning of the term *treatment* is not restricted to its typical medical connotations. The term, as used in this book, includes teaching, training, any type of remedial or rehabilitative work, and all attempts at helping people by changing their behaviors or teaching new skills. The essence of treating or teaching is to change a person. However, treatment also may be defined in a larger sense.

Historically, treatment in communicative disorders was somewhat narrowly thought of as working in clinical or educational settings with adults and children who have various speech, language, and hearing problems. It has become increasingly clear, however, that treatment work restricted to professional settings and the client, although still necessary, is insufficient.

Clinicians have repeatedly discovered that skills taught in the professional setting involving only themselves and their clients are not readily produced and maintained in natural settings. This problem of maintenance, discussed further in Chapter 7, has created a need for a redefinition of treatment. The various concepts and distinctions described thus far contribute to a more comprehensive definition of treatment that particularly suits the work of the specialist in communicative disorders.

Communication is social action and interaction, which involves other people. Similarly, disorders of communication involve other people, not only the client. Although neither communication nor its disorders typically involve the clinician, treatment is usually restricted to the client and the clinician. In restricting treatment to themselves and their clients in professional settings, clinicians may have violated the essence of communication itself. Therefore, to remediate disorders of communication, the clinician or the educator must broaden both the scope of treatment and its setting. The focus of treatment should be social action and interaction.

Treatment in communicative disorders may be defined as a rearrangement of relations between speakers and their environment (Hegde, 1988). The most important feature of this environment is the people who interact with the client. Therefore, in treating communicative disorders, the clinician rearranges social relations between speakers and listeners. In this definition of treatment, the focus is on interactions that take place in natural settings with people other than the clinician.

Traditionally, the clinician is the sole audience for the newly acquired communicative behaviors. Clinically established communication, such as it is, is limited to a small, controlled, nonsocial treatment room. People normally involved in communication with the client are not a part of this treatment. Because the clinician is not a part of the client's family and social environment, newly acquired communicative behaviors are restricted to the clinical setting. To extend these behaviors to natural settings, the clinician should include in the treatment process those people who typically interact with the client.

In the initial stages of treatment, it may be efficient for clinicians to establish behaviors in a restricted setting, involving only themselves and their clients. But soon the clinicians should involve other persons and expand the treatment setting to make it more naturalistic. When others are involved, treatment becomes a rearrangement of communicative relations between the client and the people with whom he or she interacts. In this view of treatment, a new pattern of interaction emerges.

This new pattern can result only when the client and the people with whom the client interacts are both changed by the treatment. Because of this change, people in the client's life behave differently toward the client. Before the treatment, people may have behaved in such a way as not to support appropriate communicative behaviors. Their actions may have supported the problematic communicative behaviors. When treatment changes this and the people acquire new behavior patterns, the client's newly learned behaviors may be better supported than before treatment. Thus, clinicians treat both the client and the people surrounding the client. This concept of treatment is discussed further in Chapters 7 and 9.

SOME LEGAL CONSIDERATIONS

In public schools, specialists in communicative disorders are a part of special educational services. During recent years, various laws passed by the United States Congress have had a significant impact on the delivery of special educational programs, including speech, language, and hearing services in public schools. Public Law (PL) 94-142, called the Education for all Handicapped Children's Act (EHA), was signed into law in 1975 and went into effect in three stages starting in October 1977. The law mandated clinical and educational services to school-age children who needed them. During its first phase, the law required that each state government begin the development of a comprehensive program for the education of all children with handicaps. Perhaps the most important requirement under the law was that an Individualized Education Program (IEP) be developed for each child in need of special educational services. In addition, the law required that the rights and the confidentiality of the child and the family be protected, and that the parents be involved in implementing the special educational programs designed for their children.

During the second phase, which went into effect in 1978, the law was extended to cover all children with handicaps between 3 and 18 years of age. It required each state government to submit revised annual plans specifying its special educational programs. The last phase, which went into effect in 1980, extended the age range to 21 years.

In general, the law specifies that each child with handicaps initially must be assessed to determine the type and extent of the problem. The assessment should include multiple and nondiscriminatory tools. Each child should have access to free and public education designed to suit his or her special needs. Each child should be placed in the least restrictive environment and, whenever possible, should be mainstreamed. Finally, needed supplementary services should be provided.

Several amendments have been made to the EHA. The 1986 amendment, PL 99-457, requires that services be offered to infants and toddlers (birth through 2 years). The amendment requires that for each infant or toddler with a disability, the special education specialists develop an Individualized Family Service Plan (IFSP), sometimes referred to as Individual Family Support Plan. This law also requires that children with disabilities in the age range of 3 to 5 years receive services comparable to those received by school-age children. When the provisions of EHA were reauthorized in 1990, the name of the law was changed to the Individuals with Disabilities Education Act (IDEA).

Besides federal laws, various state laws and regulations affect special education services, including those of specialists in communicative disorders. In addition, school districts formulate policies and guidelines within the scope of the various laws. It is not the purpose of this chapter to review the full scope of various laws, regulations, and local guidelines that affect communicative disorders. The reader should consult other sources (e.g., American Speech–Language–Hearing Association [ASHA] Congressional Relations Division, Government Affairs Department, 1989; ASHA Government Affairs Review, 1990; Arena, 1978; Lerner, Dawson, & Horvath, 1980; McCormick & Schiefelbusch, 1990) and policies of specific school districts.

In developing clinical speech, language, and hearing programs for school-age children, IEP guidelines are important. In essence, an IEP describes an educational program specific to a given child. Based on the assessment results, the IEP contains statements concerning the child's current communicative behaviors. It then specifies the target behaviors in operational terms, the procedures to achieve them, the program's initiation date, the program's predicted duration, and the objective criteria to be used in judging the program's success. How often the evaluative criteria will be applied should also be specified. Under the law, the effects of the program should be evaluated at least once a year. The entire program should be developed as a team effort involving the educational agency, teachers, parents, and other professionals. Whenever needed and considered appropriate, the child may also participate in the process of developing an IEP.

PL 99-457, which requires the IFSP for infants and toddlers, places a special emphasis on involving the family members, especially the parents, in developing and implementing special educational services. An IFSP includes an analysis of the strengths and needs of the family that might affect the infant's development. Therefore, an IFSP describes not only the special educational services an infant or toddler needs, but also the social services the family members may need. The objectives of an IFSP must be reviewed every 6 months. A case manager is responsible for coordinating services offered to the infant and the family.

Although an IEP and an IFSP are required under the law, they are not legal contracts. The development of special educational and family services remains a scientific and professional task. The clinician working in the public schools is certainly bound by the requirements of the law. But it is a mistake to think that what the law requires is merely a matter of governmental and administrative bureaucracy, which it often is. Many of the requirements of the law are also the requirements of science. Therefore, the professional requirements of the laws are relevant to any professional setting.

The laws are expected to make effective and appropriate services available to children and their families; however, the laws do not remove the aspect of clinical judgment based upon scientific facts and observations. Selection of target behaviors, development of treatment procedures, documentation of the effectiveness of treatment or changes in client behaviors, and specification of evaluative criteria are all matters of scientific and professional judgment. For example, when a child's treatment program will be terminated is stated not in terms of certainty, but in terms of probability, which reflects the best clinical judgment. It is a scientific statement, not a legal promise. When the child will complete the program depends upon many uncontrolled factors, including the child's rate of learning, family's cooperation, frequency and duration of treatment sessions, and severity of the disorder being treated. The treatment program will be terminated only when the target behaviors are learned and maintained.

It is often thought that one of the most important effects of the laws is to make clinicians more accountable. This means that clinicians must objectively demonstrate that the client behaviors showed systematic and positive changes under the treatment program. Subjective statements such as "the child has improved tremendously" or "the child has benefited from the services" are not acceptable when they are not substantiated by objective data. In addition, the target behaviors must be defined in measurable terms, so that changes in the frequency of those behaviors can be documented. It should be noted, however, that the need for legal mandates in matters such as these is somewhat ironic. Science has always required that the target behaviors be measurable, the procedures be specific to the client, and the treatment effects be measured in terms of changes in the frequency of those behaviors. Scientifically oriented clinicians have always done these things, but unfortunately, not all clinicians in the past based their clinical methods on scientific principles.

The experimentally based treatment paradigm presented in this chapter, and elaborated on throughout the book, antedates the legal requirements but is in full compliance with them. The treatment paradigm considers each individual as unique and requires that the individual behaviors be objectively measured. There is little emphasis on evaluating the individual's behaviors in relation to some group performance. The paradigm suggests that the target behaviors selected for clinical training be appropriate and useful to the particular client. It requires that the treatment procedure be described in objective and specific terms so that it can be replicated by other clinicians. There is a great deal of emphasis on documenting the treatment effectiveness. In the coming chapters, many of these issues and procedures are discussed in some detail.

SUMMARY

Some aspects of treatment are common across disorders and clients, and some are unique. The treatment principles are common, whereas certain procedures may be unique.

Treatment principles are data-based empirical rules that are conceptual, broad, and abstract. Treatment procedures are specific clinical operations derived from those principles. There are fewer principles than procedures.

A paradigm is an overall philosophy of a subject matter. A treatment paradigm is a philosophy of treatment, based on the methods of science. The paradigm presented in this book suggests that communicative behaviors and disorders are a function of (caused by) both genetic or neurophysiological contingencies and environmental contingencies. The treatment paradigm suggests that a management of the contingency between stimuli, responses, and consequences is treatment.

In communicative disorders, the only currently manipulable contingencies are environmental. The contingency includes measurable response rates as target behaviors.

Logical validity is assumed when statements are internally consistent and do not violate the rules of logic. In contrast, empirical validity is assumed only when statements are based upon research evidence. Statements that are logically valid can be empirically false.

Treatment targets are the client behaviors, whereas treatment procedures are clinician behaviors.

A treatment program is an overall clinical strategy. Treatment variables are technical operations performed by the clinician.

Treatment is defined as a rearrangement of relations between speakers and their environments. Both the clients and people surrounding them must be treated.

Public Law 94-142 and its various amendments, including Public Law 99-457, mandate clinical or special educational services to all children with disabilities. In the case of infants and toddlers, Individualized Family Service Plans are required. In the case of school-age children, Individualized Education Programs are required. Among other things, the laws require that an individual educational and service plan be developed for each child and the treatment effects be documented objectively. The various requirements of the law are consistent with clinical and educational practice based on the methods of science.

STUDY GUIDE

Answer the following questions in technical terms. Check your answers with the text. When necessary, rewrite your answers.

1. Why do some clinicians tend to believe that different disorders are treated differently?

2. Define treatment principles.

3. Define treatment procedures.

4. Give examples of treatment principles.

5. Give examples of treatment procedures.

6. Compare and contrast treatment principles and treatment procedures.

7. What is a treatment paradigm?

8. What are the conceptual bases of the paradigm?

9. What are the procedural bases of the paradigm?

10. Define a contingency.

11. What are the two kinds of contingencies?

12. What kinds of contingencies are manipulable?

13. What are antecedents of behaviors?

14. What are consequences of behaviors?

15. Define replication.

16. What is objectivity?

17. What is empirical validity?

18. What is logical validity?

19. Are all logically valid statements empirically valid?

20. What kinds of research encourages speculation and fruitless controversy?

21. Distinguish between treatment targets and treatment procedures.

22. Give an example of confusion between treatment targets and procedures.

23. Define treatment.

24. What is the focus of treatment as defined in this chapter?

25. Justify why not only the clients, but also the people surrounding them, must be treated.

26. What is the historical view of treatment?

27. What is PL 94-142?

28. What are the requirements under PL 94-142 that affect clinical speech, language, and hearing services in the public schools?

29. What are IEPs?

30. What is meant by multiple evaluative criteria?

31. Are IEPs legal contracts? Why or why not?

32. How do you state when a treatment program will be terminated?

33. Describe the three phases of PL 94-142.

34. What are nondiscriminatory tools of assessment?

35. What is PL 99-457?

36. What is the main focus of PL 99-457?

37. What are IFSPs?

38. How are IFSPs different from IEPs?

39. What is the role of a case manager?

40. How does the treatment paradigm relate to the legal requirements of the law?

2

Documenting Treatment Effectiveness

- What is science?

- Science and clinical practice

- Improvement versus effectiveness

- Documenting treatment effectiveness

- Generality of treatment effects

- Selection of treatment procedures

I n recent years, the issue of clinician accountability has received much public and professional attention. This is partly because of PL 94-142 and the subsequent amendments. Regulations of speech, language, and hearing services by state and local governments, professional organizations, and insurance companies that pay for services have also pushed the concept of clinician accountability. As pointed out in the previous chapter, various laws and regulations require objective documentation of the effectiveness of clinical and special educational services rendered to children and adults served by specialists in communicative disorders. Understandably, society will not continue to support services whose effects are questionable or are based upon subjective evaluations.

21

Independent of legal requirements, there is a growing recognition within the profession of communicative disorders of a need to strengthen the scientific basis of clinical activities. To gain better public recognition as a scientific profession, specialists in communicative disorders must provide services within the framework of science and its methodology. The education of these specialists should include a thorough understanding of the philosophy and methodology of science. Unfortunately, many graduates in communicative disorders may not have had significant coursework in scientific concepts, philosophies, and methodologies.

Some stereotypic notions of science may have had a negative impact on the education of specialists in communicative disorders. There is an implicit belief that "science" within the profession is restricted to such subject matters as anatomy, physiology, neurology, and acoustics. Study of language, articulation, stuttering, hearing impairment, rehabilitation, and special education may not be considered very "scientific." A related belief is that, for a certain subject matter to become recognized as a branch of science, the word "science" or the suffix "–ology" is simply added to it. Thus, empty phrases such as "language science" and "aphasiology" have been created. Unfortunately, under the relabeled subject matter, research and writing may continue to be just as nonscientific as before.

WHAT IS SCIENCE?

Science is no particular subject matter. It is not to be defined as physics, neurology, acoustics, or anatomy. In fact, **science** is a certain philosophy, a particular disposition, and a set of methods. When those who study a given subject matter adopt that philosophy, learn those dispositions, and use those methods, they have a branch of science. How a subject matter is approached and studied will determine whether it is a science.

Science as a Philosophy

Science is a certain philosophy that takes a unique approach to the study of physical and biological nature, including human beings and their behaviors. Several philosophical concepts underlie science. One of these, **determinism**, states that nothing happens without a cause. Events are determined (caused) by prior events, and it is possible to analyze those prior events. Human behaviors also may be determined by their consequences. Established behaviors may be a function of (determined by) both antecedent and consequent events. Extended to communicative disorders, the philosophy of science would assert that all communicative behaviors and their disorders have antecedent and consequent events that partly determine those behaviors and disorders.

Another important philosophical concept of science is **empiricism**, which means that statements must be supported by observational evidence. Unless scientists can observe and verify, their statements and explanations of events are not valid. Empiricism also maintains that sensory experience is the basis of all verifiable knowledge. Presumed events that cannot be observed, measured, and experienced in some way, are outside the realm of science.

Other philosophical concepts of science include understanding, predicting, and controlling events or phenomena. These are often described as the goals of science. Scientists **understand** an event when they know what caused it. In this sense, to explain an event is the same as to understand it. An event is explained when its causes are pointed out. For instance, hearing impairment is both understood and explained when its causes are specified. To say that phonological disorders in many children cannot be explained means that their causes are not understood.

When scientists can explain events by understanding their causes, they can **predict** them. In predicting an event, scientists point out the conditions under which it happens, and state that, when those conditions are present again, the event will happen again. For example, a scientist studying hearing impairment might predict an increase in conductive hearing loss when ear infections are on the rise. Another scientist might predict an increase in aphasia associated with increased risks of cardiovascular accidents or accidental head injuries.

When causes are known, the effects can be modified. When scientists are able to modify a phenomenon, they have gained **control** over it. Clinicians, too, gain control over a problem when they can change it in some way. Some similarities between this philosophy of science and that of clinical professions are discussed in a later section.

Science as a Disposition

Science requires a certain disposition on the part of those who practice it (Bachrach, 1969; Skinner, 1953). Scientists tend to behave in ways that may be unique to them. Science is what scientists do. The products of science are also the products of scientists' behaviors.

Scientists value evidence more than opinions, and objective demonstrations more than subjective statements. A scientist believes that it is the subject matter that knows best, not any person—including himself or herself (Skinner, 1953). Scientists tend to accept evidence, not authorities. Although they have feelings and opinions about the nature and causes of events, they are always willing to have them replaced by what has been experimentally demonstrated.

Although most people are eager to offer and accept explanations of events that puzzle them, scientists are inclined to go without an explanation rather than accept a bad one. Scientists tend to reject explanations without evidence they can evaluate. Good scientists find it perfectly acceptable to say, "I don't know."

Science as Methods and Procedures

Science is a set of methods and procedures. This definition is better known than that of science as a philosophy or disposition. The methods and procedures of science are rules that regulate the activities of a scientist. Scientists are usually careful not to violate those rules. In conducting their business—understanding, predicting, and controlling natural phenomena—scientists use the methods of science.

Some methods of science are essential to establishing clinician or educator accountability. Therefore, clinicians and educators should follow most of the rules the scientists follow. An understanding of the methods of science is necessary not only to establish accountability, but to improve the quality of services offered to people with communicative disorders.

Scientific methods are procedures of answering research questions. The procedures offer structures within which investigations can be conducted. The scientific procedures are **objective**, meaning that other scientists may verify the procedures and their results. Also, scientific procedures are based on **measurement**. Unless objectively measured, a phenomenon cannot be further analyzed. It is especially difficult to perform experiments on phenomena that are not measured. Objective and measurement-based procedures are necessary to (1) manipulate variables and (2) find out causes of events.

Scientists measure variables or factors. Two kinds of variables are important for this discussion. **Dependent variables** are the effects of some causes. In communicative disorders, dependent variables include normal and disordered speech, language, fluency, vocal behaviors, nonverbal behaviors, and sign language and other symbolic communicative behaviors. Any behavior or skill a clinician or educator teaches a child is a dependent variable. In the natural environment, communicative behaviors are a product of known or unknown causes, whereas in clinical and educational settings, acquired skills may be the product of teaching.

Independent variables are the causes. In communicative disorders, causes of normal and disordered communication are independent variables. In science, causes must be experimentally demonstrated. In practice, many causes of normal and disordered speech, language, and hearing are suggested, hypothesized, or inferred. Although nothing is wrong with initially suggesting, hypothesizing, or inferring causes, they should eventually be verified through scientific procedures.

If it is demonstrated, for example, that a child's language behaviors are determined by certain parental reactions, then those reactions are the independent variables and the child's language behaviors are the dependent variables. Similarly, if it is shown that stuttering is due to some genes a person inherits, then those genes are the independent variables and stuttering is the dependent variable. If it is shown that certain kinds of ear infections cause conductive hearing loss in children, then those infections are the independent variables. All effective treatment and teaching techniques are independent variables. Skills taught to children and adults are dependent variables.

Scientists often begin with dependent variables or effects of some unknown variables. The effect may be an eclipse, an earthquake, a chemical reaction, a behavioral problem such as a crime, or a disorder of communication. A scientist in communicative disorders may wish to find out what causes stuttering, hearing impairment, or language delay; another may wish to find out how normally speaking children acquire language or how hearing impaired children naturally acquire sign language. In these examples, stuttering, hearing impairment, language delay, normal language acquisition, and acquisition of signs are all dependent variables. They are the effects that need to be explained by finding their causes. Starting with those effects, scientists begin their investigation of causes.

Most effects do not have a single cause. This is the concept of **multiple causation**. An articulation disorder, for example, may be the result of several factors, including low intelligence, an organic defect, poor environmental stimulation, and faulty contingencies of reinforcement. Stuttering may be due to a genetic predisposition combined with situational stress, anxiety, punishment of some aspects of speech, or reinforcement of dysfluencies.

Delayed language may result from neural damage or lack of environmental stimulation. Many chemical (toxic), structural (physiologic), and environmental factors cause hearing impairment. It is important to note that most of these are only potential independent variables that have not been demonstrated to be definitive causes of those communicative disorders. The examples serve only to show that there may be numerous potential independent variables for a given dependent variable.

An important task of scientists is to show a cause–effect relation. To demonstrate that a certain variable is indeed an independent variable, one must rule out all other variables that may cause the effect under investigation. In a clinical situation, for instance, a clinician may wish to find out if a new treatment technique is effective in teaching language skills to children who have language disorders. The clinician will use the new technique in teaching these children. If the children do learn the target language skills, the clinician may be tempted to conclude that the treatment was effective (i.e., that the treatment was the cause of the newly acquired language skills) and that, without the treatment, the children would have acquired no skills.

However, other clinicians might question the conclusion. They might point out that some other factor—perhaps the classroom teacher's efforts to stimulate language or the parents' work at home—may be responsible for the children's new language skills. The research clinician must show that all other potential independent variables were not the cause of the children's new skills.

Experimentation is the standard method of showing that only what the scientist did produced the results, and not some other factor. In essence, experiments help to rule out extraneous, but potential independent variables, thus helping to establish a cause–effect relation between two specific events.

Experiment

The concept of *experiment* captures the essence of scientific methods. An **experiment** may be defined as a systematic manipulation of an independent variable under controlled conditions to produce changes in a dependent variable. An experiment is a means of establishing cause–effect relations. It is designed to rule out the influence of potential independent variables the experimenter considers to be *extraneous* to the purposes of his or her experiment. The two important aspects of an experiment are manipulation of an independent variable and controlled conditions.

In the new language treatment example, the treatment (the independent variable) is applied in a specific quantity, such as twice a week for 30 minutes each time. Both the duration and the frequency of sessions may be increased or decreased, and the amount of reinforcement for correct responses may be higher or lower. Changes such as these constitute **manipulations** of an independent variable. The independent variable must be manipulated under **controlled** conditions to rule out the influence of potential extraneous independent variables, such as the teacher's language stimulation program or coincidental developmental changes.

Scientists use either a group or a single-subject experimental strategy to establish a cause–effect relation between any two variables and to rule out the influence of extraneous independent variables. In clinical and educational research, the same two strategies are used to establish the effectiveness of treatment or teaching programs. These strategies are described in a later section.

SCIENCE AND CLINICAL PRACTICE

Historically, there has been an unfortunate division between clinical or educational practice and scientific research. Several misconceptions seem to underlie this artificial division. Scientific research is often thought to be basic and clinical activity to be applied. Scientific research is rigorous, and clinical practice is more or less informal. Scientists find out what the clinicians ought to do, and clinicians then do it. Speech–language pathology is a humanistic and helping profession, whereas scientific research is cold and mechanical. Clinicians need not spend much time studying the concepts and methods of science, because clinical practice is inherently different from scientific work. Misconceptions such as these have affected the training of specialists in communicative disorders and, in turn, the nature of clinical and educational practices. A closer look at these practices, however, shows significant similarities between the works of scientists and clinicians.

Similarities Between Scientific and Clinical Activities

The starting point of either scientific or clinical activity is a problem, a question, or a situation that demands analytic attention. Whether the problem is basic or applied, clinical or nonclinical, it requires an answer. The question may concern the movement of stars or the causes and treatment of a speech disorder. Once the scientist or clinician has identified a phenomenon or problem for investigation, the next step usually involves gathering whatever information is available on the phenomenon. This stage of description also is common to both scientific and clinical work. A scientist reviews past studies and their results, identifies the need for further work, and refines the problem in need of investigation.

A clinician who wants to treat a client's problem or disorder either knows the previously researched information on the disorder or finds out. The clinician then assesses the problem by measuring and describing the behaviors the client exhibits (or does not exhibit). These initial clinical activities of taking the client's history and making an assessment are similar to scientific activities of reviewing the literature and describing the problem to be investigated. In this process, both the scientist and the clinician will have specified a dependent variable: the effect the scientist wishes to explain, and the disorder the clinician wishes to treat.

Once the phenomenon or disorder has been described, the scientist may proceed to conduct an experiment and the clinician may proceed to treat the client. In an experiment, the scientist will try to isolate the independent variable of the phenomenon. The scientist typically arranges an experimental situation under controlled conditions and then manipulates an independent variable to see if the dependent variable changes. If it does, the scientist will have isolated the cause of the event.

The clinician also seeks to identify and manipulate independent variables. The independent variables that are manipulated in treatment may or may not be the original causes of the disorder. They may be maintaining factors that, when changed, will change the disorder. New skills may be taught to replace the old noncommunicative behaviors. In any case, treatment or teaching methods used by the clinician are similar to the independent variables manipulated by the scientist.

In scientific research, when causes of an event are isolated under controlled conditions, and the same causes have been replicated by other scientists, the event will have been explained. Most scientific disciplines try to gain control over an event studied. If the event can be reproduced or changed by the scientist, then it is being controlled. Similarly, in clinical practice, when effectiveness of the same treatment variables is replicated by different clinicians across different clients, then the disorder is being manipulated or controlled. Successful treatment of a disorder can eventually lead to an explanation of that disorder.

When scientific events can be successfully controlled and explained, they can also be predicted. This chain of control and prediction is one of the highest goals of scientific activities. Similarly, successful control (treatment) and prediction (prognosis and prevention) are among the highest of clinical goals.

An Important Distinction Between Scientific and Routine Clinical Work

Despite their similarities, routine clinical work and scientific research have at least one important difference. This difference is the amount of care taken to rule out the influence of extraneous independent variables. In scientific research, a great deal of care is taken to ensure that the only independent variable active in an experiment is the one in which the scientist is interested. Steps are taken to rule out the influence of causes extraneous to the purposes of the study.

In routine clinical work, however, the clinician rarely takes steps to rule out the influence of other variables on client learning. Typically, clinicians use procedures whose effects have been demonstrated in controlled clinical research. Not much is done to ensure that the client is not simultaneously exposed to other formal or informal treatment procedures. In fact, beneficial extraneous treatments may be promoted by the clinician. For instance, the clinician may ask a child's regular classroom teacher or parent to work on the child's communicative behaviors. The purpose of routine clinical work is not to show that certain treatments are effective, but to provide the most effective and economical services to the client. Therefore, clinicians often seek the help of others in promoting faster learning and maintenance of target behaviors, whereas scientists, in evaluating the effectiveness of a treatment procedure, must convince others that no other variable can explain the effects produced in an experiment.

The distinction is valid only when routine clinical work is compared with controlled laboratory research. The distinction is not as clear when clinical research is compared with basic or nonclinical research. In fact, there are no significant procedural differences between controlled clinical and laboratory research. Both kinds seek to isolate a cause–effect relation between two events. The clinical researcher may wish to isolate the original or the maintaining cause of a disorder, or an effective treatment for it. To do this, the clinical researcher must follow the same procedures the scientist follows. Like the scientist, the clinical researcher should rule out extraneous independent variables, manipulate a specific independent variable (treatment), produce changes in a dependent variable (communicative behavior or disorder), and thus establish a cause–effect relation between the treatment and the client behavior.

IMPROVEMENT VERSUS EFFECTIVENESS

Because little is done in routine clinical work to rule out the influence of other potential treatment variables, an important distinction between improvement in client behaviors and effectiveness of treatment techniques is created. These two concepts should not be confused.

Through assessment, the clinician establishes whether the client produces certain communicative behaviors. Baselines of target behaviors strengthen such assessment results. Typically, treatment follows. After a period of time, the client may begin to produce the target behaviors that he or she did not produce before the treatment. Throughout the treatment period, the clinician measures the target behaviors for systematic changes. Before treatment is terminated, an additional measure is taken to show that the client has mastered the target behaviors. With this, the clinician usually concludes that the client has improved with the help of clinical services. As long as **positive changes** in the client behaviors were documented, the clinician can appropriately claim that the client improved under treatment. Therefore, **improvement** is defined as positive changes in client behaviors under treatment. Documented improvement demonstrates clinician accountability.

That the client improved while receiving treatment does not necessarily mean that the treatment was effective. Improvement is a necessary, but not a *sufficient,* condition for claiming effectiveness of treatment techniques. In routine (uncontrolled) treatment, there is no assurance that clients could not have produced the target behaviors without treatment. Normal developmental changes and potential influence of formal or informal teaching done by people other than the clinician cannot be ruled out. Therefore, clinicians normally cannot claim effectiveness for treatment programs used in routine clinical work.

To be accountable, clinicians need not establish the effectiveness of procedures they use. They need only to show that their clients improved by documenting positive changes. If clinicians use only procedures that have been evaluated in controlled experimentation, they need not use time-consuming control procedures.

The distinction between client improvement and treatment effectiveness highlights the importance of controlled clinical research. Treatment techniques can be advocated only on the basis of controlled evidence. Unfortunately, many "treatment procedures" are recommended in the absence of such evidence. In due course, some of those procedures begin to be used in routine clinical work without ever having been evaluated experimentally.

DOCUMENTING TREATMENT EFFECTIVENESS

As noted earlier, legal, social, scientific, and professional considerations point up the need for the profession of communicative disorders to demonstrate the effects of treatment techniques. It is often thought that clinical researchers will establish the effectiveness of treatment by following the methods of science, but that clinical practitioners need not be concerned with these methods. Although a majority of clinical activity will always remain uncontrolled, clinicians cannot ignore the process of treatment evaluation.

All clinicians must thoroughly understand the basic set of procedures by which systematic observations are made, measurements are taken, and cause–effect relations are established. Demonstrating treatment effectiveness is a matter of establishing a cause–effect relation between certain procedures implemented by the clinician and changes in the client behaviors. Even if most clinicians are not going to do research, they are expected to be consumers of scientific information. Unless clinicians have a good grasp of the methods of science and experimentation, it is doubtful whether they can be informed consumers of technical information. One consequence of lack of knowledge of science and its methods is that the clinician will continuously lag behind the developments in the profession. Another consequence is that the clinician, although unable to critically evaluate new procedures, may nonetheless use them to be "current in the field."

Clinicians need to be *critical* consumers of research. It is not enough for a clinician to merely understand research studies; he or she also must evaluate the results of those studies in light of the concepts and methods of science. Critical evaluation of treatment procedures in communicative disorders is especially important because of many untested suggestions, programs, and procedures that are routinely offered to clinicians. The clinician must be able to judge whether each treatment procedure has been tested in a controlled study and, if so, what evidence is available regarding its effectiveness. An uncritical clinician is endlessly swayed by faddish developments in the profession. Every profession has its share of such developments that may be considered revolutions and breakthroughs. A critical clinician can distinguish those treatment procedures whose effects are experimentally demonstrated from those that are based merely on logic, rational arguments, and uncontrolled clinical applications.

A by-product of having a clear understanding of experimental procedures is that some clinicians may gather controlled evidence to support their clinical practice. Clinicians may then help evaluate untested but established treatment procedures. There are experimental treatment evaluation procedures that clinicians may use while treating or teaching their clients. These procedures are described under the single-subject strategy.

There are two major approaches to evaluating treatment effectiveness: the group design strategy and the single-subject strategy. They are described in the following sections.

The Group Design Strategy

The traditional method of documenting treatment effectiveness is based on group comparisons. It is variously known as the group design method, between-groups strategy, statistical research design, and so forth. The underlying idea is that the clients who are treated will change, whereas those who are not treated will remain unchanged. In a group research design, there are at least two groups of subjects: the **experimental group**, which receives treatment, and the **control group**, which does not.

The experimental and control groups must be comparable for a treatment or teaching method to be proven effective. The only difference between the two groups is treatment, which is given only to the experimental group. The subjects in the two groups must be similar on all variables that could potentially affect the treatment outcome. For example, age could affect the outcome of stuttering treatment. Children who stutter may show more rapid and more permanent improvement than adults who have been stuttering for years. Therefore, the researcher cannot have children in one group and adults in the other. Also, because the researcher wishes to extend the results to people who stutter, the subjects selected for study should represent this group. If people who stutter are of different ages and come from varied socioeconomic levels, occupations, and educational status, the subjects selected for the study should be similarly varied.

Most researchers try to select subjects who are comparable in age, gender, intelligence, family and social background, educational level, occupation, and the type and the severity of the disorder being treated. To achieve two groups of comparable subjects, the researcher may use one of two methods: random procedure or matching.

The Random Procedure

The random procedure is based on the statistical theory of probability. The theory states that if a small number of persons are selected without any bias from a large group of people, then those few persons will represent the larger group. The larger reference group is called a population, and the selected smaller group is called a sample. A **population** is a defined group in which all members possess certain characteristics. All language handicapped children in public schools, all hearing impaired adults in the United States, all persons who stutter in a state, all children in the second grade, and so on, are defined populations. Note that the term population, as defined, is a technical term. It does not mean people at large, which is the meaning of the term in ordinary usage. In a research study, a population is a large but special group that a researcher defines.

Because it is impractical to observe all persons in a defined population, researchers select a **sample** of individuals from that population for study. Also, because the results of the study must be applicable to the entire population, not only to the selected persons, special procedures must be used so that the sample is representative of the population.

The representativeness of a sample is assured when every subject in the population has an equal chance of being selected into the study. Experimenter bias cannot influence subject selection. Thus, the subjects are selected randomly. Each individual in the population may be assigned a number, for example, and all odd-numbered persons may be selected for the study. Such a random procedure gives samples that represent the population.

The random approach requires the availability of a large population of subjects from which a sample can be drawn. For clinical research, patients or clients with a specific disorder must be available in large numbers. For example, in establishing the effects of a new treatment program for school-age children with a language disorder, the clinician must have access to a large group of children with that disorder, all of whom are willing to participate in the study. The needed number of children can then be selected on a random basis.

After the subjects are selected randomly, they are **randomly assigned** in equal numbers to the experimental or control group. Random assignment helps avoid experimenter bias in deciding who gets treatment and who does not. Random assignment of subjects to the experimental and control groups creates two comparable groups. Thus, the random procedure must be used at two levels: first in selecting the subjects from the larger population, and then in assigning them to the experimental or control group. The clinician can then assume that the subjects in the two groups are comparable on such relevant variables as socioeconomic status, intelligence, family background, type and severity of the disorder to be treated, and so on.

Matching

Another method of forming two comparable groups for research is **matching**, in which the clinician selects specific *types* of comparable subjects. Whereas randomly drawn samples are larger and representative of the population, matched groups are smaller and do not represent the population. However, the subjects in the two groups are comparable to each other. For example, if the 15 language disordered subjects in an experimental group are 5-year-olds with average intelligence, coming from middle class families, and living in suburbs, the control group should consist of 15 children with the same characteristics. Note that such matched groups do not represent all children with language disorders (population). The matched groups do not represent children with all levels of age, intelligence, and socioeconomic status, living in inner cities and rural areas.

In treatment research, the duration, specific types, and severity of the disorder are factors considered in matching subjects. For example, in a study involving articulation disorders, if the subjects in the experimental group have functional articulation disorder, those in the control group cannot have neurologically based articulation disorder. If the experimental group subjects have been stuttering for 5 years, the control group subjects should also have been stuttering for 5 years. If the children in one of the groups are nonverbal, those in the other group should also be nonverbal.

Experimentation

The formation of two groups, either randomized or matched, sets the stage for the experimentation. Before the treatment is begun, the relevant dependent variables are measured. For example, if a study involves teaching sign language to nonverbal or hearing impaired children, the clinician should find out whether the children produce any signs and, if so, how many. Such measures of behaviors established before starting an experimental teaching program are called **pretests**.

The new treatment is then given to subjects in the experimental group. The control group subjects go without treatment until the experiment is over.

After the experimental group has received treatment for a duration considered appropriate, the communicative behaviors of subjects in both groups are again evaluated. This second evaluation, which follows treatment of the subjects in the experimental group, is known as the **posttest**. Note that, although treatment is given only to the experimental group, pretests and posttests are given to both groups.

The effects of the treatment procedure are determined through statistical analysis. Such statistical procedures as analysis of variance or a *t* test may be used to find out if the treatment produced a significant effect. In general terms, if the treatment was effective, the persons in the experimental group will show significant improvement, but those in the control group will show no changes or only minimal changes. The pretest and posttest results of the control group will be comparable, but those of the experimental group will be different.

When the posttests indicate that only the experimental group learned the target behaviors, the clinician may assume that the treatment, not some extraneous variable, produced the beneficial effects. If some other variable were responsible for the positive changes in the experimental group, then the control group should show similar changes from the pretest to the posttest. In this case, the effects of the treatment procedure would remain questionable. The underlying assumption of such a study is that the subjects in the two groups have similar experiences except for treatment.

The experimental group–control group design is only one of many basic group designs. Each design also has variations. It is not the purpose of this chapter to review clinical research designs. Rather, it is to provide some basic information on the need to establish treatment effectiveness and to point out the importance of studying research methods in some detail.

Limitations of the Group Design Strategy

For several reasons, group designs are difficult to use in clinical sciences. First, it is not easy to find a large number of persons (population) with a given disorder who are accessible and willing to participate in a study. It is difficult to gain access to populations of children who have language disorders; persons who stutter, have aphasia, or hearing impairment; or people who have undergone laryngectomy. When such populations are not accessible, the clinical researcher cannot draw random samples. Therefore, the researcher is forced to use persons who happen to seek professional services. For instance, hearing impaired children in a special school or classroom, stroke patients in a hospital, or stutterers seeking help from a speech–hearing clinic may be requested to participate in treatment evaluation studies. Those who agree to participate may be randomly assigned to the experimental or control groups, but the initial pool of subjects is not randomly selected.

Second, the matching procedure is very difficult to implement. It may not be possible to find subjects with specific clinical disorders of the same type and severity who also have the same personal, social, family, and educational characteristics. Therefore, very few experimental clinical studies are done with matched subjects.

Third, the requirement of a control group that does not receive treatment may pose some practical and ethical problems. It may be undesirable to deny or postpone treatment for the sake of research. In some clinical research, patients on a clinician's waiting list have served in a control group, but many researchers may not find a large number of patients waiting for services. Regardless, the waiting list–based control group is not a matched or randomly selected sample.

Fourth, sufficient numbers of clients needed to form two groups of subjects simply may not be available, irrespective of the random procedure. The clinical researcher might never find 30 or 40 persons who have dysarthria; share similar personal, social, health, and other characteristics; and are simultaneously available for research.

Fifth, group designs are not conducive to intensive observation of individual subjects, which is often needed in clinical sciences. Performance of the individuals in each of the two groups is averaged to derive two mean scores, one for each group. Such average performances do not give a clear picture of individual differences that are typically noteworthy. Not knowing how individual subjects in a research study performed, a clinician reading a published group study will find it difficult to decide whether his or her client will also benefit from the researched procedure.

Sixth, the group design strategy does not provide a complete picture of changes in the client behaviors across treatment sessions. Because only two measures are normally obtained (once before and once after the treatment), there is no record of changes as they occur during or between treatment sessions. Therefore, the clinician cannot monitor the techniques or modify them during treatment sessions.

For these reasons, few experimental studies in clinical sciences use the group design method in an appropriate manner. Many researchers who use this method ignore random selection or subject matching. Therefore, in practice, the most important aspect of the group design method is omitted.

The Single-Subject Strategy

An alternative to the group strategy is the **single-subject strategy**, in which individual subjects are intensively studied. The single-subject strategy has been used extensively in teaching new skills and changing behaviors under controlled conditions to show that the methods used are indeed effective. The method is especially suited to clinical sciences and education, which study individual clients intensively to change behaviors or generate new skills.

In the single-subject approach, a large number of subjects are not observed only once or twice, as is frequently done in the group strategy. Instead, fewer individuals are observed repeatedly. Because clinicians tend to see the same few clients repeatedly, this method has been found to be highly suitable to answering clinical and educational research questions. Additionally, because this approach is not based on the random procedure, there is no need to have access to a large clinical population that is willing to participate in a study.

Single-subject designs rarely require matching, since the approach is not based on group comparisons. Normally, there is not a control group that receives no treatment. Therefore, the problems associated with a no-treatment control group are avoided. Instead of comparing the performance of subjects who do and of those who do not receive treatment, each subject's performance under treatment is compared with the same subject's performance under no treatment. Because there is no need to compare one subject's performance with that of another subject in the single-subject method, each individual is treated as unique.

In single-subject designs, a subject's behaviors are measured continuously. Treatment effects are not determined only on the basis of pretest and posttest measures. To see how behaviors change when treated, the researcher measures them in all experimental treatment sessions.

It is not possible to review all the single-subject designs used to evaluate treatment effectiveness. This chapter reviews the three most frequently used single-subject designs: the ABA, the ABAB, and the multiple baseline design.

A common feature of most single-subject designs is the establishment of baselines before the application of treatment. **Baselines** are pretreatment measures of behaviors. Although they are similar to pretests used in the group designs, there are important differences. Unlike pretests, baselines are repeated to establish a reliable measure of behaviors before introducing treatment. Only when the behaviors show a stable trend across a few sessions does the clinician introduce treatment.

For example, suppose a clinician wishes to find out if a certain training program will be effective in teaching certain morphologic features to language delayed children. First, the clinician determines the frequency with which the children produce the selected features. The children may not produce the features at all (zero frequency), or they may produce them at some low frequency. Through language samples or other means, the clinician determines this frequency (between 0 and 100%). To establish baseline reliability, the clinician takes two or more language samples. The baserate is stable when multiple measures are consistent with each other. If the measures differ widely, then the language sampling is continued until the frequency of morphologic use across two or three samples is stable. Detailed procedures of establishing baselines of communicative behaviors are described in Chapter 5.

After establishing the baselines of target behaviors, the clinician initiates treatment. Because the phases subsequent to treatment can be somewhat different across designs, the designs are discussed separately.

The ABA Design

The ABA is one of the first experimental designs developed for the study of single individuals. In clinical and educational research, the design is used to show that a new treatment or teaching method is effective. To begin with, the researcher takes the baserate of the behaviors to be taught (the initial A condition of the design). When the baserates are stable, the new treatment is applied (the B condition). The behaviors are measured continuously as treatment is continued until the subject shows a dramatic improvement in the target behaviors. When the treatment is ineffective, the experiment is terminated. When the treatment is effective, the clinician withdraws treatment (the final A condition).

The logic of the design is simple. If the behaviors were either not produced or produced only at some low frequency during the baserate condition (A), but improved dramatically during the treatment (B), and returned to the baserate when the treatment was withdrawn (second A), then the treatment was probably effective. If extraneous variables were active, then the changes would have continued even after withdrawal of treatment.

This design is used when a new treatment must be evaluated. The design can clearly show if a treatment was effective. Because the design ends in no treatment, it should not be used if the objective is to have the treatment effects last. The behaviors acquired in the B condition are reduced in the final A condition. A variation of this basic ABA design can be used to offer extended treatment that may produce lasting effects. This is the ABAB design, described next.

The ABAB Design

The ABAB design has two versions: withdrawal and reversal. The first three conditions of the **ABAB withdrawal design** are identical to the basic ABA design: (1) the target behaviors are baserated, (2) the treatment is applied to those behaviors, and (3) the treatment is withdrawn. As in the ABA design, these three conditions demonstrate the effectiveness of the treatment. Then, after demonstrating the declining trend in the behaviors after treatment withdrawal, the clinician *reapplies* the treatment in the final B condition of the design. The treatment is typically continued until the target behaviors are reliably produced in nonclinical settings. Thus, in the ABAB withdrawal design, the treatment is withdrawn once, and applied twice to show that the behaviors changed when the treatment was initially applied, changed again when it was withdrawn, and changed a third time when it was reapplied.

The **ABAB reversal design** is identical to the ABAB withdrawal design except for the second A condition. After the initial baselines are established (A), the treatment is first applied to the target behaviors (B); then, the treatment is not simply withdrawn, but is applied to the incompatible or error responses (second A). This is done only briefly to demonstrate that when the treatment is applied to the error responses, they increase in frequency while the target behaviors simultaneously decrease. In the treatment of an articulation disorder, for example, the correct production of the selected target phoneme may be baserated initially and reinforced in the first B condition. In the second A condition, the incorrect productions may be briefly reinforced to see if the correct production decreases and the incorrect production increases. If such results are seen, the clinician may conclude that the reinforcement contingency was an effective treatment method. In the final B condition of the ABAB reversal design, the target behaviors are again treated until the final clinical goals are achieved.

Figure 2.1, reproduced from a language training study (Hegde & McConn, 1981), illustrates the ABAB reversal design. In this study, "probes" were conducted between experimental conditions to assess generalization of treatment effects. (The probe procedures are described in Chapter 5.) Note that although the trained production (auxiliary *are*) was reversed for a brief duration, the study was terminated only when the target feature was produced and generalized at a high level. Incidentally, the graph shows that the experimental manipulations of the auxiliary had corresponding effects on the copula *are* as well. This means that teaching auxiliary was sufficient to have the subject produce the copula.

Both versions of the ABAB design rule out the influence of extraneous independent variables, including maturational factors. If some extraneous variables were to be responsible for the treatment effect, then the target behaviors would not decrease when the treatment is either withdrawn or reversed.

A problem with the ABAB design is that, to rule out extraneous independent variables, the treatment effect is neutralized (withdrawn) or reversed (incorrect responses reinforced). Although this is done only briefly, it can still be somewhat inefficient. In some cases, it may be totally undesirable to withdraw or reverse treatment. In certain clients, it may be difficult to reduce or eliminate a trained behavior within short durations. In such cases, reversal training may have to be extensive, which is obviously undesirable. Normally, behaviors are reversed during early stages of training when they are not yet firmly established, but reversing a target behavior can still be difficult.

A design that avoids the problem of the ABAB designs is the multiple baseline design. It permits conclusions about the effectiveness of treatment

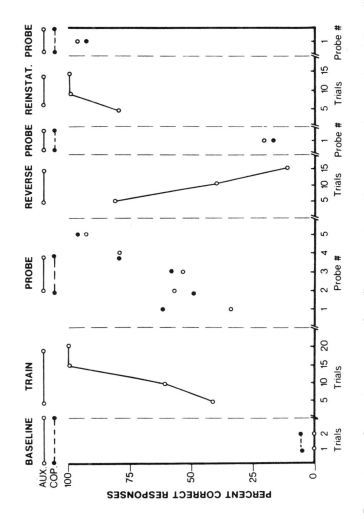

FIGURE 2.1. Percentages of correct responses of auxiliary *are* and copula *are* across the experimental conditions when only the auxiliary was trained, reversed, and reinstated in a 22-year-old female subject. The graph shows the baseline, experimental, probe, reversal, and reinstatement conditions of an ABAB design. From "Language Training: Some Data on Response Classes and Generalization to an Occupational Setting" by M. N. Hegde and J. McConn, 1981, *Journal of Speech and Hearing Disorders, 46,* p. 356. Reproduced with permission.

without reversal or withdrawal of treatment. In several respects, it is one of the best clinical research designs.

The Multiple Baseline Design

The multiple baseline design has three variations: across behaviors, across settings, and across subjects. The multiple baselines refer to several target behaviors, treatment settings, or clients.

In routine clinical situations, the **multiple baseline across behaviors design** is probably easier to implement than the other two variations. The design requires that at least three target behaviors be treated in a given client. This rarely poses a problem to the clinician because most clients need to acquire more than one target behavior. This is especially true of clients with language and articulation disorders and students in regular and special education who need to learn multiple academic or other skills.

In using the multiple baseline across behaviors design, the clinician first establishes baselines on all the selected target behaviors. If a child with an articulation disorder is to receive treatment on four phonemes, these are base-rated with a certain number of words each. Then the treatment is started on the first phoneme, which may be taught at the word level to a specified performance criterion. When the child reaches this criterion, the clinician *normally* moves to the next phoneme. Within the multiple baseline design, instead of immediately starting the treatment on a different phoneme, the baselines of the remaining three untrained phonemes are repeated. If only the treatment and no other factor was responsible for the changes in the first phoneme taught, the percentage of correct production of the three untrained phonemes would not show significant change from the initial baseline.

The next step is to train the second phoneme to the performance criterion. When this is accomplished, the baselines of the remaining two untrained phonemes are reestablished. Once again, these baselines are expected to be comparable to the first two baselines. The third phoneme is then trained, followed by another baseline of the last phoneme, which is then trained to the criterion. In this manner, baseline and training are alternated until all target behaviors are trained.

Figure 2.2, reproduced from a language training study (Hegde & Gierut, 1979), illustrates the multiple baselines across behaviors. Note that four grammatic features were sequentially trained in the same subject. Each subsequent behavior had more baseline trials, and none of the behaviors under baseline changed.

In the **multiple baseline across settings design**, the same behavior(s) of the same client are baserated and sequentially trained in different settings. For example, a hearing impaired child's production of selected manual signs

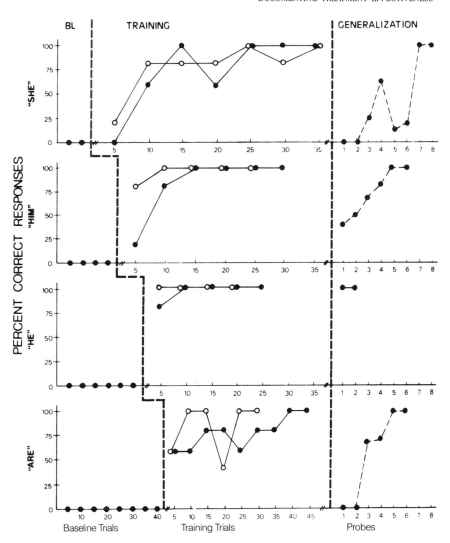

FIGURE 2.2. Percentages of correct verbal responses on baseline, training, and probe trials for the four behaviors trained in a language delayed child (aged 4.9 years). The training segments of the graph represent responses given to two training items in the case of each behavior. The graph illustrates the use of the multiple baseline across behavior design. From "The Operant Training and Generalization of Pronouns and a Verb Form in a Language Delayed Child" by M. N. Hegde and J. Gierut, 1979, *Journal of Communication Disorders, 12,* p. 30. Reproduced with permission.

may be baserated in the clinic, in the regular classroom, and in the special classroom the child attends for a few hours each day. Assuming that the target signs are not produced in any of these settings, the training is started in one of the settings. After the behaviors reach the training criterion in that setting, the sign productions are baserated a second time in the remaining two "untrained" settings. The training is then started in the second setting, followed by the last baseline in the third setting. Finally, the training is given in the third setting. If the signs are produced only in the setting(s) where they were trained, but absent in setting(s) in which training was not yet given, then the clinician will have demonstrated the effectiveness of the teaching procedure.

In the **multiple baseline across subjects design**, the same behavior(s) are treated in different individuals. Reduction of hypernasal speech production, for example, may be the treatment target in four children with repaired cleft. The production of nonnasal speech sounds with nasal resonance is initially baserated across these children. One of the children is then trained to the training criterion in the nonnasal production of target speech sounds in words. The target behavior in the other three subjects is baserated a second time, followed by training of the second child. In this manner, training and baselines are alternated across children until all are trained.

Of the single-subject designs, the multiple baseline across subjects design comes closest to the matched-subjects group design. Subjects who do not receive treatment serve the control function the way they do in many group designs. Therefore, the selected subjects should be comparable on relevant characteristics. Also, the design shares some of the problems associated with the matched-group design.

With the multiple baseline design, the clinician hopes to show that the frequency of a given target behavior will increase only when treated. In the across behaviors version, the frequency of each behavior of the same client should remain unchanged until the clinician teaches it. In the across settings version, the trained behavior should not be produced in untreated settings. In the across subjects version, the untreated subjects should not show changes in the target behaviors. In this manner, potential extraneous variables are ruled out.

An attractive feature of the multiple baseline design is that it can be used in routine clinical work. It does not alter clinical service to any significant extent. The components of the design are a part of responsible clinical work. For example, the design requires that the target behaviors be baserated. This is a normal clinical procedure used to document the need for clinical services. The repeated baselines are also necessary in everyday clinical practice because a baseline established earlier must be repeated immediately before the training is initiated on that behavior.

Other single-subject strategies include the alternating treatments design and interactional design. In the former, the relative effects of two or more treatments can be assessed, whereas in the latter, independent and interactive effects of more than one treatment can be established. For more information, interested clinicians should refer to other sources on single-subject designs (Barlow, Hayes, & Nelson, 1984; Barlow & Hersen, 1984; Hegde, 1987; McReynolds & Kearns, 1983). In addition, clinical studies published in professional journals can be helpful in understanding these and other methods of establishing treatment effectiveness. Throughout this book, clinical studies documenting treatment effectiveness are cited.

GENERALITY OF TREATMENT EFFECTS

The effectiveness of a treatment program is initially demonstrated by one or a few researchers using a certain number of clients. Either the between groups or the single-subjects strategy may be used. Once this is done, the researchers need to show that the technique can be effective with other clients, when used by other clinicians, and in other professional settings. The **generality** of a technique is the extent to which it may be applied in a wide range of situations by different clinicians who treat different clients.

Replication is the method of establishing the generality of treatment effects. In replicating the effects of a treatment procedure, different researchers repeat the study in different settings. The researchers use the same treatment procedure to treat different clients to see if the technique is as effective as it was in the original study. If it is, the researchers conclude that the technique has generality.

Initial replications use subjects similar to those used in the original study. Subsequent replications may include clients who differ in some respects from those in the original study. For example, if the original study had demonstrated effectiveness of a language training procedure with 5-year-old children, a replicated study may try to find out if similar results can be achieved with older or younger children, or even with adult clients.

Generality of treatment effects is important for clinical practice. Unless it is known that different clinicians have obtained favorable results in such divergent professional settings as university or private clinics, hospitals, and public school settings, a technique may not be recommended for general use. An initial failure to establish generality of a technique does not always suggest that it is ineffective. Those who tried to replicate the study may not have applied the technique correctly. Sometimes, however, lack of generality means that a technique may be used only in certain settings, only by those clinicians who have established its effectiveness, or only with certain clients. This limits the usefulness of a technique.

SELECTION OF TREATMENT PROCEDURES

Clinicians must select from many available treatment procedures. A review of treatment literature in communicative disorders reveals a variety of procedures to treat the same disorder. Some of the standard controversies in the field are concerned with how to train clients with language and articulation disorders, stuttering, or hearing impairment. Sometimes, contradictory approaches seem equally appealing, especially when each is considered alone. The descriptions of multiple procedures may have logical or face validity; that is, they appear logical and seem like they should work. The descriptions may be scholarly, and hence impressive. Although the clinician may find it difficult to select one technique over the other, when alternative treatment procedures are available, the clinician must select.

In some cases, subjective factors may influence a clinician's selection of treatment techniques. The clinician may know and like an author or may be impressed with descriptions of a technique. The clinician may consider a technique easy to use, or find it inherently appealing. The author may be well known and considered an authority on the subject. Factors such as these, however, should be irrelevant to the treatment selection process.

Probably the single most important criterion of treatment selection is the presence or absence of **controlled** and **replicated evidence**. Ideally, the technique selected must have been experimentally evaluated to show that it is effective in the absence of other potential treatment procedures. It must have been used by different clinicians in different settings with similar results. The (presumed) effectiveness of the technique should not depend upon such vague factors as the personality of the clinician or the clinician–client rapport. These factors are often lame excuses for ineffective techniques.

In selecting a treatment procedure, then, the clinician should ask three basic questions: (1) Has the technique been experimentally evaluated? (2) Have the results been favorable? (3) Has the technique been replicated across settings, clinicians, and clients? If the answer is positive to all three questions, the clinician is justified in using the technique in routine clinical situations.

Answers to these questions are not always clear, however. Although different techniques may be supported to different degrees, supportive evidence can often be found on a hierarchy. At the lowest level are those techniques based purely on speculative but logically consistent and scholarly reasoning. These are the most suspect of the techniques and should be avoided in routine clinical practice. Next are those techniques based on uncontrolled case studies. Data show that when these techniques are used systematically, the clients improve, but there is no assurance that the techniques are effective. Such techniques may be used on a tentative basis. At the next level are treatment procedures that have been experimentally evaluated and are found to be effective. There may not be replicated evidence, however. The clinician can use these techniques with a certain degree of confidence, while being watchful of possible replications that may be published. The most desirable techniques are those that present favorable, controlled, and replicated evidence with known limits of generality.

The emphasis placed upon the use of experimentally evaluated techniques is not meant to discourage creative clinical work. Clinicians should always be willing to try new techniques. While doing this, however, a clinician should remain fully aware that something unproven is being tried. The clinician must be scrupulously careful in measuring the client behaviors, keeping objective records, and systematically (even if informally) evaluating the effects of the technique on individual clients. The clinician who uses some of the single-subject designs can evaluate a technique while providing clinical services. Multiple baseline designs are especially helpful in generating controlled evidence.

SUMMARY

There is a growing recognition in the profession of communicative disorders of the need to strengthen the scientific bases of the profession.

Specialists in communicative disorders must adopt the philosophy of science, learn scientific dispositions, and apply the methods of science to the study of communication and its disorder. Increased use of the method of experimentation is especially needed.

Scientific and clinical work share several common characteristics. Both science and clinical work seek to analyze phenomena, determine cause–effect relations between events, modify the effects of certain variables, and predict and control events. Unlike science, however, most clinical activity is uncontrolled.

Client improvement refers to changes in behaviors under treatment. Treatment effectiveness, which is not the same as improvement, is documented only when the influence of other potential treatment variables is ruled out.

Clinicians should understand the philosophy, methodology, and dispositions of science so that they can be critical consumers of technical information. They must know the methods by which treatment effects are established.

There are two methods of establishing treatment effectiveness: the group design strategy and the single-subject strategy. The former approach is based on the statistical theories of probability, random or matched samples, and group performance differences that are evaluated statistically. The single-subject approach is based on intensive study of individual clients. Each strategy, however, has strengths and weaknesses. By and large, the single-subject strategy is more suitable for clinical research.

Replication is the method by which the generality of treatment effects is demonstrated. Eventually, generality across settings, clinicians, and clients must be established for each treatment technique.

The degree to which a treatment technique is based upon controlled evidence, replicated evidence, or both should determine its selection or rejection.

STUDY GUIDE

Answer the following questions in technical language. Check your answers with the text. Rewrite your answers when necessary.

1. Define science.

2. What are some of the popular misconceptions of science?

3. What are some of the assumptions of science as a philosophy?

4. What is the meaning of objective procedures?

5. Define dependent variables.

6. Define independent variables.

7. Are communicative disorders typically dependent or independent variables?

8. What kinds of variables are treatment techniques?

9. Give at least two specific examples each of independent and dependent variables.

10. What is an experiment?

11. What is meant by "manipulations of an independent variable"?

12. Define control.

13. What are extraneous independent variables?

14. Describe the similarities between scientific and clinical activity.

15. Compare and contrast scientific experiment and clinical treatment.

16. When is an event "explained"?

17. What are among the highest scientific as well as clinical goals?

18. What is an important distinction between scientific research and routine clinical work?

19. Are there critical distinctions between clinical research and nonclinical research?

20. Distinguish between improvement and effectiveness.

21. State the reasons why a clinician cannot claim effectiveness even though the client improved under treatment.

22. Specify why a clinician who does not wish to do research should still understand the methods of science by which treatment effects are established.

23. Who is a critical consumer of research information?

24. Describe the group design strategy.

25. Define the single-subject strategy.

26. What is a random procedure?

27. Define population and sample.

28. Distinguish between random selection and random assignment.

29. What is matching?

30. Distinguish between experimental group and control group.

31. How are the results of the group experimental designs analyzed?

32. State the limitations of the group design strategy.

33. What are the general characteristics of the single-subject strategy?

34. What is an ABAB design?

35. Describe the reversal design.

36. Define a withdrawal design.

37. What are the limitations of the ABA and ABAB designs?

38. What is a multiple baseline design?

39. What are the variations of a multiple baseline design?

40. What are the problems with the multiple baseline across subjects design?

41. Why are single-subject designs more applicable to clinical research?

42. Define generality.

43. What are the three major kinds of generalities?

44. What are some of the subjective factors that might influence the treatment selection process?

45. What are the specified objective criteria for the selection of treatment techniques?

46. Describe the hierarchical arrangement of clinical evidence.

47. How should a clinician use treatment techniques that are not verified?

48. What kind of knowledge or expertise will help in evaluating treatment effectiveness?

3

Selection and Definition of Target Behaviors

- An overview of assessment strategies
- Selection of target behaviors
- Response classes as target behaviors
- The normative strategy
- The client-specific strategy
- Definition of target behaviors

Clinicians should carefully select target behaviors to be taught to persons with communicative disorders. The kinds of behaviors selected for training may have an impact on how long training must last, whether trained behaviors will generalize to the clients' everyday situations, whether generalized responses will be maintained over time, and whether clients or parents who seek help will consider the training successful. In the case of language and articulation disorders, the issue of what to train has been about as controversial as the treatment techniques. For example, recent literature on stuttering suggests that an important factor in therapeutic success is the type of target behavior selected for treatment (Hegde, 1985). Thus, it is important for clinicians to know how to select behaviors for training.

Once a clinician selects a behavior for training, how he or she defines it may affect clinician accountability. In establishing accountability, some definitions of target behaviors are more useful than others. Therefore, this chapter examines the issue of defining target behaviors.

Before target behaviors are selected and defined, however, a client's communicative behaviors must be assessed. Therefore, it is necessary to take an overview of assessment strategies and philosophies.

AN OVERVIEW OF ASSESSMENT STRATEGIES

Assessment (sometimes referred to as diagnostics) of a client's communicative behaviors is the initial step in providing clinical services. As soon as they receive a request or referral for professional help, most speech and hearing centers send out a case history form that the clients or parents of young clients complete and return. Soon thereafter, an appointment is made for an assessment.

Assessment includes a set of clinical procedures with which information is obtained on a client's existing communicative behaviors, communicative problems, nonexisting but desirable communicative behaviors, and potential factors associated with these problems. Relevant medical, personal, educational, social, and occupational information also is obtained. This information is evaluated to understand the client's problems and to design a treatment program.

The assessment typically begins with an interview in which additional information on the client's problem is obtained. Also, vague or unclear information supplied by the client or parent on the case history form is clarified. Generally, the background information obtained through the interview and the case history covers such areas as the client's birth and developmental history; health, medical, and educational information; family history; details on speech and language development; the onset and the course of the disorder; information on prior assessment, treatment, and their results; and occupational and marital information, if relevant. The focus of the interview depends on the disorder, the client's age, additional medical or behavioral problems the client may have, and so on. Because it is not the purpose of this chapter to give detailed information on assessment areas and procedures, the clinician should consult other sources (Emerick & Haynes, 1986; Peterson & Marquardt, 1990).

The actual assessment procedure depends to some extent on the information obtained through the case history and interview. An orofacial examination is done to evaluate the oral structures. If structural deviations, such as a cleft palate, are noticed, the client is referred to a medical specialist.

During the initial few minutes, the clinician makes informal observations of client behaviors to help determine which assessment procedures to select. This observation will help the clinician decide what types of standardized tests are useful and what kinds of client-specific procedures may be needed. For example, if a child barely produces single words, there is no use administering an advanced syntactic test. Also, the clinician may notice signs of hearing impairment that were not suggested by the case history or interview, indicating a need for audiological assessment.

Also as part of the assessment, the clinician records the client's language sample, administers selected standardized tests, screens the client's hearing, and uses any special procedures needed to assess the specific disorder. Because of certain limitations of standardized tests, it is desirable to use additional procedures. I shall shortly address some of the limitations of standardized tests and suggest alternatives.

Language samples are more useful than standardized tests because they are more naturalistic, and the number of opportunities to produce given aspects of language can be increased to the extent necessary. Because language samples can involve conversational speech, they reflect the natural communicative behaviors of the client more accurately than the results of standardized tests. If the client is a young child, the clinician usually arranges a controlled situation in which pictures, toys, and other stimuli are manipulated to evoke specific responses. With adult clients, the more typical conversational speech can serve the purpose.

Taking an adequate language sample from a young child requires some planning and skill on the clinician's part. The *clinician,* not the child, should control the stimulus materials. Often, toys and objects more readily evoke play activity than verbal responses. Therefore, the selected stimulus materials must be used to evoke speech, not to keep the child "happy" during the assessment.

While evoking speech from the child, the clinician should not talk too much. When the clinician spends much time talking, the child may not have enough opportunities to speak. The clinician's speech should serve merely as verbal cues for speech from the child. Therefore, it is not useful to ask questions that can be answered "yes" or "no." Yes–no questions tend to evoke nonverbal behaviors (e.g., nodding or shaking the head) from many children. Questions must be open-ended. For example, questions and requests such as "What is this?" or "Tell me about this picture" or "What did you do yesterday?" may be more effective than "Is this a car?" or "Is the cat jumping?" or "Do you like it?"

The extent to which the clinician must manipulate the stimulus material in a language sampling procedure depends upon the child's verbal level and the complexity of the language structures to be evoked. If the client is fairly verbal, not much concrete stimulus manipulation may be needed. The child may then be engaged in conversational speech. Generally, the less verbal the child, the greater the need for stimulus manipulation. In addition, the more complex the structure to be evoked, the greater the extent of stimulus manipulation required. For example, pictures of two or more objects may be sufficient to evoke certain regular plural inflections, but a greater degree of verbal and concrete stimulus manipulations may be needed to evoke past tense *ed* inflection or passive sentence forms.

The information obtained through case history, orofacial examination, observations of the client's general behaviors, interview, tests, and language samples are analyzed and integrated to obtain a total picture of the client's communicative behaviors. The case history and interview provide the background information. The tests, language samples, and other observations help determine the client's current communicative behaviors. The test results and language samples are analyzed to find out the types of speech, language, voice, or fluency behaviors that are present and those that are not. For example, the phonemes the child can and cannot produce accurately may be determined. Various language structures, including grammatic, semantic, and pragmatic features, that are and are not present may be identified. Similarly, normal and abnormal voice characteristics, percentages of fluency and dysfluency rates, and rate of speech may be determined for individual clients. Use of nonverbal behaviors, including manual signs and gestures, may be noted. The presence of hearing loss and other problems that need further assessment by appropriate professionals also are noted.

Limitations of Traditional Assessment Procedures

Traditionally, soon after an analysis of the assessment data is completed, the client is considered ready for intervention. However, this is a questionable assumption because of the limitations of assessment procedures routinely used in speech–language pathology. Many of these limitations center around the concepts of reliability and validity of measures taken during assessment. These limitations are especially noteworthy in the context of standardized tests.

Reliability is defined as consistency of repeated measures of the same event. When the same phenomenon is measured two or more times, the results should agree. Therefore, there is no reliability without repeated measures. The reliability of a single measure of speech–language behaviors taken during an assessment session is unknown. The clinician cannot know whether similar results would be recorded when the same client's communicative behaviors were measured again.

Assessment is intended to document the need for clinical intervention by showing that the client does not produce certain communicative behaviors. To later demonstrate the effects of treatment or improvement in the client behaviors, the initial assessment data must be reliable. If not, the need for, or the results of, clinical treatment may become questionable. For instance, in measuring language behaviors, at least two language samples should be obtained to make sure of the presence or absence of behaviors. Nevertheless, it is not uncommon for clinicians to initiate treatment as soon as the traditional assessment procedure is completed.

Validity is defined as the degree to which a measuring instrument measures what it purports to measure. A measure of speech and language should sample speech and language skills, and not something else. In a limited sense, most tests and language samples can be considered valid because they do seem to sample speech and language behaviors. When a test appears to measure what it is supposed to measure, it is said to have face validity; however, this is only a superficial kind of validity. There are other, more appropriate means of establishing a measure's validity.

The question of validity is especially serious when certain inferences are drawn from measures of communicative behaviors whose validity is questionable, or is limited to face validity. On the basis of such measures, the clinician may infer the communicative behaviors of the client in his or her natural environments. For instance, a language sample taken in the clinic may not accurately reflect the client's language behaviors at home, at school, or in the occupational setting. Additional inferences may be drawn regarding response modes that were not tested. Such inferences may also be questionable. For example, responses given on test items may not reflect conversational speech or oral reading skills. Similarly, imitative responses may not reflect productive skills.

Because the purpose of an assessment is to find a client's typical communicative behaviors, those behaviors must be sampled adequately and repeatedly. The behaviors should also be sampled in multiple settings, and in different response modes if relevant.

Other than lack of multiple measures, most problems associated with the traditional assessment procedure stem from an overdependence on standardized tests. Often, assessment is equated with testing, and the ensuing report on the client is full of test results whose reliability and validity may be unknown. The fact that the test was "standardized" does not mean that a given client's performance is reliable. Reliability must be established for the particular measure, taken on a specific client.

Because of the problems of reliability of a given client's tested behaviors, standardized test results may not suggest appropriate target behaviors for clinical intervention. If a test cannot firmly establish whether the client indeed does or does not produce various types of communicative behaviors, the target behaviors will not have been identified.

Probably the most significant methodological problem with standardized tests is that they do not sample behaviors and response modes adequately. Test developers tend to point out the large number of subjects (sample) who were tested during standardization. Such a sample may be an adequate, but local, sampling of *subjects*. Unfortunately, most test developers tend to ignore the issue of sampling *behaviors* adequately. A test of articulation, for example, may give a client one or two opportunities to produce a phoneme in a given word position (initial, medial, or final). Phonemes may be tested not at all or only inadequately in conversational speech. Yet the test results may be an important, if not the sole, basis to conclude whether the child produces the tested phoneme. On a test of language, a child may be asked to produce a given grammatic morpheme in the context of one or two sentences. Whether the child produces the morpheme in those limited contexts may lead to the conclusion that the child does or does not produce the morpheme in all contexts. Such conclusions are often true of many aspects of language included in a variety of tests. These and other conclusions based on extremely limited sampling of behaviors are inevitable when one relies exclusively on standardized tests.

There are some equally significant philosophical problems with the use of standardized tests. First, tests encourage the use of limited and standardized stimulus materials to evoke responses. In many cases, it may be more appropriate for a clinician to design stimulus materials that are appropriate to the individual client. Stimuli selected for specific clients may be more meaningful training materials that better promote maintenance of target responses.

Second, all standardized tests are based on the notion of norms, which reflect the performance of a typical group. Norms are statistical averages of group performance. However, performance of individuals within groups typically varies, and such individual variations get lost in the statistical averaging process. Thus, norms do not do justice to individual uniqueness or differences. One cannot adequately predict individual performance from group norms, but this difficulty in the use of test results is usually overlooked.

Assessment as Measurement of Client Behaviors

An alternative way of viewing assessment is as a process of **measuring** the client behaviors. In many cases, assessment or diagnostics rarely involves the discovery of the instigating (original) cause of speech–language disorders. Before the treatment is started, the clinician should determine the client's current communicative behaviors, which is the accepted function of an assessment. This goal can be achieved by measuring those behaviors. In obtaining reliable and valid measurement of communicative behaviors, the following four criteria may be used.

First, all relevant **response modes** must be measured. Measures of imitative and evoked ("spontaneous") behaviors must be obtained. Also, conversational speech and, whenever appropriate, oral reading modes should be measured. In most cases, response topography (form of a response) also should be considered. For example, the rate of stuttering or correct production of phonemes must be measured at the levels of single words, phrases, and sentences.

Second, the behaviors to be measured must be **sampled adequately**. Whether the clinician is measuring a client's articulation, language, stuttering, or voice characteristics, the number of observations must be sufficient to establish reliability. In the assessment of articulation, phonemes must be tested with multiple words, phrases, and sentences. Several opportunities must be given for each position in which the phonemes are tested. Language structures should also be evaluated with multiple linguistic contexts. For example, if the present progressive *ing* is to be measured, it must be presented in the context of at least 15 to 20 words, phrases, or sentences. The rate of stuttering must be measured with extended conversational speech and oral reading samples. Vocal behaviors (voice characteristics) also must be measured with extended speech samples, oral reading samples, or both.

Third, all measurements must be **repeated** to establish the reliability of measures obtained on a given client. The fact that the measurement procedures used by the clinician, such as standardized tests, were reliable with other subjects assessed somewhere by someone at another time is no basis to conclude that the given client behaviors were also measured reliably. The relevant behaviors must be measured on at least two occasions. If the two measures do not agree, additional measures must be obtained. The basic requirement is that, across two or more measures, the behavior being measured meets some criterion of stability. Criteria used are more or less stringent, depending upon the purposes of the measurement. In most cases, a criterion of no more than 2% variation in behaviors across two measures can be adequate. It is better to use a specified criterion consistently.

Fourth, it is desirable to obtain measures of behaviors in **extraclinical situations** because reliability must be established across settings. Also, because the target behaviors must be produced and maintained in nonclinical situations, pretreatment measures established in those situations will help evaluate the eventual success of treatment. This is probably the most difficult of the measurement requirements, because it needs the cooperation of parents and other persons. The clinician may have to go to those situations to measure behaviors, or train either the client or the parents to record them. The clients or parents may be requested to tape-record language samples at home and submit them for evaluation. In Chapter 9, I discuss in some detail the issue of parent training designed to accomplish these and other objectives.

During assessment, it is rarely possible to measure the target behaviors according to the four criteria specified here. In most cases, the clinician will have barely sufficient time to take the history, interview the client or the parents, complete an orofacial examination, administer selected tests (if any), and take conversational and (if appropriate) oral reading samples. More detailed measurement takes time. Consequently, the typical assessment can only help identify a range of potential target behaviors that need to be measured further. Even this limited purpose can be better served if the clinician does not spend most of the assessment time in administering standardized tests. Extended observations, conversational speech–language samples, and simple interactions will be more useful in identifying behaviors that must be measured in some detail. Then, before the treatment is started, a limited number of potential target behaviors may be selected and measured appropriately. These pretreatment measures of target behaviors, called baselines, are described in Chapter 4.

SELECTION OF TARGET BEHAVIORS

There are two major reasons for selecting target behaviors. First, most clients with communicative disorders need treatment on multiple targets. A majority of children with articulation disorders need training on more than one phoneme. Typically, language disordered children may not produce a variety of language behaviors, described as grammatic, semantic, or pragmatic structures, or different classes of verbal behaviors. Some clients may have more than one kind of communicative disorder. A child, for example, may misarticulate multiple phonemes and not produce several language structures. A child with a repaired cleft may have articulation problems, as well as some voice disorders of resonance. In each of these cases, the clinician must decide which behaviors should be treated, and in what sequence.

Second, when a client has several disorders, theoretical considerations dictate the selection of certain target behaviors. In the treatment of stuttering, for example, many target behaviors have been used over the centuries. Some of the behaviors targeted for training in modern times include self-confidence, self-image, anxiety, muscular tension, psychosexual aberrations, psychological role conflict, negative attitudes, motor integration, "fluent" stuttering, rhythmic speech, reduced rate, gentle phonatory onset, prolonged speech, and regulated breathing. To a certain extent, the target selected for treatment depends on the theory of stuttering adopted by the clinician.

In language disorders also, researchers with differing theoretical viewpoints have advocated different targets for training. Over the years, clinicians have been encouraged to train auditory and visual processing, comprehension of spoken language, rules of grammar, syntactic and morphologic features, semantic notions, pragmatic structures, and response classes. In the treatment of articulation disorders, such targets as auditory discrimination, isolated practice of sounds, production of phonemes in nonsense syllables or meaningful speech, distinctive features, and phonological rules or processes have all been suggested as treatment targets.

It is obvious that when theories change, the target behaviors also change. When language was viewed primarily from the standpoint of universal transformational grammar, rules of grammar were the advocated clinical targets. When the theoretical emphasis shifted from grammar to meaning, semantic features were the recommended treatment targets. When the theory shifted again from semantics to pragmatics, rules of language usage were considered more appropriate targets. Similar changes in the study of articulation have resulted in shifting target behaviors. The trend is perhaps common to most if not all disorders of communication.

A Practical Approach to the Selection of Target Behaviors

Shifting theories sometimes suggest scientific progress, and the clinician should be able to change the target behaviors accordingly. However, theoretical shifts do not always suggest advances in the study of a subject matter. Many new viewpoints may turn out to be short-lived. In only a few years, there have been several "revolutions" in the study of language. The frequency of changes suggests that new theories were premature, could not be sustained by research, and therefore were discarded in a hurry. Sometimes theories seem to die down, only to be revived again after some years. Frequently advanced "new" theories of stuttering testify to this trend. Such frequent "revolutions" and shifts in emphasis create an ever-changing bandwagon effect: Many clinicians who earnestly wish to keep abreast of changes may find themselves climbing somewhat bewildered onto such bandwagons almost as frequently as they get off them.

Clinicians need an approach to the selection of target behaviors that is based, not on speculative and theoretical reasoning, but on clinical and experimental research. The approach should be flexible enough that it can accommodate changing viewpoints that are experimentally based and clinically verified. Also, the approach should be based on some long-standing, repeatedly tested principles so that inconsequential shifts in emphasis and viewpoints do not undermine clinical practice.

Principles and results of experimental clinical science will fulfill these requirements. Experimental clinical research has shown that nontheoretical but personally and socially meaningful target behaviors may be identified. This research can verify the usefulness of target behaviors suggested by new theories or empirical research. A concept that has emerged from experimental clinical research is known as *response classes*. This concept provides a means of identifying experimentally verified target behaviors.

RESPONSE CLASSES AS TARGET BEHAVIORS

Target behaviors selected for clinical intervention must be empirically valid; that is, they must be real. Although this is not a controversial statement, many communicative behaviors that clinicians plan to teach their clients may not be empirically valid. Many behaviors are suggested based on theories that describe structures of language. The problem is serious in the case of language and articulation. Most popular linguistically based theories of language and phonology are based on structures of language and speech. For instance, syntactic, morphologic, semantic, and pragmatic aspects are based on structural analysis of language. Distinctive features and phonological processes also are based on structural variables.

Because of the influence of structural theories, target behaviors are typically distinguished on the basis of their structures. For instance, regular and irregular plural words differ because of their structures. Similarly, a question and a passive sentence are identified on the basis of their structures. Final consonant deletion differs from fronting because of structure. If an utterance takes one shape, it belongs to one linguistic category, and if it takes another shape, it belongs to another category.

Purely structural analysis may suggest responses that are unreal because it does not take into account the independent variables of those responses. This means that categories of responses formed strictly on the basis of their structures may not be valid. The problem arises because the structural analysis is not sensitive to the possibility that (1) behaviors that have the same structure or form may have different independent variables, and (2) the behaviors that have different structures may have the same independent variables.

The statement that behaviors that have the same structure may have different independent variables means that behaviors that look or sound the same may be produced under different conditions, for different reasons. For instance, a speaker may say "water" when thirsty or when seeing water running in the street. Although the same structure (the word "water") is produced, the statements are different behaviors because they are caused by different conditions producing different effects on the listener. In examining the structure, there is no difference; both have the same structure (word). In one case, the speaker's response is due to thirst and the listener is likely to offer water to the speaker. In the other case, the speaker's response is due to the sight of running water and the listener may say, for example, "Yes, what a waste!"

The statement that behaviors that have different structures may have the same independent variables means that behaviors that look or sound different may be produced under similar conditions, for similar reasons. The active and passive sentence forms may differ structurally, but are produced under the same stimulus condition producing similar effects on listeners. A speaker might say,

"The boy hit the ball" or "The ball was hit by the boy." The two utterances have different structures, but the reason for saying them is the same. Listeners are likely to react similarly to these structurally different utterances.

Experimental clinical research has shown that responses grouped according to their independent variables may not necessarily follow structural distinctions. Such research has shown that response classes are better treatment targets.

A few examples will illustrate the concept of response class and the limitations of structural analysis. First, take the example of the grammatic feature *plural.* Linguistic analysis classifies the plural feature into two categories: regular and irregular. Accordingly, if a language delayed child does not produce the plural, then the clinician has those two target behaviors to teach. However, some clinicians who taught the regular plural with /s/ inflections found that clients overgeneralized to plural words with /z/ inflections (see Guess & Baer, 1973, for a description of these studies). It was then necessary to teach the regular plural /z/ separately. Furthermore, other allomorphic variations of the regular plural (/əz/ as in *dresses* and /vəz/ as in *leaves*) were also to be taught separately. Thus, although the structural analysis suggests one target behavior (regular plural), there are several target behaviors, each corresponding to an allomorphic variation of the grammatic morpheme.

An absence of the irregular plural, which according to the structural theory is a single category, suggests a single target behavior. But if a client needs training on the irregular plural, the clinician does not have a single target behavior to teach, but as many targets as there are irregular plurals in the English language (Hegde & McConn, 1981). For instance, a client taught to produce such words as *women, men,* and *children,* will not produce other such irregular plurals as *teeth* or *feet.* Each irregular plural is a separate target behavior.

The past tense poses similar problems. The regular past tense inflection breaks into several independent target behaviors, depending upon whether the inflected word ends with /d/ (as in *buzzed*), or /t/ (as in *baked*), or *ed* (as in *counted*). In addition, each irregular past tense is a unique target behavior to be taught separately. These examples make it clear that a single grammatic category may turn into a collection of different target behaviors, each in need of separate training. Therefore, a grammatic category is not a functional response class; it is a collection of responses produced under different conditions having different effects on listeners.

Clinical research also has documented that behaviors that are separate within the structural analysis may indeed be the same empirically. Take the example of subject noun and object noun phrases. McReynolds and Engmann (1974) selected some children who did not produce either the subject noun phrase or the object noun phrase. The children were then taught the production of subject noun phrases. Without additional training, the children began to produce the object noun phrases as well. The experimental control was established within a reversal design, as described in Chapter 2. These results demonstrate that subject noun and object noun phrases, although separate grammatically, are not separate empirically. They form a single response class, requiring only one teaching condition.

A second example of structurally different but empirically the same response category can be found in the distinction between verbal auxiliary and copula. A study by Hegde (1980) demonstrated that when children who have produced neither auxiliary *is* nor copula *is* are trained to produce only one of them, the other untrained feature may be produced without specific training. A study by Hegde and McConn (1981) obtained similar results with the auxiliary *are* and copula *are*. In both studies, extraneous independent variables were controlled within a reversal design. Again, what were considered to be different behaviors within a structural analysis turned out to be the same in clinical research.

The clinical research designed to identify true response classes in normal and disordered language is still in its early stages. Most of the studies have been concerned with grammatic features. Whether semantic notions and pragmatic structures or rules are different targets (response classes) has not been researched. Although pragmatic analysis is supposedly concerned with why people say what they say and under what conditions, the research itself has not been experimental. The reasons for producing different kinds of utterances are inferred from the structure of utterances, not demonstrated experimentally. Therefore, even pragmatic categories may or may not be empirically valid.

Only a few studies have been reported on response classes in articulation disorders and stuttering. In recent years, the study of articulation has become very structurally oriented, as illustrated by the distinctive feature theories and the more recent phonological theories. In either theory, responses are grouped according to their topographic (form-related) characteristics. There is not enough experimental evidence to show that all sounds that share common distinctive features belong to the same response class or that the sounds that do not share features belong to different classes.

Currently popular phonologic processes present similar difficulties. It is not clear that different phonological processes are systematically related to empirical response classes. For example, such phonological processes as *cluster reductions* and *final consonantal deletions* (Bernthal & Bankson, 1988; Stoel-Gammon & Dunn, 1985) may not be anything more than inferred, logical concepts. If cluster reduction is a general response class, then training on a few clusters should eliminate all other cluster reduction problems in a given client. Clinical–experimental evidence does not support this possibility, however (McReynolds & Elbert, 1981). Under experimental scrutiny, responses grouped under a process or a distinctive feature may turn out to be independent of each other. Also, some of the multitudes of features and processes may collapse into fewer empirically valid response classes.

In the case of stuttering, the question is whether different forms of dysflu-encies (e.g., part-word repetitions, interjections, prolongations) and associated motor behaviors (e.g., an eye blink) belong to the same or different response classes. Despite some conflicting results, it appears that most forms of dysfluen-cies can be reduced or increased by similar methods. If this is sustained by further research, dysfluencies may be classified as one response class. Perhaps different associated motor behaviors of stutterers form a single response class, although this question has not been researched adequately.

What Are Response Classes?

Responses that have the same or similar antecedents and consequences form a class. Therefore, a **response class** is a group of responses created by the same or similar contingencies. Responses within a class are functionally similar, but they may not be structurally similar. Thus, if structurally different responses are produced under similar conditions, for similar reasons, produc-ing similar effects on listeners, then those structural differences are not impor-tant; the responses form a single class. Also, if structurally similar responses are produced under different conditions, for different reasons, producing different effects on listeners, then those structural similarities are not important; the responses belong to different classes. Responses within a class are produced for the same reason; responses belonging to different classes are produced for different reasons.

Why speakers produce certain responses and what effects the responses have on listeners must be determined experimentally, not by speculation. Teach-ing behaviors under controlled conditions is the best method of finding response classes. Therefore, it is the clinician, not the theorist or the structuralist, who has the best chance of discovering response classes. A clinician who teaches a few responses and finds that responses thought to belong to a different struc-tural category are produced without training will have identified a potential response class that includes responses of different structure. Similarly, a clini-cian who teaches a few responses and finds that responses thought to belong to the same structural category are not produced without training will have iden-tified potentially different response classes that include responses of similar structure.

For example, a clinician wishing to train the production of the auxiliary *is* in a language disordered child selects several sentences in which that feature is used (Hegde, 1980). Some of these sentences are then trained with appropriate stimulus conditions and response consequences (contingencies). After training a few sentences, the clinician might present the remaining untrained sentences to see if the production of the auxiliary *is* is generalized. If the amount of training was adequate, the child might produce the target feature in those untrained sentences. Then all of the trained and untrained sentences with the auxiliary *is* would belong to a single response class. If, as a result, the child begins to produce the copula *is* as well, then the production of the copula *is* is under the control of the same contingency that created the production of the auxiliary *is*. This possibility is strengthened when the copula is trained and the auxiliary is produced without additional training.

To further confirm the effects of teaching one behavior upon another behavior, the clinician may conduct an experiment. For a brief duration, a child who has been taught the auxiliary may then be taught to produce sentences without the auxiliary. This is the reversal of training. If the results are that when the auxiliary is taught, the previously nonexistent copula is also produced, and that when the auxiliary is reversed, the production of the copula is also reversed, then auxiliary and copula most likely belong to the same response class. The structural or grammatic distinctions between them do not matter, at least for teaching purposes. Furthermore, if teaching and reversing the copula result in the production and reversal of the auxiliary, the clinician might conclude that the probability of the two belonging to the same response class is high.

The clinician who selects linguistically based categories of semantics, grammar, and pragmatics for the target behaviors is taking a certain amount of risk. Some of those categories may contain no empirical responses, and other categories may contain more than a single response entity. The problem is that the clinician would not know the number of target behaviors that need clinical training. A given feature (e.g., plural /s/) may be more than one target, and two features (e.g., auxiliary and copula) may be actually a single target. If the experimental methods are used to determine empirically valid response classes, this problem may be avoided.

Because the experimental procedure used in identifying response classes is based on the methods of science, it is not limited by a particular theory. If new response categories are suggested by nonexperimental research, the clinician can put them to experimental test. Any structural or other kind of category that proves to be empirically real can be a target behavior.

Many target behaviors (semantic notions, pragmatic rules, distinctive features, phonological processes) that have been suggested in recent years have not been experimentally tested. We know that many grammatic features may not be empirically valid. It would be helpful if the tendency to categorize behaviors on the basis of their structures is tempered by the experimental method.

It can be expected that continued research on response classes will identify empirically valid clinical target behaviors. Even then, there would be a need to select target behaviors. As stated earlier, most clients need training on multiple targets, and only a few targets can be trained at any given time. Therefore, with most clients, clinicians are likely to face the problem of selecting target behaviors.

A problem closely related to the selection of target behaviors concerns the sequence with which multiple targets should be trained. Multiple behaviors can be trained in one of several sequences, and what sequence to follow is a question the clinician needs to answer. There are two approaches to these interrelated problems of selection and training sequence, one based on normative information and the other on client-specific considerations.

THE NORMATIVE STRATEGY

Clinicians have traditionally used the normative strategy in selecting both the target behaviors and the sequence in which they are trained. In the **normative strategy**, target behaviors are selected from the norms that are established for different age groups. This strategy is most relevant to disorders of language and articulation in which multiple target behaviors are selected and taught on the basis of normative information.

It is generally believed that clinical training must follow the behavior sequence found in normally developing children. Behaviors that are normally mastered earlier in the sequence should be taught before those that are mastered later. Studies of normal language acquisition are supposed to have established norms that specify ages at which children master different phonologic, grammatic, semantic, or pragmatic features. The normative studies are also supposed to have determined the sequence in which various language behaviors are acquired. If the client is a 4-year-old child, then the sequential norms for 4-year-olds will dictate the targets and the treatment sequence.

The normative strategy is probably one of the most widely accepted of the clinical strategies in speech–language pathology. The strategy is based on three assumptions that are not critically examined. The first assumption is that there are age-based norms that will serve as target behaviors for individual clients. The second is that there is a fixed sequence in which speech and language behaviors are learned by most if not all children. The third is that the sequence found in normally developing children is the best sequence to use in clinical training. A careful examination of these assumptions will show some serious problems.

Are There Valid and Useful Age-Based Norms?

Norms refer to the average performance of a typical group of persons of certain age and other defined characteristics. Two critical questions are what is a typical group and has it been adequately sampled in establishing norms. Most frequently, norms are established with the method of cross-sectional sampling of a group of children. Such norms often are established by those who standardize tests of speech and language behaviors. When a new test of articulation or language development is constructed and standardized, it is administered on a sample of children at selected age levels. The performance of children in the study becomes the norm for the age groups sampled.

Norms are rarely established on a large enough sample to make them representative of children seen in clinics across the country. Often, they are local norms relevant only to children in the area sampled. Even then, due to practical problems, samples are not always drawn strictly according to the random procedure. Therefore, to what extent the performance of the sampled children represents the performance of unselected children in the local or distant areas may remain doubtful.

A different kind of problem exists with norms based on samples drawn randomly from a large population. This problem arises because norms are a statistical representation of the mean (average) performance of the entire group. As noted before, the mean usually does not accurately reflect an individual subject's performance. Variations in individual performance will have been masked by the mean. As a result, the clinician cannot use norms to determine the particular communicative behaviors of a given child. Indeed, the larger the sample, and hence the more representative it is of the population, the less relevant the results are for predicting an individual's performance. This is because very large samples have included subjects of varied social, educational, and personal backgrounds, with the result that a given individual's performance is likely to be even more different from the statistical mean.

The concept of norms negates individual variations, differences, and uniqueness. The concept typically ignores cultural and social variables that create differences in children and adults. The notion of norm often is confused with a standard to which all clients of a certain age or other characteristics are held. In culturally and socially diverse societies, the notion of norms can create more problems than it can solve.

It is often said that lack of norms for various speech and language behaviors is a major problem for the clinician. However, in view of the problems associated with norms, the lack of norms is not as handicapping as the basic concept itself.

Another method can provide more useful information than can statistical norms. This method involves repeated observations on a single child or a few children. Brown's (1973) now classic study of three children's language learning process illustrates this method. Brown recorded the same children's speech and language samples periodically to see how the behaviors changed over time. This is the well-known longitudinal method. Only a few studies of this kind have been done because they are expensive and time-consuming. Since a few children are studied intensively, individual variations and unique patterns are readily recognized. This type of information can be more useful than the statistical mean for clinicians who want to be sensitive to individual variations and unique patterns of behaviors in their clients. Because the longitudinal method typically involves small numbers of subjects, it is less likely to yield statistical norms of speech and language development. Instead, these studies describe the sequence with which some subjects learn different language behaviors. This leads us to the second assumption of the normative strategy.

Is There a Fixed Sequence of Language Acquisition?

The question of sequence of acquisition is more often debated in the context of language, but the basic logic applies to speech and all other aspects of communication. The assumption that there is a sequence in which children normally learn communicative behaviors is about as widely accepted as the concept of norms. Any statement regarding the sequence in language learning can be more or less controversial depending upon how the statement is interpreted. If the statement refers to a broad and variable pattern in learning language, it is probably least controversial. By and large, children tend to master certain behaviors before they learn certain other behaviors. However, if this is interpreted to mean that the sequence is *invariable* across children (Brown, 1973; Gleason, 1989; Owens, 1988), and that there may be an innate mechanism that universally determines the sequence, then the statement is highly questionable. Known sequences of language acquisition are not invariable. Children differ widely in the sequence in which they acquire speech and language behaviors. Sequences also are based on average performances of groups, and hence are not always applicable to individual children. A clinician, however, is always concerned with individual children.

If there are sequences, they are not necessarily innate. Some sequences may simply be due to the nature of language. For example, the child would have no use for an auxiliary *is* until the present progressive *ing* is learned. A child who does not yet say such words as *walking* and *eating* cannot use the auxiliary. This suggests that some language "structures" may be elements of a chain, but different elements may be acquired at different times. More importantly, most sequences researched thus far have shown individual differences.

Any sequence observed is frequently explained on the basis of such inferred mental variables as innate mechanisms and cognitive stages. However, known sequences in behaviors do not automatically rule out the influence of external (manipulable) independent variables. Normative research may show the average sequence, but it does not explain why there is such a sequence. When we begin to manipulate certain environmental events to which children are exposed, we may find that the sequences can be changed. This can be done only by experimental research on the acquisition of communicative behaviors in children. Mere observational technique, which is so commonly used in the study of language, does not support or refute hypotheses concerning the manipulability of observed sequences or patterns. Some experimental evidence indicates that children who are learning the language normally can be taught grammatic structures out of the known sequence (Capelli, 1985; De Cesari, 1985; Nelson, 1977). Reversing the sequence recorded by Brown (1973), both Capelli and De Cesari taught grammatic morphemes to children ahead of their known sequences. Their results clearly show that sequences found in language acquisition may be altered by systematic teaching.

Should Clinical Training Follow Normative Sequences?

The third assumption of the normative strategy—that it is best to follow the developmental sequence in teaching behaviors—is one of the most untested of the common assumptions of clinical practice. Clinicians generally believe that it is difficult or impossible to teach behaviors out of their normative sequence. They also believe that clients learn or generalize faster when the training is based on the normative sequence. However, these beliefs are not based on controlled experimental evidence; they are merely cherished beliefs that clinicians hold but rarely question. As noted before, there is evidence that behaviors may be taught out of known normative sequences, and there is no evidence that a normative sequence is superior to a non-normative sequence of teaching.

A clinical science should be based on clinical evidence. Therefore, the best training sequence must be determined by clinical research. The sequence in which children normally learn language may indeed be the best strategy to teach target behaviors to clinical populations; however, a sequence not consistent with normative information may be just as effective, or even more so. The best sequence of teaching must be determined by controlled clinical data, not by the argument that children normally show a particular sequence. Clinicians should be free to experiment with different sequences and carefully record the results of such manipulations to determine the relative effectiveness of following different sequences. In essence, better sequences in which to train target behaviors will be determined not by identifying the normal sequence, but by clinical experimentation with different sequences.

Because of its fundamental philosophical assumptions, the normative strategy is unlikely to encourage experimentation with different sequences in which the target behaviors can be trained. Therefore, normative strategy is not self-corrective. The clinician who always follows the normative sequence will not discover a better sequence. The clinician who experiments with other sequences may find sequences that are efficient with different clients. If it is wrong to experiment with training sequences, the only one who finds out is the one who experiments. Ironically, if normative sequence is indeed more effective than other sequences, only the clinician who experiments with different sequences is likely to show that. This may be the best reason to experiment and determine the sequence of teaching multiple behaviors.

THE CLIENT-SPECIFIC STRATEGY

An alternative to the normative strategy is the client-specific strategy, which is based upon the philosophy that both the selection of target behaviors and the sequence in which they are trained must be client specific and based on clinical experimentation. Although normative information can provide some broad guidelines, it can hardly suggest specific target behaviors. Within the client-specific strategy, target behaviors for a given client are selected based on such factors as the client's environment, the relevance or usefulness of the behaviors selected, the potential for generalization and maintenance, and the potential for behavioral expansion.

The first consideration within the client-specific strategy is the client's **environment**. Before selecting target behaviors, the clinician should study the client's environment to find out what kinds of behavioral demands are placed upon that client. Age-specific norms play only a minor role, if any, in the selection process. For example, a 10-year-old child in need of clinical services may be "functioning more like a 6-year-old," to use a typical expression, but this does not mean that the target behaviors should be the typical (if known) behaviors of a 6-year-old. In many ways, the 10-year-old might differ from most 6-year-olds. The child may be in a special educational program, the demands of which may differ from those faced by normal 6-year-old children. At home and on the playground, the child may be expected to do things other than what would be expected of a 6-year-old. The client's physical development may be far ahead of his or her language behaviors, which might also lead to different kinds of demands made upon the child. In cases such as these, it may be more appropriate to select target behaviors that are specific to the particular client. The selected behaviors may or may not be consistent with norms.

The need to study the client's environment becomes even more critical with older children and adults who are mentally retarded. It is probably inappropriate to select the typical language behaviors of a 10-year-old because a retarded adult client's "language age" is 10 years. This client may be working in a sheltered workshop or in a special job training program, or may be enrolled in an adult literacy course. The best speech–language services for clients such as these are not the age-based normative behaviors, but the particular kinds of language that would make them more efficient in their occupational or educational situations. In selecting the target behaviors, an analysis of the sheltered workshop situation, the job training program, or the education program is more appropriate than checking out the norms. The client may be better off learning the vocabulary and the language responses needed for his or her particular situations. Adult persons who have aphasia are in similar situations. That a man with aphasia has lost most of his speech, and thus his communicative behaviors resemble those of a child, does not mean that the target behaviors should be selected on the basis of the client's "functional age."

The second consideration is that the language behaviors taught must be **useful or relevant** to the client. Many target behaviors typically taught in clinical situations may not be useful to the clients. Some clinicians routinely select target responses that label color, shape, size, and body parts. Although these are useful in some sense, they may not be for individual clients who do not have other language responses in their repertoire. A child going around the house naming colors and identifying shapes and sizes of objects does not exhibit relevant or useful verbal behavior. In some cases, even counting numbers or reciting days of the week and months of the year may not be very useful. Because speech is a means of affecting other persons' behaviors, a child who is able to say "mommy," "juice please," "hi," or "cookie" can exert more precise control over other persons than the one who points to objects or says nonfunctional words. Mands (demands, requests) that result in specific reinforcement for the client with limited language are more useful than some other kinds of target behaviors. The child who is able to ask for things needed, tell about personal experiences, and indicate internal states of pain and motivation, has a more effective repertoire of verbal behavior than does a child who can only name colors or recite days of the week.

The third consideration is that the target behaviors must have a **potential for generalization and maintenance**. Traditionally, generalization and maintenance were considered only after the target behaviors were established. However, clinical research suggests that some target behaviors have better potential for generalization and maintenance than other behaviors. For instance, behaviors that are useful to the client and are likely to be exhibited in the natural environment may have a better chance of getting initially generalized to the client's everyday situations. Once generalized, those responses are more likely to be reinforced at home. For instance, a child who learns to say "mommy" in the clinic is more likely to say it at home, and the child who says "mommy" at home is more likely to be reinforced than the child who says "sofa." Responses reinforced at home are likely to be maintained over time. The concept of generalization and strategies for promoting maintenance are discussed in Chapter 7.

The fourth consideration is that the behaviors trained must serve as **building blocks for new behaviors** that the client can produce without additional training. This potential for behavioral expansion is called response generalization or induction, which means that untrained and more complex responses can be produced without further teaching. When mastered, various grammatic features permit response induction. For example, a child taught to use the copula *is* in the context of the personal pronoun *he* ("he is good") may produce that copula in the context of other pronouns such as *she* ("she is nice"). Similarly, a client taught to produce the possessive inflection in the context of a given set of nouns, such as "man's paper" and "man's hat," may produce the inflection in the context of other nouns, such as "lady's hat" and "lady's purse" (Hegde, Noll, & Pecora, 1979).

Expansion possibilities of some types of responses are limited. Simple labeling of objects or colors, routine responses such as reciting the days of the week, or questions such as "What is that?" may be limited. This does not mean that such responses should not be taught at all, but that they should be taught only after more meaningful responses that can be readily expanded are taught.

In summary, clinicians have typically adopted the normative strategy in the selection of target behaviors. This strategy has certain limitations that are both philosophical and methodological. An alternative strategy involves client-specific considerations. In selecting the target behaviors, the clinician should consider the environment of the client, the usefulness of the behaviors, the potential for generalization and maintenance, and response expansion possibilities.

DEFINITION OF TARGET BEHAVIORS

Selected target behaviors should be clearly defined. Initially, the selected behaviors may be described in general terms; soon, however, the behaviors must be defined precisely. There are several reasons why the target behaviors must be defined in certain ways. First, to be accountable, the clinician must measure the target behaviors before, during, and after treatment. Behaviors may be continuously measured only when the responses are defined precisely, as vague definitions do not permit objective measurements. Second, objective definitions allow other clinicians to replicate treatment procedures in teaching the same target behaviors to other clients. Third, objective definitions make it possible for an external observer to verify the results of clinical services. For these and other reasons, it is necessary to define target behaviors in an appropriate manner.

There are two basic ways of defining target behaviors: constituent and operational. The most important distinction between the two is that constituent definitions may not suggest procedures of measurement, whereas operational definitions do.

Constituent Definitions

Constituent definitions, also called conceptual definitions, come close to everyday definitions of words. Dictionaries offer **constituent definitions**, in which words are defined with the help of other terms that refer to other concepts. If one did not know the meaning of these other concepts, the definitions may not help. For example, to define language as linguistic competence is to define that term constituently. If the meaning of linguistic competence is unclear, the definition is not helpful. But more importantly, the definition does not say how language can be measured. To take another example, to define intelligence as mental capacity is to define it constituently. The term mental capacity may be as vague as the word intelligence, and therefore may not permit measurement. If stuttering is defined as a disorder of rhythm, one must know normal and disordered rhythm before the definition can make sense. Similarly, an articulation disorder may be defined conceptually as an inability to acquire phonological rules, but before this definition can be used in measurement, it must go through a series of translations.

Constituent definitions not only are used in describing disorders and general behaviors, but often are used in defining target behaviors taught during treatment. For example, the treatment target for a language disordered child may be defined as linguistic competence, but this definition does not specify how the behavior can be measured to show that the client who did not have that target began to show it after treatment. Another clinician might define the goal of an articulation treatment program as teaching phonological rules, but this definition does not specify how to demonstrate whether the client has learned those rules. Other treatment goals may be defined as an increased level of self-confidence, better self-image, increased communicative competence, stimulation of language abilities, facilitation of communicative behaviors, enrichment of language, better cognitive abilities, perceptual processing of linguistic information, and so forth. Each target behavior (treatment goal) makes conceptual sense, or so it is generally thought, but none tells the clinician how to measure those behaviors.

Operational Definitions

Operational definitions define behaviors in terms of measurement procedures. In a sense, operational definitions are not definitions per se. They are descriptions of operations that are necessary to measure behaviors being defined. A clinician who comes across an operational definition should be able to measure the behavior by simply following the descriptions. To take an extreme example, intelligence may be defined as a persons's score on the Stanford–Binet test of intelligence. To determine a person's intelligence, all a clinician must do is administer the Stanford–Binet test and score the client's performance according to the standard procedure. A child's language behavior may be defined as his or her score on a particular language test, although no comprehensive test is available. As discussed shortly, behaviors can be more meaningfully defined operationally without the help of test results.

Operational definitions are more useful in describing clinical targets than in describing behaviors at a global and theoretical level. Clinical targets usually have limited scope. A clinician wishing to train the language competence of a client would probably have a very long way to travel, and would not know when and whether the destination has been reached. Therefore, treatment targets are more narrowly defined so that they can be observed and measured.

Training considerations also require that the target responses be limited in scope, defined narrowly, and observable. A well-defined response of limited scope has a better potential of getting trained than a global language competence or communicative ability. In addition, the clinician can manipulate only a few independent (treatment) variables at a time. Therefore, at any given time, only a few specific dependent variables (responses) can be handled efficiently.

Several examples of operational definitions can be considered. In treating a child who is minimally verbal, a clinician can select certain words as target behaviors. The treatment target can be defined as "the production of the following 10 words at 90% accuracy when asked to name appropriate pictures across two consecutive sessions" and include a list of the selected words.

If the training is expected to involve morphologic features, the treatment targets can be specified in terms of selected morphemes. For example, the target behavior may be defined as "the production of the regular plural morpheme /s/ at the level of single words while naming 20 pictures with 90% accuracy." Eventually, the plural morpheme may be trained at the level of conversational speech. Then the target behavior may be redefined as "the production of the regular plural morpheme /s/ in conversational speech at 90% accuracy across two consecutive sessions each, with a minimum of 20 opportunities to produce the target behavior." The final or dismissal criterion may be defined as "the production of the regular plural morpheme /s/ in conversational speech exhibited in the child's home at 90% accuracy across two separate language samples, with each sample containing at least 20 opportunities for the morpheme production." These examples make it clear that the target behaviors are defined somewhat differently depending upon the level of training.

If treatment involves certain types of sentences (syntactic structures), the targets may be defined as "the production of three- to four-word sentences in conversational speech across three home samples, each containing at least 100 utterances." Various syntactic structures can then be specified in the description of the treatment targets. For a particular client, the selected syntactic structure may be declarative sentences, requests, or passive forms of sentences.

The treatment targets in articulation disorders are also narrowly defined. Typically, the speech sounds are trained in the initial, medial, and final positions of words. For example, the phoneme /s/ may be trained in words such as *sun* and *soup* (initial), *muscle* and *hassle* (medial), and *toss* and *boss* (final). The initial treatment target for a given child may be defined as "the correct production of /s/ in the initial position of words evoked on a set of 20 discrete trials at 90% accuracy." A subsequent treatment target may be defined as "the correct production of /s/ in the initial position of words used in two-word phrases evoked on a set of 20 discrete trials at 90% accuracy." Similar definitions would be required at the level of sentences and conversational speech. The final dismissal criterion may be defined as the "correct production of /s/ in conversational speech at home and other situations at 90% accuracy across three language samples, each containing a minimum of 20 opportunities for the production of /s/." Production of sounds in the medial and final positions of words can be similarly defined.

Patterns of sound productions targeted for treatment should be defined in measurable terms. For example, if the pattern final consonant deletion—a phonologic process—is the target of intervention, it must be defined in terms of specific sounds that need to be taught to eliminate that process. Because no phonological pattern is eliminated without teaching specific sounds, the definition of a process elimination is still a description of target sounds. For instance, the pattern target may be defined as "the elimination of final consonant deletion by teaching the following sounds in the word final positions" and include a list of sounds to be taught.

In the treatment of stuttering, it is necessary to distinguish the final outcome of the treatment program and the specific target behaviors that must be taught to achieve that outcome. The final outcome of a stuttering treatment program may be defined as a "reduction in dysfluencies to less than 1% in conversational speech in clinical settings, and no more than 5% in everyday situations." The definition may also specify the length of speech samples in which the fluency is measured (e.g., three 300-word samples). Alternatively, the outcome may be defined as "99% fluency in conversational speech containing a minimum of 300 words produced in clinical settings on at least three consecutive occasions." The final outcome may be defined as "95% or better fluency in conversational speech containing a minimum of 300 words produced at home and other nonclinical settings recorded on at least three consecutive occasions." As in the treatment of any other communicative disorders, the initial, intermediate, and final outcome must be defined separately. The initial outcome in the modification of stuttering may be a "fluency rate of 99% or better at the level of single-word responses, or during oral reading of isolated words." In either mode, fluency must be measured in multiple and consecutive samples. As the response complexity increases from the single-word level to phrases and sentences, additional definitions are required.

In most stuttering treatment programs, to achieve the final treatment target or outcome, the clinician must teach specific skills of fluency. The following target responses are commonly taught: (1) inhalation and slight exhalation before the production of an utterance, (2) maintenance of airflow throughout the utterance, (3) soft and gentle initiation of sound, (4) reduced rate of speech through stretching of the syllables, (5) soft articulatory contacts, and (6) normal prosodic features (Hegde, 1985). The normal prosodic features are a clinical target because the other targets, when mastered, alter the pattern of speech. Although stutter-free, the speech is unusually slow and monotonous. Therefore, the typical intonation patterns and socially acceptable rate must eventually be shaped. Except for the normal prosody, which is shaped in the latter stages of treatment, all the target responses are initially trained at the level of single words or short phrases, and in successive steps the length of utterances is increased. Finally, the skills of fluency are practiced in conversational speech in clinical and nonclinical settings.

Treatment targets in voice disorders often are defined in terms of the clinician's judgments or evaluations. Sophisticated electronic instruments that measure and display various parameters of voice are available and are becoming increasingly affordable. When these instruments are not available, the clinician usually judges whether the client's voice is of acceptable pitch and intensity, and whether it is free from harshness, hoarseness, hypernasality, and so forth. Instruments such as Visipitch make this task easier by providing immediate feedback in the form of an electronic display. For example, in treating pitch disorders, electronic instruments may be used to assess the client's habitual pitch before starting treatment. In treatment sessions, the clinician and the client experiment to vary the pitch. Through such experimentation, a desirable target pitch is identified and described. The target itself can then be defined operationally. For example, the treatment target for a given client can be defined as "the maintenance of a level of pitch judged appropriate by the clinician with 90% accuracy in conversational speech exhibited in everyday situations." As in the case of other disorders, the number and length of speech samples should also be specified.

Similar instrument-assisted or judgment-based measurement procedures can be established in treating hypernasality, hyponasality, and other vocal characteristics. An operational definition would essentially specify the absence of undesirable vocal qualities in particular speech productions evoked initially in the clinic and eventually in the client's natural environments. Also, if vocally abusive behaviors must be changed to reduce undesirable vocal qualities, the reduction of those behaviors becomes a treatment target. The frequency of such behaviors as excessive yelling and talking in noisy environments can be measured for a few days before those behaviors become the operationally defined treatment target. For example, for a child who yells too much on the playground, the treatment target may be defined as "an absence of yelling in a 30-minute play activity." If a client is known to visit noisy bars frequently, a reduction in such visits, measured on a weekly basis, may be the treatment target.

For some clients, the targets to be taught may be nonoral or nonverbal communicative behaviors. Persons who are deaf and those who have multiple sensory and physical deficits may be candidates for nonoral means of communication training. These targets also may be defined operationally. For example, for a child who is deaf, the clinician may wish to teach American Sign Language. In this case, the clinician may define target behaviors as "the production of selected manual signs with 95% accuracy in conversational interaction produced in nonclinical settings." Whether the mode of nonverbal communication is sign language, an abstract symbol system, or electronic or manual display boards, the target behaviors may be defined in the same objective manner.

The Five Criteria of Operational Definitions

The examples given earlier illustrate the basic concepts underlying operational definitions of target behaviors. An operational definition should fulfill at least the following five criteria:

1. Specify the response topography. The topography or the form the behaviors take must be specified. Response forms include the production of the present progressive *ing*, the production of /s/ or /z/, such dysfluencies as part-word repetitions, nasal resonance on non-nasal sounds, hoarseness of voice, manual signs, and so forth.

2. Specify the mode of responses. In what mode the responses will be measured must be specified. Response modes include oral reading, conversation, imitative speech, or nonimitative (evoked, "spontaneous") productions.

3. Specify the level of responses. Whether the target responses will be measured at the level of single words, two-word phrases, or complex sentences must be specified. At different stages of training, targets are measured at different levels.

4. Specify the stimulus and setting conditions. Under what stimulus conditions and under what environmental settings the behaviors will be measured must be described. The responses may be measured when the client is shown pictures or asked questions, in the clinical situations, at the client's natural environment, and so on.

5. *Specify the accuracy criterion.* For the most part, a 90% accuracy rate is used. However, some behaviors may be held to a higher criterion. In some stuttering treatment programs, dysfluencies are held to a criterion of less than 1% (fluency of 99% or better). The number of consecutive observations for which the criterion is applied also must be specified (across three speech–language samples, over a set of 20 trials, in 10 consecutive responses, etc.).

Limitations of Operationalism

The operational approach has encouraged clinicians to define what they teach in objective and measurable terms. Although such definitions have been useful in documenting client improvement in treatment, the approach has limitations. When carried to its extreme, operationalism can turn complex concepts into meaningless definitions.

For example, when intelligence is defined as a person's score on a certain test, intelligence is reduced to a number that may mean nothing, or at least nothing important. This operational definition provides no better understanding of intelligence than before it was "operationalized."

Sometimes operationalism gives an air of scientific credibility to questionable concepts. It can dress up mentalistic and essentially unobservable concepts by redefining them in "measurable" terms. Simply because something is measured does not mean the underlying concept is valid. "Attitudes" are an excellent example. There are scales of measurement that "operationalize" attitudes. The resulting statistical analyses may give an impression of a valid scientific concept because it was measured; however, such measurement procedures may not validate the concept of attitudes. Attitudes are often inferred from certain kinds of behaviors; it may be more appropriate to measure those behaviors directly.

When the operational approach is used prudently, it can serve the clinician well. Although the operational approach is acceptable in defining somewhat concrete and specific behaviors of limited scope, the approach is not useful in defining broader and abstract concepts.

For example, the concept of language is not easily defined operationally, but the production of a morphologic, syntactic, or phonologic feature is easily defined operationally. To establish his or her accountability, the clinician needs to measure behaviors. Operational definitions make such measurement possible. An operational approach also can help avoid vague descriptions of treatment procedures. To this extent, operationalism is useful to clinicians.

SUMMARY

Assessment of clients' communicative behaviors is the first step in providing clinical services. Traditionally, in assessing a client, the clinician takes a case history, interviews the client, records a speech–language sample, completes an orofacial examination, screens the hearing, administers standardized tests, and conducts a closing interview.

The traditional assessment tends to overemphasize the use of standardized tests. Tests are limited in terms of questionable statistical notions of norms, lack of reliability of measures, limited sampling of behaviors, and so forth.

Assessment is better defined as reliable and valid measurement of clients' communicative behaviors. During the assessment, (1) all response modes must be measured, (2) the behaviors must be sampled adequately, (3) all measures must be repeated, and (4) extraclinical measures ideally must be obtained.

Multiple target behaviors and theoretical considerations create a need for selecting target behaviors. Structural categories are often selected as treatment targets. A better alternative is to select clinically verified response classes.

Responses that have the same or similar antecedents and consequences form a class. Such structural categories as grammatic morphemes, semantic notions, pragmatic structures, distinctive features, and phonological processes may or may not be empirically valid response classes.

Structurally similar categories may form different classes, and structurally different categories may belong to the same class. Response classes are found only through controlled treatment research.

The normative and the client specific are the two approaches to the selection of target behaviors. The normative strategy suggests that age-based norms are the appropriate targets for treatment. The client-specific strategy suggests that the client's environment, the relevance of the behaviors, the potential for maintenance, and the potential for response expansion must be considered in selecting target behaviors.

The normative strategy suggests that selected targets must be taught in the normal sequence with which they are acquired, whereas the client-specific strategy suggests that the best sequence of teaching multiple targets must be determined by clinical research in which different sequences are evaluated.

Target behaviors can be defined either constituently or operationally. The former does not specify measurement procedures, but the latter does. In defining the target behaviors operationally, the clinician must specify (1) the response topography, (2) the mode of responses, (3) the level of responses, (4) the stimulus and setting conditions, and (5) the accuracy criterion.

STUDY GUIDE

Define, describe, or answer the following questions in technical language. When you are not sure, reread the text and, when necessary, rewrite the answers.

1. Describe the traditional approach to assessment.

2. What is the recommended definition of assessment?

3. What was emphasized in the recommended assessment procedure?

4. Describe the need for selecting target behaviors.

5. What are norms?

6. Define reliability and validity.

7. Describe the language sampling procedure.

8. What are some of the things a clinician should not do while taking a language sample from a child?

9. What are the limitations of traditional assessment procedures?

10. What are the four criteria of measurement?

11. Distinguish between subject and behavior sampling.

12. What are the limitations of standardized tests?

13. How are theories related to the selection of target behaviors?

14. What is the normative strategy of selecting target behaviors?

15. Describe the client-specific strategy of selecting target behaviors.

16. What are the questionable assumptions of the normative strategy?

17. What are response classes? How are they determined?

18. Why should you be concerned with the sequence of training?

19. How should you determine the best sequence of training?

20. Describe two language response classes that do not correspond with structural (grammatic) categories.

21. What are structural categories? What critical variable is missing in pure structural analysis?

22. What are constituent definitions?

23. What are operational definitions?

24. Operationally define target behaviors for a client in the following categories:

- Language.
- Articulation.
- Fluency.
- Voice.
- Manual signs.

25. What are the two limitations of operationalism?

4

Contingencies as Treatment Variables

- Reinforcement and reinforcers

- Positive reinforcers

- Types of positive reinforcers

- Negative reinforcers

- Schedules of reinforcement

- Clinical use of reinforcement schedules

The professional task of clinicians who work with persons who have communicative disorders has been variously described as remediating communicative disorders, treating speech–language problems, reducing communicative deficits, helping people realize their communicative potential, teaching communicative skills, and so on. Although all these descriptions may be appropriate, some are not measurable. In Chapter 1, treatment was defined as a rearrangement of communicative relations between a speaker (client) and his or her environment. In this rearrangement, the clinician performs two basic tasks.

The clinician's first basic task is to **create** certain kinds of communicative behaviors, **increase** them, or both. Clients seek professional help either because they cannot produce certain communicative behaviors or because they produce the behaviors at very low frequencies. A child with a language disorder may not produce certain grammatic or semantic features or some response classes, or the child may produce those behaviors at only a very low rate. The child then needs to either learn those responses or learn to produce them more often. Similarly, a person who stutters exhibits less than the desirable level of fluency, and he or she wants this increased. A client who cannot maintain a desirable pitch level wants this vocal behavior increased. A child who is deaf may produce a few manual signs inconsistently. In this case, the frequency of sign production must be increased. Another deaf child may not produce any manual signs, in which case the signing behavior must be created.

New behaviors must be created or increased not only in clients, but also in people surrounding the client. The client's new behaviors may not be maintained if the people surrounding him or her behave in old ways that do not support the new behaviors. The same techniques that are used to create or increase behaviors in the client are used to create or increase behaviors in the people surrounding the client.

The clinician's second basic task is to **decrease** certain behaviors considered undesirable by the client, society, or both. This is often a counterpart of the first task of increasing desirable behaviors. A child who has a language disorder may be using gestures that need to be decreased while verbal behaviors are increased. A stutterer's dysfluencies need to be decreased while fluency is increased. In treating a child with an articulation disorder, faulty production of certain speech sounds needs to be decreased while the correct production is increased. In addition, clients may exhibit interfering behaviors that are nonverbal (e.g., out-of-seat behaviors) and they, too, must be reduced.

Certain existing behaviors that interfere with communication also should be decreased in people surrounding the client. Parents and spouses may offer suggestions that do not help a stuttering person. People may offer noncontingent and indiscriminate criticisms of faulty articulation of a child or language problems of a person with aphasia. Family members may react emotionally and in emotionally hurtful ways to the client's communicative problems. These types of actions by persons surrounding a client must be decreased.

To accomplish the two basic tasks, the clinician needs two sets of procedures, one to create and increase desirable target behaviors and a second to decrease or eliminate undesirable behaviors. A clinician's expertise is the efficiency with which these two sets of techniques are managed. This chapter focuses on techniques that increase behaviors that exist at low levels of frequency. Chapter 6 is concerned with creating new behaviors, and Chapter 8 with techniques of decreasing undesirable behaviors.

I pointed out in Chapter 1 that the most significant aspect of the treatment program within the paradigm is a contingency between certain stimulus variables, a response of certain topography, and consequences arranged by the clinician. The clinician manages the interdependent relation between these three elements of the contingency. Technically, **treatment variables** are the clinician-arranged response consequences, and **treatment** is a successful management of the contingency.

REINFORCEMENT AND REINFORCERS

While biologic contingencies select and shape the behaviors of species, environmental contingencies select and shape the behavior of individual members of a species (Skinner, 1989, 1990). Reinforcement is the most important element of an environmental contingency; therefore, reinforcement is essentially a selection process. Reinforcing consequences select and strengthen behaviors of individuals, just as biologic factors select and strengthen traits of species. Reinforcement is a broad concept of significant implications and the only highly researched concept that helps change behaviors, teach new behaviors, and shape more adaptive behaviors.

The clinician's job is to select and strengthen certain communicative and academic behaviors. Through this selection process, the clinician shapes such desirable behaviors as fluency, language skills, nonverbal communicative skills, vocal qualities, and academic skills. Therefore, it is essential to understand the broader concept of reinforcement as a means of environmental selection and shaping of behaviors. The essence of all remedial work and forms of education is this selection and shaping of behaviors.

The terms reinforcement, reinforcers, and reinforce must be distinguished. **Reinforcement** is a process of selecting and strengthening individuals' behaviors under specified stimulus conditions. It is a process of arranging events such that certain behaviors are more likely in the future. Reinforcement is the process of operant conditioning. **Reinforcers**, on the other hand, are events and objects that follow behaviors and increase their frequency. While reinforcement is abstract, reinforcers are concrete. We do not see or hear reinforcement; we only see its effects on behaviors, which are to increase their frequency. But we can see or hear reinforcers; we can hear a verbal praise or see a token. There is only one principle of reinforcement, but there are many kinds of reinforcers. Therefore, in Chapter 1, reinforcement was described as a principle and specific reinforcers as procedural examples of that principle. The verb **reinforce** means to strengthen and increase. We reinforce behaviors with specific reinforcers.

This means that certain events or objects, presented as consequences for behaviors, increase the frequency of those behaviors.

Decades of research on human behavior has established that consequences generated by behaviors shape the future course of those behaviors. Consequences of behaviors determine (1) whether a behavior will be initially learned; (2) if it is learned, whether it will be maintained over time; and (3) the strength and frequency of maintained behaviors. Therefore, in teaching and learning, response consequences are important. Both laboratory and applied human research has produced extensive information on how to program response consequences so that behaviors are selected, shaped, and maintained at high frequency. There are two kinds of consequences that help learn, increase, and maintain behaviors: positive reinforcers and negative reinforcers.

POSITIVE REINFORCERS

Positive reinforcers are those events that, when made contingent upon a response, increase the future probability of that response. Events that follow a response and thereby increase its frequency are positive reinforcers.

To reinforce, an event should follow a response *immediately.* This is described as a **response-contingent** occurrence of a consequence. A much delayed consequence is not contingent on a response. A temporal gap between the response and its consequence reduces the effectiveness of the consequence. In everyday life, consequences "naturally" follow responses. These consequences usually are the responses (reactions) from other people. In treatment settings, the clinician's reaction to a client's behaviors is the consequence. In the form of his or her behavior, the clinician carefully selects and arranges certain consequences such that they follow the target behaviors immediately. Then, to find out if the consequences so arranged are acting as reinforcers, the clinician carefully monitors the frequency of the client's behaviors.

In communicative disorders, a number of misunderstandings prevail about the definitions of basic behavioral terms. The definitions of positive and negative reinforcers and punishment procedures often are misrepresented by both clinicians and researchers. To use them correctly in treatment, research, and discourse, it is necessary to understand the technical meaning of these terms.

Positive reinforcers have a few critical features. First, reinforcers are *not* defined in terms of subjective feelings. How the clinician feels about a consequence or subjectively evaluates it is irrelevant to the definition. The clinician cannot determine that a piece of candy or verbal statements such as "Excellent!" are reinforcers because people want them, like them, or feel good about them. Giving something to a client because he or she "likes it" is no assurance that a reinforcer has been used. Such feeling states associated with reinforcers are not critical in the definition of reinforcers. Reinforcers must increase responses they were presented for.

Second, whether a given consequence is a reinforcer is not determined beforehand. A clinician should not say that candy will be used with a client because it is a reinforcer. It may or may not increase the client's response rate. Only after having demonstrated the positive effects of candy on a client's behavior should a clinician say that candy was used as a positive reinforcer. This means that there is no standard list of positive reinforcers from which the clinician may select reinforcers for given clients. There are no "presumed positive reinforcers." Therefore, the term is a misnomer.

Third, what is a reinforcer for one client may not be a reinforcer for another client. Indeed, an event that increases (reinforces) a behavior in one client may decrease (punish) it in another client. Therefore, it is important to determine objectively the effect of a given consequence on a particular person's rate of response. This requirement is consistent with the clinical concept that each client is unique, despite many common characteristics across clients. Therefore, every time a clinician uses a certain consequence as a potential reinforcer for a client, the rate of response must be measured continuously to see if it increases.

Fourth, an event that reinforces a client's behavior at one time may not reinforce the same client's behavior at another time. Therefore, the same event may not reinforce the same client across treatment sessions. In fact, an event that reinforces a client at the beginning of a treatment session may not reinforce toward the end of the same session. Again, an event is not a reinforcer unless it increases the frequency of a response. This also emphasizes the need to measure the response rates continuously. Thus, to be measured precisely, target responses must be objectively defined as described in Chapter 3.

TYPES OF POSITIVE REINFORCERS

There are two main types of positive reinforcers: (1) primary or unconditioned and (2) secondary or conditioned. Several varieties of conditioned reinforcers are described here, including (a) social reinforcers, (b) conditioned generalized reinforcers (c) informative feedback, and (d) high-probability behaviors.

Primary or Unconditioned Reinforcers

Reinforcers whose effects do not depend on past experience are called **primary** or **unconditioned**. The effects of unconditioned reinforcers are not learned. Primary reinforcers have their effects because they promote biological survival of the individual and the species. Genetic and neurophysiologic mechanisms of species predispose their members to react in certain ways to certain stimuli. When stimuli that promote survival are used to teach new behaviors that may or may not be related to biological survival, individuals take advantage of the natural effects of certain stimuli.

Food is a major form of primary reinforcer. Other edible or consumable items that may or may not have a significant food (nutritional) value are also grouped under this category. Most primary reinforcers have survival value, but some consumables do not. Cigarettes and chewing gum are examples of this sort. These reinforcers may not be totally unconditioned because there usually is a history of learning (experience) associated with them.

Food is used more often with certain populations than with others. Young children, children who are nonverbal or minimally verbal, and persons who are profoundly retarded often respond well to food. Food is almost indispensable in teaching or stimulating early speech and language behaviors to infants who have a high risk for developing communicative disorders. Normally intelligent adults who seek clinical services may be sufficiently motivated, however, to have their communicative disorders remediated that they may react favorably to secondary reinforcers.

When used appropriately, food can be an effective reinforcer. Because its effects are free from past conditioning, clients who have little learning history behind them can be expected to be sensitive to food. This may be especially true of nonverbal or minimally verbal clients for whom verbal praise, including "good" and "excellent," may not mean much. In working with such clients, both research clinicians and those providing routine services have used foods, including cereal, ice cream, milk, candy, fruits, cookies, cheese, and so on.

Strengths and Weaknesses of Food as a Reinforcer.   Food is a strong reinforcer. Clients who do not respond to conditioned reinforcers will usually respond to food. When it is needed, there are very few alternatives; therefore, it is used only when needed.

Although food can be a powerful reinforcer, it has certain limitations that the clinician should know how to overcome. First, food may be effective only when persons are **deprived** of it and motivated for it. If not, food may not reinforce behaviors. Therefore, it makes no sense to use cereal for a reinforcer in a session conducted soon after the client had breakfast. If a child ate plenty of candy during the not-too-exciting ride to the clinic, candies may not reinforce target responses in the treatment sessions. Therefore, the clinician must plan ahead when using food items as reinforcers. Most parents will cooperate if asked to withhold certain food items for several hours prior to the treatment sessions. Although unethical deprivation must be avoided, a snack of cookies, for instance, may be delayed for a brief duration until the client arrives at the clinic. In the case of infants, treatment sessions can be arranged close to breakfast or lunch times. Parents may bring food to these treatment sessions that the clinician can use for reinforcers.

Second, food may not promote **generalization** and **maintenance** of communicative behaviors the clinician teaches because food is not a natural reinforcer for many classes of speech and language behaviors. Most language response classes are more likely to be reinforced by conditioned (social) reinforcers in the form of verbal and nonverbal responses from other people than by food. Therefore, when food is used during training sessions, the language behaviors so learned may not easily generalize to other situations. This problem can be handled by simultaneous presentation of food and conditioned reinforcers. Food can be withdrawn gradually while continuing social reinforcers. This was done in most clinical studies in which food was the reinforcer.

Some classes of verbal behaviors are reinforced only by primary reinforcers, however. These behaviors are called *mands* in behavioral analysis (Skinner, 1957; Winokur, 1976). Mands (commands, demands, requests) are made because of certain motivational states, such as hunger or pain, and are reinforced by the presentation of food or termination of the aversive event that caused pain. For example, if the clinician were to train a response such as "May I have some juice please?" the most appropriate reinforcer would be some juice (primary reinforcer). Therefore, the frequent criticism that food is not a natural reinforcer for speech and language behaviors is not totally valid.

Third, food is susceptible to the **satiation effect**. Even following deprivation, the client may soon cease to work for food simply because of having had enough. This is the main reason why food, which worked fine in the beginning of a session, may be ineffective toward the end of it. This problem can be handled by the use of an intermittent reinforcement schedule in which food is given only for certain responses while certain other responses go unreinforced.

Fourth, it is not always convenient to present food **response contingently**. Because dispensing food can be messy and time-consuming, a delay between the response and the reinforcer may result, especially in group therapy situations. It is difficult to reinforce correct responses given simultaneously by a group of clients (Kazdin, 1984).

Fifth, clients and parents may **object** to the use of foods or certain kinds of foods in clinical sessions. The clinician wishing to use food as a reinforcer should consult with the clients, parents, or both beforehand. The clinician should select healthy food items. Medical conditions (e.g., diabetes and obesity) that restrict the consumption of certain kinds of foods must be ascertained before selecting food items for reinforcers. In such cases, the clinician may consider avoiding food altogether and select only secondary reinforcers.

Sixth, food can **interrupt** the sequence of training trials. If a child insists on eating every bit of cereal presented on each trial, the presentation of the training stimuli is slowed down. The clinician must wait until the child chews and swallows the food before presenting the next trial. However, during the latter stages of treatment, children may be persuaded to save their reinforcers until the end of the session, or eat only some of them periodically.

Seventh, food reinforcers **cost money**. Many clinics do not have funds to buy food items for reinforcers. Clinicians sometimes have to spend their own money to buy food. If family members agree to bring food that the clients would have consumed anyway, there is no extra cost to any party.

When prudently selected and used in such a way as to overcome its limitations, food is an acceptable reinforcer. When motivation seems to be a problem, the clinician should not hesitate to use food items in the early stages of training and then fade their use.

Secondary or Conditioned Reinforcers

Events that select and strengthen behaviors because of past conditioning are called **secondary** or **conditioned reinforcers**. Whereas primary reinforcers are biological, conditioned reinforcers are social and cultural. Without the benefits of a social and cultural environment, conditioned or secondary reinforcers are not effective. Conditioned reinforcers are especially important for specialists in communicative disorders because a large class of these reinforcers consists of verbal responses. Communicative behaviors not only are behaviors that are strengthened, but are tools of reinforcement. For example, verbal praise, a form of conditioned reinforcer, is both a powerful reinforcer and a class of verbal behavior.

Food may reinforce instantaneously, but most conditioned reinforcers are neutral in the beginning; they do not reinforce without some past learning or experience. For example, a smile or phrases such as "Fine job!" and "I like that" may not be reinforcing until a child has had certain experiences with them. Tokens are not reinforcing until they are associated with other kinds of reinforcers. When neutral stimuli become reinforcers, they have acquired conditioned reinforcement value. Neutral stimuli acquire such value because they are associated with other reinforcing events. While feeding, bathing, holding, and playing with the child, the caregiver might smile and say nice words. Later on, a smile and nice words may suggest such other tangible reinforcers as feeding and being picked up. Because of their association with already established reinforcers, neutral stimuli become conditioned reinforcers.

Among the varieties of conditioned reinforcers that are useful in the treatment of communicative disorders are social reinforcers, conditioned generalized reinforcers, informative feedback, and high probability behaviors. These are described in the following sections.

Social Reinforcers

As a form of conditioned reinforcers, social reinforcers are especially useful in teaching communicative behaviors. As suggested earlier, excluding mands, verbal behaviors are strengthened by social reinforcers. Therefore, it is natural to use them in teaching verbal responses. The most frequently used social reinforcers include verbal praise, attention, touch, eye contact, and facial expressions. For most individuals, these can be powerful reinforcers. Among these, the effects of verbal reinforcers in teaching communicative behaviors are particularly well documented. Verbal praise has been an especially useful social reinforcer.

Even when other reinforcers are used, social reinforcers should always be used. Verbal reinforcers may be combined with tokens and primary reinforcers. Verbal praise includes such statements as "You are working hard today," "That is right!" "I like that!" "Good job!" and "Excellent!" When paired with tokens and primary reinforcers, social reinforcers can become more powerful than they would otherwise be. Later, the target behaviors may be maintained only on social reinforcers.

Strengths and Weaknesses of Social Reinforcers. Social reinforcers have many strengths that the clinician can exploit. First, they are **not susceptible to satiation**, as primary reinforcers are. Apparently, people do not easily tire of verbal praise. Verbal praise may continue to be effective long past the point where food has ceased to be effective.

Second, social reinforcers are **more natural** than primary reinforcers. Because more verbal behaviors are reinforced verbally, social reinforcers may better promote generalization of target behaviors to extraclinical situations.

Third, social reinforcers **do not interrupt** the sequence of target behaviors. Verbal stimuli such as "Good girl" and "Excellent job" take little time and the treatment process need not stop. Treatment trials or conversational speech may be continued in an almost uninterrupted manner while using social reinforcers, especially verbal praise.

Fourth, social reinforcers can help **fade out** primary reinforcers. Initially, the two kinds of reinforcers may be paired. Later, the primary reinforcer can be gradually withdrawn, maintaining responses on social reinforcers alone.

Despite their strengths, social reinforcers may not always work. As noted before, they tend to be least effective with clients who do not have a past history of verbal behavior. Persons who are profoundly retarded, nonverbal clients, some autistic children, and other populations without much language experience may not initially react to smile and verbal praise. In such cases, the clinician should establish the reinforcing value of social stimuli by systematically pairing them with primary reinforcers. If this is done in the initial stages of training, the social reinforcers will acquire reinforcing value.

Conditioned Generalized Reinforcers

Conditioned generalized reinforcers are a powerful class of reinforcers. They are **conditioned** because they depend on past experiences to be effective; they are **generalized** because they are effective in a wide range of situations. Tokens, check marks on sheets of paper, marbles, stickers, points, and so forth, can be conditioned generalized reinforcers because, once earned, they can be used to gain a variety of "true" reinforcers. Their effects do not depend upon a particular state of motivation.

Money is a conditioned generalized reinforcer. People work hard for it because it does what a generalized reinforcer does: It gives access to many other kinds of reinforcers. In the beginning, however, conditioned generalized reinforcers may not be reinforcing by themselves. Their reinforcing value depends upon past experience. Eventually, they may be reinforcing in their own right. For those who hoard money, it is reinforcing by itself.

Much research has been done on the effects of tokens on various behaviors. Tokens were originally used in modifying behaviors of institutionalized mental patients. Since then, tokens have been used in a variety of clinical and educational settings to change a wide range of behaviors. Speech–language pathologists and audiologists have used tokens in modifying many aspects of communicative disorders.

Some clients, especially those who are institutionalized or developmentally disabled, may not initially work for tokens because the reinforcing value has not been established. In such cases, tokens are simply given to the client whose specific behavior is targeted for change. This is the initial noncontingent presentation of tokens. The client is given a choice of backup reinforcers for which the tokens can be exchanged. Soon, the tokens are made response contingent; that is, the client must perform the target behavior before the clinician presents tokens. Studies have shown that this procedure can change behaviors rapidly (Kazdin, 1984).

A common mistake in using tokens is not to have a backup system of reinforcers. Some clinicians who claim to use tokens may simply dispense marbles and plastic chips without backup reinforcers. Stickers given at the end of a session for being a "good girl" or "good boy" may or may not be reinforcers. Tokens must be exchanged for preferred reinforcers. These backup reinforcers may be small gifts or edible reinforcers, or they may be opportunities for various activities, including free play, listening to music, looking at comic books, listening to stories, taking a walk on campus, going to a store, and so forth.

Tokens are effective in treating all forms of communicative disorders. For instance, in treating articulation disorders, each time a client produces a target sound correctly, the clinician may place a mark, dot, or sticker on a chart, or a marble or plastic chip in a cup placed in front of the client. A client who earns a certain number of tokens may exchange them for a preferred backup reinforcer. The same procedure may be used in teaching language structures, skills of fluency, and various vocal behaviors. In teaching sign language, symbolic communicative behaviors, and academic skills, tokens may be used in the same manner.

Clinicians who have used various recording symbols for measuring target behaviors may have noticed that different symbols used for correct and incorrect responses sometimes acquire reinforcing and punishing values. When a plus mark (+) has been used for correct responses that are reinforced, the client may begin to react to it as he or she would to an actual reinforcer. Similarly, the client may react to minus signs (–) that may have been associated with punished responses as though they were punishing stimuli, even in the absence of the actual punishing consequence. These observations are suggestive of the way the conditioned reinforcers develop. A neutral stimulus becomes a conditioned stimulus because of its association with other reinforcing or punishing stimuli.

Strengths and Weaknesses of Conditioned Generalized Reinforcers.   Conditioned generalized reinforcers have several advantages. First, their effects do not depend upon a single state of **deprivation**. Because tokens or points can be exchanged for various reinforcers, the client is likely to "work for" a backup reinforcer. There is always something a client wants to which the tokens can give access. Therefore, conditioned generalized reinforcers are not susceptible to satiation effects.

Second, tokens and points are **easy to administer** in individual and group situations. Tokens are especially useful in reinforcing behaviors of individuals in a group. Tokens help personalize back-up reinforcers. Individuals can exchange tokens for reinforcers of their choice.

Third, tokens **do not interrupt** the treatment sequence. Time-consuming reinforcers that would normally interrupt treatment trials may still be used as backup. For example, short durations of play activity or food consumption may be used as backup reinforcers without interrupting every trial.

Fourth, tokens are useful when a client must work hard to obtain a **valuable reinforcer**. For example, if a cherished visit to a nearby zoo is a backup reinforcer, the clinician may require a large number of tokens or points to be accumulated before the trip is allowed. Only a token system will allow a large reinforcer to be earned in stages by cumulative work.

The limitations of a token system are mostly practical. First, a **variety** of backup reinforcers must be available all the time or there is no particular advantage in using a token system and, worse, there are no reinforcing stimuli. Because an effective backup system can be expensive to maintain, some institutions may not have funds to support a token backup system.

Second, when tokens are withdrawn, behaviors may **decline** suddenly (Kazdin, 1984), although this problem is not unique to tokens. Any system of reinforcement should be withdrawn gradually. Whenever tokens are given, social reinforcers also should be administered. Tokens can then be withdrawn in gradual steps while maintaining the behaviors on social reinforcers.

Informative Feedback

Another form of conditioned reinforcer, **informative feedback** reinforces responses by giving the client information about his or her performance. Persons who strive to achieve a certain level of proficiency in performing a skill would like to know how they are doing. Information that they are moving in the right direction can reinforce their efforts and keep them working toward achieving the criterion. Informative feedback provides such specific information to the client.

Some forms of informative feedback are similar to verbal reinforcers, but others are not. For example, feedback need not be verbal, as in the case of biofeedback. Mechanical feedback of information regarding a client's performance can be as reinforcing as verbal feedback. Also, verbal feedback need not be in the form of praise. It can be an objective statement regarding the level of performance in relation to a previously specified target criterion. The clinician can praise the client by saying "Good job!" or "Excellent work!" or the clinician can provide informative feedback by saying "Your dysfluencies were 15% last time; they are 10% this time." Informative feedback can be combined with verbal praise and other kinds of reinforcers.

Feedback is most efficiently and instantaneously provided by sophisticated electronic instruments. Many computerized instruments can give feedback on pitch, loudness, nasal resonance, oral resonance, phonatory onset, syllable durations, and other aspects of speech production. The feedback may be visual, auditory, or both. For instance, voice pitch may be visually represented in graphic form. Higher and lower pitch levels may be shown in corresponding bar or line graphs. Auditory feedback may represent higher and lower levels of pitch with tones of higher or lower pitch. Many such instruments are now commercially available. For example, such instruments as Visi-Pitch and Nasometer give feedback on vocal characteristics or nasal resonance. This feedback may be used to modify pitch, loudness, nasal resonance, and so forth.

One of the most researched aspects of informative feedback is **biofeedback**, in which the clinician uses mechanical devices to give information regarding the client's various physiologic functions, such as blood pressure and heart rate.

For example, in the treatment of stuttering, researchers have measured various muscle activity by electromyography (EMG), electrical conductance of the skin by galvanic skin response (GSR), and electrical activity of the cerebral cortex by electroencephalography (EEG). Of these, EMG has been monitored most frequently, presumably because stuttering seems to be associated with some degree of tension in speech-related muscles.

In biofeedback, the physiologic function of interest is measured and displayed in visual or auditory form. The client is instructed to maintain the display or change it in some manner. For example, the stutterer might be asked to reduce the level of muscle activity from the basal level in gradual steps. As the activity level decreases, a tone of progressively lower pitch may be heard. If muscle tension increases, the pitch of the tone will increase. In visual feedback, lights of different color may signal movement in the desirable or undesirable direction.

Direct feedback of muscle activity has not proven to be very effective in the treatment of stuttering. Because clinical studies done thus far have had methodological problems, it is unclear whether poor results were due to faulty studies or to some inherent weakness of informative feedback. However, a special form of feedback, known as **delayed auditory feedback**, is effective in reducing the speech rate, and thus inducing stutter-free speech. Several kinds of electronic delayed auditory feedback instruments are now available. As persons who stutter speak, these instruments provide feedback of what they said to them, but only after a brief delay. The clients do not immediately hear what they said. This delayed feedback causes clients to slow down their speech, thus eliminating most dysfluencies. The duration of delay may be gradually reduced and eventually faded out. Normal-sounding fluency is then shaped.

Strengths and Weaknesses of Informative Feedback. An outstanding strength of mechanical feedback is that it is objective and can be almost instantaneous. Verbal feedback by the clinician is easy to administer, but may not be as instantaneous as mechanical feedback.

The weakness of feedback procedures is the lack of controlled and replicated data on their effectiveness, especially long-term effectiveness. The use of recently developed, computerized, electronic feedback devices is becoming more common. However, controlled studies on their effectiveness are badly needed. This is especially true of mechanical feedback of information regarding physiological activity in clients with speech disorders.

Because of the lack of replicated data, feedback should be combined with other kinds of reinforcers, including verbal praise and tokens backed up with other reinforcers. When a clinician sets a performance criterion for the client and reinforces verbally, information regarding the performance is given to the client automatically. Eventually, any kind of reinforcer provides such feedback to the client. This might suggest that pure feedback regarding performance levels may be less effective than the feedback inherent in other kinds of reinforcers.

Informative feedback, including biofeedback, has been tested extensively in the treatment of behavioral disorders, including headaches, hypertension, anxiety and phobic reactions, cardiac arrhythmias, and epileptic seizures. However, questions have always been raised about the durability of pure feedback effects (Kazdin, 1984). Until supportive data are published, exclusive use of feedback procedures in communicative disorders may be considered experimental. Feedback is most applicable in the treatment of voice disorders and stuttering.

High Probability Behaviors

Reinforcers described thus far are things and events. Immediately following a response, some object, statement, or mechanical stimulus is presented. A reinforcer, however, need not be a stimulus or a thing presented by someone else. It can also be an opportunity to engage in some type of activity. The reinforcer in this case is a client's own behavior, which is something other than the target behavior the clinician is trying to establish. Because this type of reinforcer was originally described by a behavioral scientist named Premack, the underlying principle is sometimes described as the Premack principle.

The Premack principle states that a behavior of high probability can reinforce a behavior of low probability. It is important to note that both the response to be reinforced and the reinforcer are behaviors of the same person. The clinician controls the opportunities for the high probability behaviors, which are made contingent on the low probability behaviors.

Behaviors targeted for treatment are of low probability. Whether the target behaviors are the correct productions of certain speech sounds, oral language features, or specific signs of the American Sign Language, the behaviors are not exhibited at high probability. If they were, there would be no need for professional help. At the same time, the client who seeks help exhibits certain other behaviors at very high frequency. If these behaviors can be made contingent upon clinical targets, then a potential reinforcer will have been found. This means that the client should produce the clinical target to gain an opportunity to do what he or she very much wants to do.

The Premack principle is at work in everyday life. Whenever possible, people control access to desirable behaviors so that certain less preferred actions are performed first. Parents know that watching television is a high probability behavior for most children, whereas doing homework may be a low probability behavior. Many children are less likely to engage in solving math problems or reading history text books on their own than they are to watch television. If parents wish to increase such academic behaviors, they can make the television watching contingent upon finishing certain homework. Similarly, parents might ask the child to eat vegetables before eating meat. A man might be required to mow the lawn before watching a football game on television.

The clinician must observe the client in an unrestrained situation to discover the "natural" and relative frequencies of various behaviors. If one behavior is exhibited very consistently and at a high rate, and if opportunities for that behavior can be controlled by the clinician, then the Premack principle can be used in treatment. Typically, information gathered from a client's family members can be used in selecting potential high probability behaviors. Observation of children's preferred activities during early treatment sessions also may reveal potential high probability behaviors. For example, a child who frequently requests opportunities to draw or look at pictures in books may be reinforced if the clinician makes opportunities for such behaviors contingent on the child's producing the target behaviors.

Various activities that children exhibit can be programmed to act as reinforcers. Typical high probability behaviors in children include such activities as looking at comic books or pictures, reading books, listening to music, coloring and pursuing other artistic activities, playing with specific toys, and playing imaginary games with other children.

A word of caution is in order regarding the use of high probability behaviors. Some speech–language pathologists may use free play as a form of treatment. Often, such free play is simply an uncontrolled and noncontingent activity that may not reinforce anything. Such activities are a waste of time. There is a difference between free play and play activity as a response-contingent event. When play is response contingent, the clinician controls the child's opportunities to exhibit play activities by first requiring the child to perform in the treatment sessions. Also, the clinician measures the frequency of the target behaviors to see if the high probability behavior is acting as a reinforcer.

In most individual treatment sessions, high probability behaviors are parceled out depending upon the number of correct responses produced by the client. Clients typically earn and accumulate tokens and check marks that they exchange for an opportunity to engage in the selected high probability behavior.

Strengths and Weaknesses of High Probability Behaviors. The major strength of high probability behaviors is that they can be **powerful reinforcers** as long as they are made contingent on the production of target responses. They may be more effective than primary or social reinforcers. Another strength of high probability behaviors is that they reduce the **monotony** of treatment sessions. When the treatment sessions are long, brief breaks during which earned activity is permitted can make the treatment sessions more interesting to children. Often, different high probability behaviors can be identified for a given client so that a "pool of reinforcers" is constantly available to the clinician.

Weaknesses of this concept of reinforcement are mostly practical. First, it may not be possible to make the high probability behavior **contingent** upon target behaviors. An opportunity for a client to play for a few minutes, for example, cannot be made available for every correct production of a target phoneme or grammatic morpheme.

Second, high probability behaviors are perhaps the most **time-consuming** of reinforcers. Therefore, high probability behaviors cannot be used during the initial stages of training when every response must be reinforced. A solution to these two problems is to give tokens for correct responses and use high probability behaviors for backup reinforcers. Thus, a child is reinforced with tokens for every correct response, and the play activity is made available when tokens have accumulated.

Third, some high probability behaviors are **presented either in total or not at all** (Kazdin, 1984). If the child must earn 25 tokens to listen to music at the end of the session, but the number of tokens falls short of the criterion, the child may go totally unreinforced.

To avoid this problem, a low criterion of correct responses may be required in the beginning. This criterion may be gradually raised as the client's response rate improves. Backup reinforcers are made available to the client in each step of the treatment.

Multiple Contingencies

A variety of positive reinforcers have been described for use in treating communicative disorders. It is the clinician's responsibility to select an event that is reinforcing to a given client. The events described are not expected to act as reinforcers for all clients, for all behaviors, and across time. The clinician must remember that an event or stimulus is a reinforcer only when it increases a response rate. Measurement of the frequency of target behaviors is the key to determining whether an event is a reinforcer.

In most treatment sessions, it is desirable to use multiple contingencies. A combination of verbal and conditioned generalized reinforcers backed up with a variety of reinforcers, including opportunities for high probability behaviors, will be more effective than any one type of reinforcer.

As noted previously, primary reinforcers are also combined with other reinforcer types. In addition to positive reinforcers, response reduction procedures made contingent on interfering and undesirable behaviors also may be necessary.

NEGATIVE REINFORCERS

Positive reinforcers comprise only one category of events that increases response rates. The second category of events that increases response rates is known as negative reinforcers. In the positive reinforcement procedure, an event or a stimulus is *presented* contingent on a response. In **negative reinforcement**, a response removes, reduces, postpones, or prevents a stimulus, and, as a result, the response increases in frequency (Iwata, 1987). The events that are removed, reduced, postponed, or prevented are described as **aversive**. A response that terminates, minimizes, or postpones an aversive event is likely to be repeated when the same or similar aversive event presents itself in the future.

Many people find the concept of negative reinforcement difficult to understand. It is often confused with punishment and other response reduction methods. However, in punishment and related procedures, response rates decrease, whereas in negative reinforcement, the rates increase. Although these two are opposite processes with contrasting effects on response rates, some clinicians use the term negative reinforcement when they mean punishment. It is important to note that both positive and negative reinforcement procedures have the same effect on response rates, whereas punishment has the opposite effect.

To understand negative reinforcement fully, two concepts must be clear. First, there is usually an aversive event or stimulus. Second, there is a behavior that in some way reduces, terminates, or postpones this aversive stimulus. In the future, the same or similar behavior is likely when the same aversive event is present. People minimize their experiences with aversive events in various ways. Two examples from everyday life illustrate how a behavior that successfully minimizes or eliminates aversive events increases in frequency. When a person walks into a room that feels too hot, the person walks to the thermostat and lowers the temperature setting. This physical action terminates the aversive heat and thus negatively reinforces the action of adjusting the temperature. The next time the room seems hot, the person is likely to do the same because of negative reinforcement.

A mother, while studying for her exam, asks her screaming son to go to his room. If the son obeys, the aversive noise is terminated. Next time, in a similar situation, the mother is again likely to request her son to go to his room. In this case, a verbal request terminated an aversive event. Therefore, the mother's verbal request is negatively reinforced. However, note that we know the request was negatively reinforced only when the mother repeats the request under similar circumstances in the future.

Some aversive stimuli, such as excessive heat, cold, noise, and pain, may cause immediate physical harm. Termination of such events is necessary for the biologic survival of individuals. Therefore, like primary positive reinforcement, some forms of negative reinforcement have a biologic basis. The negative effects of other aversive events may not be immediate, but delayed. Rooms filled with cigarette smoke, for example, may be immediately aversive, but their biologic effects (e.g., lung cancer) may be delayed for many years.

Some events or stimuli may not have any undesirable physical or biologic effects, but may still be aversive enough that people would prefer not to experience them. The sight of a boring person, telephone calls from salespersons, screaming children, noisy neighbors, and excessive talkers are some stimuli that people tend to terminate. Those actions that are successful in terminating specific aversive events tend to be repeated.

Escape and Avoidance

Actual or potential experiences with aversive stimuli shape two kinds of behaviors: escape and avoidance. These behaviors are of interest to speech–language pathologists because they are frequently seen in persons with certain communicative disorders. In **escape**, a person comes in contact with an aversive event and then terminates it or reduces it. When neither termination nor reduction of the event is possible, the person may move away from it. In **avoidance**, the person prevents the occurrence of an anticipated aversive event so that the event is not experienced at all. In everyday life, persons typically move away from anticipated aversive events. Generally, first there is escape, and soon there is avoidance. For example, if a man who invites himself to your cafeteria table starts to ruin a pleasant lunch hour, you and your friends may hurriedly finish your lunch and leave. This is escape behavior, since you did come in contact with the aversive person and then you terminated or reduced the duration of the contact.

Escape may eventually lead to avoidance. For instance, if you learn that the aversive person regularly eats lunch at a certain time, you may decide to go to lunch earlier or later to avoid further contact with that person. As an extreme response, you may even start eating lunch at a different restaurant. These behaviors prevent the aversive experience. You escape from an aversive situation you are already in, and avoid the one you expect to get into. In either case, the behavior is reinforced negatively. The process of teaching new behaviors or increasing the frequency of existing behaviors through negative reinforcement is called **avoidance conditioning**.

In the example just given, escape behavior preceded avoidance behavior. However, one can learn to avoid a situation without first having escaped from it. In human behavior, this often happens because of the benefit of the verbal contingency. Your friend tells you not to go to a certain part of town because it is dangerous, and you do not go, even though you have never seen that part of town. This is avoidance without prior escape. When people follow safety rules, verbal advice, suggestions, warnings, and so forth, they avoid consequences of certain behaviors without having exhibited those behaviors.

Avoidance behaviors are commonly seen in some clients with communicative disorders. Persons who stutter may avoid telephone conversations, talking to strangers, ordering in restaurants, and speaking in front of groups. They also may avoid certain words and phrases. Some children and adults with articulation problems and persons who use alaryngeal speech or artificial larynges may avoid talking to persons who react negatively to their speech.

In the treatment of communicative disorders, there are few examples of negative reinforcement. To use it as a reinforcer, an aversive stimulus must be presented continuously. The stimulus is terminated when the client gives a desirable response. For instance, in reducing the rate of speech in a person who clutters, the clinician might provide continuous aversive noise through headphones and turn it off as the speech rate decreases. Such a decreased rate would be negatively reinforced.

The need to provide a constant aversive stimulus before it can be terminated response contingently makes the negative reinforcement procedure less attractive than positive reinforcement in reinforcing desirable behaviors. However, negative reinforcement plays a significant role in maintaining certain undesirable behaviors that need to be reduced. Avoidance behaviors of stuttering persons, for example, are undesirable and should be reduced. Many other kinds of undesirable behaviors exhibited by clients in clinical sessions may be negatively reinforced. When this is the case, the clinician must find ways of removing negative reinforcement for behaviors that must be decreased. Removal of negative reinforcement to decrease behaviors is discussed further in Chapter 8.

SCHEDULES OF REINFORCEMENT

Early laboratory research on ways in which responses may be reinforced produced a wealth of information on what came to be known as schedules of reinforcement (Ferster & Skinner, 1957). A **schedule of reinforcement** is a relation between (1) the number of responses and the amount of reinforcement, or (2) responses and the time duration between the delivery of reinforcers. A schedule specifies *how many* responses will be required before giving a reinforcer or *when* the reinforcer will be given. The reinforcement schedules used during training will determine to some extent whether the response will be acquired slowly or quickly, whether it will be maintained or extinguished as soon as the reinforcer is withdrawn, and whether or not the response will be maintained. Obviously, these are important treatment considerations.

There are two broad categories of reinforcement schedules: continuous and intermittent. There are several types of intermittent schedules. Each schedule has strengths and weaknesses and generates a distinct pattern of responses. The major schedules, their characteristic effects on response rates, and their clinical use are described in the following sections.

Continuous Reinforcement

In the continuous reinforcement schedule, every response is reinforced. In the early stages of treatment, however, when clients are likely to give both correct and incorrect responses, the clinician reinforces *only* the correct target responses. Incorrect responses may be presented with response reducing consequences. In clinical practice, then, the continuous reinforcement is interrupted by a continuous response reduction procedure administered for incorrect responses.

Social reinforcers can be easily administered on a continuous basis. Some other reinforcers, such as high probability behaviors, are not efficiently administered continuously. However, as noted earlier, when high probability behaviors are used as backup reinforcers, tokens may be given on a continuous basis.

A major strength of continuous reinforcement is that it can help generate a very high rate of response. When a response is totally absent or present only at a very low level of frequency, continuous reinforcement can be very useful in shaping that response or increasing its frequency. Therefore, continuous reinforcement is used in the initial stages of treatment. However, continuous reinforcement has a distinct weakness. Continuously reinforced behaviors may not be sustained when that kind of reinforcement is no longer available. Withholding reinforcers for a response is known as *extinction,* a procedure that typically results in a decreased rate of response. Continuously reinforced responses are highly susceptible to extinction. Therefore, in the latter stages of treatment, responses must be reinforced on an intermittent schedule so they are maintained in natural settings.

Intermittent Schedules of Reinforcement

In an intermittent schedule of reinforcement, some responses are not reinforced. There are several schedules in which reinforcers are delivered intermittently. Four schedules that have clinical applications to varying degrees are described earlier in this section. Two of these are dependent on the number of responses; the other two are dependent on the time interval between reinforcers. The former, called ratio schedules, have two variations: fixed ratio and variable ratio. The latter, called interval schedules, also have two variations: fixed interval and variable interval.

Fixed Ratio Schedules

Under a fixed ratio schedule, a predetermined number of responses is required before a reinforcer is delivered. For example, in treating an articulation disorder, a clinician might reinforce every fifth correct response. This would be a fixed ratio of five. The schedule is often abbreviated FR (fixed ratio), and followed by a number that specifies how many responses are required for reinforcement. An FR2 schedule would mean that every second response is reinforced, and an FR50 schedule would mean that every 50th response is reinforced.

Laboratory studies have shown that responses generated by fixed ratio schedules have certain important characteristics. First, between reinforcers, the response rate is very high. Once the initial response is made, the ratio requirement is completed rapidly. For example, under an FR20 schedule, as soon as the first response (after the last reinforcement) is made, the remaining 19 responses are made with very little hesitation between responses. Second, reinforcement typically results in a distinct pause in the response rate. The subject tends to "rest" a little each time the ratio requirement is completed and the reinforcer is received. This rest period is known as the **postreinforcement pause**. Third, the length of the postreinforcement pause is determined by the size of the ratio. The larger the ratio, the greater the duration of pauses.

The three characteristics of the fixed ratio schedule result in an all-or-none pattern of responses. The person is either working very hard or resting. There are few periods of lazy, slow, and unsure responding. High response rates and rest periods form a cyclical pattern under fixed ratios. Arrangements in many work-related situations approximate fixed ratio schedules. In agriculture, seasonal workers are typically paid on the basis of the number of bushels, boxes, or baskets that the workers fill with picked cotton, fruit, or vegetables. In the garment industry, payment may be contingent upon a certain number of dresses sewn. This type of an arrangement, known as piecework, is similar to fixed ratio schedules and can generate a very high production rate.

Ratio schedules also can make people work harder while receiving progressively less reinforcement. Laboratory studies have shown that by stretching the ratio in small and gradual steps, response rates can be maintained on very large ratios that deliver minimum reinforcement. Pigeons' pecking responses, for example, have been maintained on FR20,000. The history of industrial production shows that, in some cases, people have been made to work harder and harder while getting paid less and less.

When the ratio must be increased, it must be done gradually. An FR2 may be initially increased to an FR4, but perhaps not to an FR20. Large, abrupt shifts that result in prolonged periods of no reinforcement may cause **ratio strain**, a reduction in response rate due to a sudden thinning of reinforcement.

In several clinical studies, fixed ratio schedules have been used. Generally, very large ratios have not been used, presumably because the clients needed lower ratios. Fixed ratios of 2, 3, or 4 have been used frequently. However, when tokens are used, a large number of correct responses may be required before exchanging tokens for backup reinforcers.

Variable Ratio Schedules

A more powerful reinforcement schedule than the fixed ratio is known as the variable ratio (VR). Under this schedule, the number of responses required for reinforcement varies from occasion to occasion. However, such variations are not random. They are based on an **average** number of responses. A VR20 schedule, for example, suggests that an average of 20 responses are made before reinforcement, but the actual number of responses needed to receive the reinforcer is varied around 20. On one occasion, the reinforcer is given after only one or two responses, but on the next occasion, many more responses are required.

Persons responding under a VR schedule cannot determine when they will receive the next reinforcer. It might appear that every response has an equal chance of being reinforced. Although the response just given was reinforced, the next response also may be. Presumably because of such lack of discrimination, persons tend to respond more consistently under the variable ratio than under the fixed ratio.

Three major characteristics distinguish the pattern of responses under VR schedules. First, response rates under VR schedules are typically high. Second, there is no marked postreinforcement pause under the VR schedule. Third, a high response rate is more steady and consistent under the VR than under the FR schedule.

The absence of postreinforcement pause is probably responsible for the steady response rate under a variable ratio. In FR schedules, the delivery of a reinforcer means that the next or the next several responses will not be reinforced. Therefore, the subject often pauses in responding. Under VR schedules, on the other hand, because consecutive responses may be reinforced on occasion, the subject does not pause soon after receiving a reinforcer.

In everyday situations, reinforcers are probably more likely to occur on a variable basis than on a fixed ratio. For instance, a person may not find an interesting letter every time he or she checks the mailbox. Nor would the person consistently find a letter on every 5th or 50th try. Thus, the mailbox checking behavior is not reinforced continuously or on a fixed ratio basis. Something interesting may be in the mailbox every day for a few consecutive days, and then several days of junk mail may follow. Then suddenly, a long-awaited tax refund may show up. This kind of variable schedule produces a very strong response rate that resists extinction. Days and days of junk mail or even no mail do not deter most people from checking the mailbox regularly.

The persistence of gambling and similar behaviors may be due to the influence of variable ratios of reinforcement. A person playing a slot machine is often unable to predict the occurrence of a payoff. Any pull on the handle might make the person rich, or so it seems to the compulsive gambler. This persistence is thought to be a result of the indiscriminable (variable) reinforcement ratios built into gambling machines.

In controlled clinical studies, variable ratios have been used less frequently than fixed ratios. Administration of a variable schedule takes more planning than does a fixed schedule. In laboratory studies, electronic programming devices can be used to vary the number of responses from occasion to occasion while still maintaining a fixed average. As long as the device receives response inputs (e.g., a bar press), the reinforcer may be delivered automatically.

In routine clinical work, variable schedules are often administered more informally than in research situations. Within a narrow range, different numbers of responses may be required on different occasions of reinforcement. For example, at a certain stage in the treatment of an articulation disorder, four to seven correct responses may be required before the reinforcer is made available. At any given time, a specific number of responses would be required, but the number would vary across reinforcement opportunities. If the range of variations is relatively small, the clinician can implement a variable schedule efficiently without sophisticated programming equipment.

Just like larger fixed ratios, variable ratio schedules can also be useful in fading reinforcers given during the early stages of treatment. With proper planning, the ratio can be increased gradually, thus making it difficult for the client to discriminate the occasions of reinforcement from no reinforcement. Once again, this schedule might better approximate the natural environment and promote response generalization and maintenance.

In ratio schedules, the important factor is the number of responses a person makes. In interval schedules, the time duration between reinforcers is important. For this reason, these schedules are sometimes described as *time dependent*. Two basic time-dependent schedules are described below: fixed interval and variable interval.

Fixed Interval Schedules

In a fixed interval schedule, an **opportunity** to earn a reinforcer is made available after the passage of a fixed duration of time. The first response made following the interval is reinforced. Although time-dependent schedules specify a certain fixed or average duration, they also require a response before a reinforcer is given. The fixed duration may be over, but if the specified response is not made, the reinforcer is not given. The schedule only creates an *opportunity* to earn a reinforcer by responding soon after the duration is over. The interval of time measured is typically the duration between reinforcers.

The fixed interval schedule is abbreviated FI. An FI5-minutes schedule means that the reinforcer is given for the first response made 5 minutes after the previous reinforced response. Laboratory studies have shown that FI schedules have effects similar to the FR schedules, but have some distinct characteristics. First, overall response rates under FI schedules may be lower (less consistent) than those under FR schedules. This is probably because responses made within the interval are not reinforced. Therefore, few responses are made soon after a reinforcer is received. Indeed, a very distinct pause in the response rate usually follows the delivery of a reinforcer. The pause durations are often longer than those found under the FR schedules. The actual durations are a function of the fixed interval: The longer the interval, the greater the pause duration after the reinforcement. Thus, an FI10-minutes schedule is likely to produce a longer postreinforcement pause than an FI5-minutes schedule.

Second, under FI schedules, responses increase gradually as time passes, and they reach their highest rate just before the interval is about to end. For instance, under an FI5-minutes schedule, the responses may be nearly or totally absent soon after getting reinforced (postreinforcement pause). As the time passes, the response rate picks up slowly and increases gradually. After the fourth minute, the rate accelerates. Around the fifth minute (the end of the interval), the rate is highest because a response around this time has the highest probability of being reinforced. Thus, the typical response rates under FI schedules show a pattern of concentrated responses around the interval, a distinct pause after the reinforcer has been given, and a slow pick up of the response rate.

Although strict fixed interval schedules are not common in everyday situations, many behaviors are probably maintained by similar types of contingencies. Suppose you are expecting a job offer in the mail, and you can typically see the mailperson's vehicle approaching by looking out your window. Also, suppose that your mail is typically delivered around noon. You are unlikely to glance at the street at 10 in the morning, but you probably begin to glance at the street several minutes before noon. Initially, these glances are occasional. Soon, however, they become more frequent until at or around noon, you are constantly glancing into the street in the hopes of spotting the mailperson. Soon after the mail delivery (regardless of whether you received the expected letter), you are unlikely to look out for the mailperson until around noon the next day. This response pattern approximates the characteristics of behaviors generated and maintained by fixed interval schedules.

Another common example of everyday behaviors that approximate the effects of fixed interval reinforcement can be found in the study habits of many college students. In the beginning of a semester, when an instructor assigns a term paper due in 6 weeks, a student is not likely to rush home and burn the midnight oil. Many students give little thought to the paper during the initial week or two. Then the student begins to hear the unsettling story that some classmates have already done some work on their papers while the student was having a good time. Soon the student begins to put some time into the paper. Initially, the student may spend only a few minutes reading or thinking about it, but as the inevitable due date nears, the student starts spending more and more time on the paper. Finally, the day before the due date, the student may be missing from parties, bars, parks, beaches, and all classes as well. When the paper is finished and turned in, that student may not rush to the library to begin work on a project due in 4 weeks. He or she probably heads toward a more interesting place for an "I deserve it" type of experience.

Fixed interval schedules have not been used in applied research as frequently as fixed ratio schedules. In clinical treatment sessions, fixed interval schedules may not be as efficient as fixed ratio schedules because, during each session, the objective is to evoke responses *continuously*. A fixed interval schedule generates concentrated responses mostly around the time when the specified duration is about to expire. It does not encourage responses during the interval, which might lead to an inefficient use of treatment time during sessions.

In the treatment of voice and fluency disorders, what appears to be a fixed interval schedule sometimes may be used. For example, the clinician might require a client to speak with a certain pitch or maintain fluency for a certain duration of time. The client may be reinforced for such time-based responses. However, these are not strictly fixed interval schedules because clients are required to maintain target behaviors throughout the specified time interval.

Variable Interval Schedules

In a variable interval (VI) schedule, the time interval between reinforced responses is allowed to vary around an average. A VI5-minutes schedule means that, on the average, the first response made 5 minutes after the last reinforcement is reinforced. The duration of intervals differs from one occasion to the next. Sometimes the required duration may be more than 5 minutes and at other times it may be less; however, the variations are arranged such that the average duration between reinforcers is 5 minutes. As in the fixed interval schedule, the passage of time alone does not result in the delivery of a reinforcer. To be reinforced, the person must give the specified response.

Several characteristics distinguish the response pattern generated by variable interval schedules. First, VI schedules generate a steady (consistent) response rate. Because of this consistency, the overall rate tends to be higher under VI than under FI schedules. Second, the number of responses may be high or low depending on the specific duration of the interval. The shorter the duration, the higher the response rate, and vice versa. Third, the schedule does not generate distinct postreinforcement pauses. Instead, it shapes a persistent and evenly spaced response rate that may be somewhat lower than that found under variable ratio schedules. It is thought that those who work hard consistently, but are not especially fast, may have been exposed to variable interval schedules of reinforcement.

Schedules that are similar to variable interval schedules shape many everyday behaviors. Supervisors who check on workers at variable times might encourage more consistent work than those who check at regular intervals (i.e., at a fixed interval). With regular checks, employees work harder around the time the supervisor is likely to visit. But when the supervisor visits the workers at unpredictable (variable) intervals, workers must maintain a steady work rate. When students are taking an examination, the instructor might walk around the class to make sure that no one is cheating. If the instructor keeps changing the "route" such that he or she ends up checking each student at varying intervals, the students will be working under a schedule similar to variable interval schedules.

In the modification of communicative behaviors, VI schedules have been used infrequently. By and large, clinicians have tried to modify behaviors by directly controlling the number of responses made by clients. Ratio schedules permit a more direct manipulation of the number of responses. Also, the clinical treatment sessions are usually limited in time. Therefore, it becomes difficult to effectively arrange varying time schedules. Under gradually increasing ratio schedules, clients have to emit gradually more responses, and clinicians appropriately capitalize on this tendency.

Differential Reinforcement of Other Behaviors

A special type of reinforcement schedule that has been used in clinical settings is the differential reinforcement of *other* behavior (DRO). Most schedules specify which responses and how many responses will be reinforced. In a DRO, however, the clinician specifies a behavior that will **not be reinforced**. Several unspecified behaviors are reinforced as long as the one targeted for extinction (no reinforcement) is not produced.

Differential reinforcement is designed to increase some unspecified behavior while decreasing a specified behavior. In clinical sessions, clients often exhibit unwanted behaviors such as leaving the chair, crying, and looking away from the clinician. A given child may have a specific unwanted behavior that needs to be reduced. For instance, a child frequently chews on his or her shirt collar during treatment sessions. The clinician may use DRO to increase any or many desirable behaviors as long as the child omits the collar chewing behavior. The desirable behaviors that must be exhibited to get the reinforcer may not be specified. A variety of responses, including looking at the pictures, sitting in a certain posture, and responding to the clinician's modeling, may be reinforced. The child is told, for instance, "If you do not chew on your collar for 5 minutes, you can have an extra token." The essential feature of the schedule is that behaviors to be reinforced may be many, varied, and left unspecified, whereas what will not be reinforced is clearly specified.

Many clinicians probably routinely use the DRO schedule in controlling uncooperative behaviors by reinforcing a variety of cooperative behaviors. Possibly, the schedule is used more frequently with young children. Whenever the clinician tells the child, "If you *don't* do this, you will get this" (and follows through with expected results), the DRO schedule may be involved. One child may be given a token for not yawning during 10 training trials. Another child may be reinforced for not wiggling in her chair during the previous few minutes. Yet another child may be reinforced for not looking into the observational mirror while the clinician is trying to focus his attention upon a stimulus picture. While the child is not doing this or that specified action, any number or variety of other behaviors may be reinforced.

In the treatment of stuttering, the clinician may specify behaviors that are stutterings, and tell clients that as long as they continue to speak without those behaviors, reinforcement can be expected. Many of the currently effective stuttering treatment programs possibly make use of this schedule of reinforcement. Most clinicians try to establish a stutter-free pattern of speech. Initially, this pattern of speech may be slow and prolonged, and thus not the final target behavior. Nevertheless, this new speech pattern may be reinforced because it does not contain stutterings. Once a nonstuttering speech pattern has been learned, that pattern may be changed by shaping the normal prosody, including a rate that sounds appropriate. In this phase of treatment, the initially learned slow and prolonged pattern may itself become the behavior that would not be reinforced. To earn reinforcers, the client would then have to speak with normal rate and prosody while still not exhibiting stuttering.

Similar strategies may be used in the treatment of voice disorders. A client with an undesirable pitch may be reinforced as long as that pitch level is not exhibited while he or she is saying words or sentences. Assuming that the new pitch is in the direction of the final target, it may be reinforced simply because it is not the client's undesirable baseline pitch.

The DRO has a tremendous potential in controlling undesirable behaviors by way of increasing desirable ones. Therefore, the schedule is further discussed in Chapter 8 on reducing undesirable behaviors. It must be noted that, although the schedule may have the indirect effect of decreasing certain behaviors, it does so by *increasing* desirable behaviors. Hence, the schedule involves a positive reinforcement contingency and should not be confused with punishment.

CLINICAL USE OF REINFORCEMENT SCHEDULES

The strengths and weaknesses of different reinforcement schedules have important clinical implications. The clinician is initially concerned with either shaping a new behavior or increasing the frequency of an existing behavior. The clinician also is concerned with generalization and maintenance of newly shaped or increased behaviors. The schedule that works best in teaching behaviors initially does not generally work well in generalizing and maintaining those behaviors in natural settings.

The initial training of a target behavior is best accomplished with continuous reinforcement. Because most clients need a high density of reinforcement in the early stages of training, intermittent reinforcement schedules are not useful at this stage. However, continuous reinforcement is not efficient in promoting generalization and maintenance of trained behaviors. Therefore, after the behavior has been established by the use of continuous reinforcement, the clinician should switch to an intermittent schedule. When the target responses increase 30% to 50% over the baseline, continuous reinforcement may be discontinued. To start, an FR2 may be appropriate, and then the ratio may be increased gradually.

SUMMARY

Within the treatment paradigm described in this book, the treatment variables available to specialists in communicative disorders are known as contingencies. A contingency describes a relation between certain stimulus conditions, a specified response, and the consequences that the clinician arranges for that response. One main clinical task is to create nonexisting communicative behaviors and increase the frequency of existing behaviors. A contingency helps the clinician accomplish this task.

One part of the treatment contingency deals with the client's behavior, whereas two other parts deal with the clinician's behaviors. What the clinician does is treatment, and what the client does is the target. The clinician typically arranges stimulus conditions, which may include pictures, objects, modeling, prompting, and so forth. When the client begins to respond, the clinician arranges different consequences for correct and incorrect responses.

Consequences that help the client learn, increase, and maintain behaviors are known as reinforcers. There are two kinds of reinforcers: positive and negative.

Positive reinforcers are events that, when made contingent on a response, increase the future rate of that response. Reinforcers are not defined in terms of subjective feelings and perceptions.

There are two major types of positive reinforcers: primary (unconditioned) and secondary (conditioned). Food and other consumable items are among potential primary reinforcers. There are four types of secondary reinforcers: social, conditioned generalized, informative feedback, and high probability behaviors. Each type of reinforcer has strengths and weaknesses.

Primary reinforcers can be very effective, but they may not promote generalization of speech–language behaviors that are typically reinforced by social reinforcers. However, primary reinforcers are necessary in teaching certain kinds of mands (e.g., requests for food). They also may be necessary with clients who have limited verbal behaviors.

Social reinforcers are appropriate for reinforcing communicative behaviors. They minimize discrimination between treatment and natural environments.

Conditioned generalized reinforcers (tokens) are highly desirable because they are not affected by satiation. For them to work, a variety of backup reinforcers are needed.

Informative feedback can be useful, but it is a somewhat weak reinforcer when used alone.

High probability behaviors can reinforce low probability behaviors. In using the former as reinforcers, the clinician must control opportunities for exhibiting high probability behaviors.

Negative reinforcers are aversive events that, when terminated response contingently, can increase the rate of that response.

Escape and avoidance conditioning involves negative reinforcement. The clinical application of negative reinforcement has been limited.

A reinforcement schedule specifies a certain relation between responses, their number, or temporal characteristics on the one hand, and the reinforcer on the other.

In a continuous reinforcement schedule, reinforcers are presented for every response. This generates a high response rate that does not resist extinction well.

In a fixed ratio schedule, a predetermined number of responses is required for reinforcement. The schedule generates a high response rate with a postreinforcement pause.

In a variable ratio schedule, the number of responses required for reinforcement is varied around an average. A high and consistent response rate with no marked postreinforcement pause is the result.

A fixed interval schedule requires the passage of a fixed duration before a response can be reinforced. A relatively low response rate with distinct postreinforcement pauses is the result.

In a variable interval schedule, the time durations between reinforcers are allowed to vary around an average. The schedule generates a consistently high response rate with no pause after reinforcement.

The differential reinforcement of other behaviors is a schedule in which the behavior that will not be reinforced is specified. Many unspecified behaviors may be reinforced.

A continuous schedule must be used in the initial stages of clinical treatment, as this permits a faster acquisition of new responses. In subsequent stages of treatment, one of the several intermittent schedules is more appropriate to promote better generalization and maintenance of target behaviors.

STUDY GUIDE

Answer the following questions in technical language. Check your answers with the text. Rewrite your answers when necessary.

1. What are the two basic tasks of a specialist in communicative disorders?

2. What three factors are determined by consequences of responses?

3. Define reinforcement.

4. Define positive reinforcement.

5. What are some of the misunderstandings concerning positive reinforcers?

6. What is the single most critical criterion of defining positive reinforcers?

7. Name the types of positive reinforcers.

8. Distinguish between primary and secondary reinforcers.

9. Who might respond better to food as a reinforcer? Why?

10. What are the seven limitations of food as a reinforcer?

11. Why are social reinforcers more appropriate in the treatment of communicative disorders?

12. What are the strengths and weaknesses of social reinforcers?

13. Define conditioned generalized reinforcers.

14. What is an everyday example of a conditioned generalized reinforcer?

15. What kinds of conditioned generalized reinforcers are used in clinical situations?

16. What are the strengths and weaknesses of conditioned generalized reinforcers?

17. Define informative feedback and distinguish it from verbal reinforcers.

18. What is the most researched form of informative feedback?

19. What are EMGs, GSRs, and EEGs?

20. Describe the strengths and weaknesses of informative feedback.

21. Define high probability behaviors. What is another name for the same phenomenon?

22. Give some clinical examples of high probability behaviors.

23. What are the strengths and weaknesses of high probability behaviors?

24. What is the significance of multiple contingencies?

25. Define negative reinforcers. Give your own examples.

26. Distinguish between escape and avoidance. How are escape and avoidance behaviors reinforced?

27. What are schedules of reinforcement?

28. Define fixed and variable ratio schedules. Compare and contrast the two schedules in terms of their effects on response rates.

29. What is a postreinforcement pause? Under what schedules is it found?

30. Define fixed and variable ratio schedules. Compare and contrast the two schedules in terms of their effects on response rates.

31. Write down everyday examples of reinforcement schedules.

32. What is a DRO? Define it with examples.

33. Write down clinical examples of the way each schedule can be used.

34. Why should a clinician use intermittent schedules during the latter stages of training?

5

Treatment Program I:
The Basic Sequence

- Baselines of target behaviors
- The basic treatment program
- The basic treatment procedure
- An example of initial training and probe sequence

This chapter concerns how and in what sequence communicative disorders can be treated. By this point, the clinician should have (1) interviewed the client and taken a history, (2) assessed the client's communicative behaviors, (3) selected the target behaviors to be trained, and (4) selected the potential reinforcers to be used during the treatment sessions. The next step is to design and implement a treatment program.

Traditionally, treatment sessions are held immediately after an assessment is made. This follows the medical model in which treatment follows diagnosis. In the current model, an assessment merely suggests that there is a problem and that the client needs treatment. It can indicate potential target behaviors, but cannot determine them. Because assessment involves several activities, including interviewing and history taking, there is rarely enough time to implement additional procedures, the most important of which is reliable measurement of a client's communicative behaviors. Absence of such pretreatment measures makes it difficult to establish treatment effectiveness, client improvement over time, and clinician accountability.

One way of overcoming the shortcomings of traditional assessment procedures is to establish baselines of target behaviors before beginning treatment. The additional time spent on baserating selected behaviors is worthwhile. Not only do such baselines enhance reliability of measures and clinician accountability, but the measures are necessary to evaluate client improvement or treatment effectiveness.

An analysis of the client's assessment data might suggest that multiple speech and language behaviors are missing. All the missing behaviors might be appropriate treatment targets. However, the clinician can train only a few behaviors at a time. Because the baselines take a long time to establish, it is more efficient to baserate only those behaviors to be taught immediately. Also, baselines are valid only when established immediately prior to treatment. Long time lapses between baselines and treatment are not desirable because the clinician cannot know if the behaviors have changed since the time of baserating, and treatment effects or client improvement cannot be adequately evaluated.

BASELINES OF TARGET BEHAVIORS

Baselines can be defined as measured rates of behaviors in the absence of treatment. They can also be defined as the operant level of responses. An operant level is the "natural," typical, or habitual level of responses (Barlow et al., 1984; Kazdin, 1984). Baselines help the clinician determine the percentages of a client's correct production of phonemes, words, grammatic morphemes, syntactic constructions, pragmatic utterances, stutterings, dysfluencies, manual signs, academic skills, and many other behaviors or skills. Baselines also help determine the percentage of speaking time a client sustains a certain voice quality, fluency, topic maintenance, conversational turn taking, and other skills that may be measured in units of time. Such academic and general behaviors as the number of math problems solved, quiet sitting time, attending behavior, eye contact, cooperative behavior, and crying or whining, may also be baserated before treatment. In essence, baselines are quantitative measures of correct and incorrect productions of communicative or other kinds of behaviors before treatment is started. Any behavior the clinician plans to teach, increase, or decrease during treatment sessions must be baserated.

There are two basic reasons for establishing baselines before treatment. First, baselines give a reliable and valid measure of the client's behaviors prior to treatment. Unlike standardized tests, baselines sample behaviors adequately. Each target behavior is evoked several times to give the client multiple opportunities to produce it. Second, baselines make it possible to evaluate client improvement, treatment effectiveness, or both. The response rates measured throughout the treatment sessions can be compared against the baselines to show that, during treatment, the client's behaviors improved.

Baseline Characteristics

Acceptable baselines should have at least two characteristics. First, baselines should be reliable, that is, stable across time. To achieve this, the behaviors are measured repeatedly until some criterion of stability is reached. For example, a clinician may decide that the rate of stuttering measured in a client should not vary by more than 1% across two sessions. Similar criteria may be used in establishing baselines of articulatory, vocal, and language behaviors.

An exception to this criterion of stability is that a baseline showing a consistent worsening of the desirable target behavior may be acceptable. This **deteriorating baseline** is acceptable because the treatment has to be both convincing and powerful to reverse the deteriorating trend in the desirable behavior. For instance, if a stutterer's dysfluency rate is worsening daily, the trend is clear. Without treatment, fluency is unlikely to improve. Therefore, it is acceptable to introduce treatment without waiting for a stable baseline of stuttering or fluency. Also, it is unethical to delay treatment when desirable behaviors are deteriorating rapidly and the client needs treatment urgently.

Second, baselines should sample the target behaviors adequately. If baselines have to replace standardized test results, they must sample behaviors to a much greater extent than the tests do. For example, a standardized test of articulation may give the client two opportunities to produce the /s/ in the initial position of words. A baseline of the same behavior, however, may involve 20 words. Each word may also be presented on two trials. Thus, the actual number of opportunities to produce the /s/ may be 40, instead of the two or three on a standardized test. Similarly, the baseline production of grammatic morphemes may be evoked in the context of 20 words or sentences, each presented on multiple trials. Dysfluencies of people who stutter and abnormal vocal qualities of clients with voice disorders may be measured on repeated occasions to establish reliable baseline measures.

Typically, baselines are established in the clinic, although it is desirable to establish the baseline measures of target behaviors in the client's everyday situations. Whenever possible, extraclinical measures of target behaviors must be obtained. If the clinician cannot measure target behaviors in the client's home or classroom, parents or teachers may be requested to tape-record speech–

language samples and submit them for analysis. Nonclinicians often require some training in evoking and recording speech. Later, these measures can be used in assessing generalization.

Baseline Procedures

In establishing baselines of communicative behaviors, the following four steps may be used. Although these steps are general enough to be applied across disorders, necessary modifications can be made in the case of specific disorders. Examples of disorders are given to illustrate the applicability of the steps across disorders.

Step 1: Specify the Target Behaviors

The first step is to have a clear idea of the behaviors to be baserated. For clients with articulation problems, the specific sounds or phonologic processes may be targeted for intervention. To provide services to clients with language disorders, the clinician may target morphologic features, syntactic structures, pragmatic features, or functional response classes. For persons who stutter, dysfluencies or stutterings defined operationally may be targeted for reduction. Children with a repaired cleft may be initially trained in the non-nasal production of words that have no nasal sounds. Nonverbal or deaf clients may be taught selected manual signs. These and other target behaviors selected for treatment are operationally defined according to the criteria described in Chapter 3.

Step 2: Prepare the Stimulus Items

The second step in establishing baselines is to prepare stimulus items to evoke target responses. Although a variety of stimulus items can be prepared, pictures are probably most frequently used. Typically, a specific picture is used in evoking a particular response. Real objects, whenever appropriate and convenient to use, should be selected as stimuli. Target behaviors should also be baserated in conversational speech. In this case, the need for physical stimuli may be minimal.

To evoke speech from children, pictures or objects are typically needed. The selected stimuli should be unambiguous, attractive, and appropriate for the particular client. Whenever possible, they should be selected from the client's natural environment. Pictures used in the initial stages of training may be simple in that they may depict single objects. Eventually, more complex pictures that evoke connected speech in the form of elaborate descriptions or stories may be used.

Modeling the target responses is another form of stimulus. Frequently, clients who need speech–language services, especially some young children, may not give correct responses without the benefit of modeling. When the clinician models the correct response, the client imitates it. Because modeling is used frequently in training, it is also used on a set of baseline trials. The exact manner in which the target behavior is to be modeled must be predetermined.

When modeling is not needed, the clinician may ask questions to evoke responses. Questions designed to evoke specific target behaviors are also stimuli, and must be prepared beforehand. Many target behaviors may be evoked with such questions as "What is this?" "What do you see?" "What is the boy doing?" or "Where is the book?" Some responses may require a more careful framing of questions so that the clinician has the best chance of evoking the target behavior. Some target behaviors may need a combination of statements and questions. For example, in evoking a past tense inflection, the clinician may have to say, "Today, the man is walking. Yesterday, he did the same thing. What did he do yesterday? Yesterday he . . ." (Schumaker & Sherman, 1970). Other behaviors may require a sentence completion task instead of questions. For example, in evoking the regular plural morpheme /s/, the clinician may show a single object such as a book, and say "Here is a book," and then point to two books, and say "Here are two. . . ." The client should complete the sentence by saying "books" (Shipley & Banis, 1981).

About 20 stimulus items should be selected for each target behavior. If /s/ is to be trained in the initial position of words, 20 words and corresponding pictures should be selected. Similar sets of words and pictures are needed for medial and final positions. About the same number of stimulus items may be used in baserating most morphologic features, syntactic structures, or pragmatic utterances. In baserating various language structures, 20 words, phrases, sentences, or utterances that include the target behavior should be used. In baserating such vocal qualities as hypernasality, 20 words without nasal sounds may be used. Other vocal qualities may be measured in similar ways.

In the initial stages of treatment, most target behaviors are taught at the simplest level of words and phrases. However, as mentioned before, the final target is the production of those behaviors in conversational speech used in everyday situations. Therefore, baselines of speech, language, voice, and fluency targets must be established at this level.

In establishing baselines of target behaviors in conversational speech, the clinician may use open-ended requests or questions such as "Tell me about the picture," "What is happening here?" or "What did you do this morning?" With adult clients, topic cards often are useful in maintaining conversational speech. On each index card, the clinician writes a specific topic known to be of interest to the particular client. Several such cards can be prepared to evoke continuous speech for extended periods of time.

Step 3: Prepare a Recording Sheet

Because baselines are objectively measured rates of responses, each target response must be recorded on a recording sheet. This is the most important step the clinician takes in establishing his or her accountability. Objectively recorded baselines can be compared later with response rates during and after treatment. They also can be used by independent observers to verify client improvement or treatment effectiveness. Therefore, it is necessary to design a recording sheet on which all responses are entered and scored.

Each clinician can design his or her own recording sheet and use it routinely. The format of the sheet should be flexible to accommodate differences in the way certain target behaviors are measured. A basic recording sheet contains essential information about the client and the clinician, a listing of the target behaviors, and spaces in which to record each client attempt (trial) of every required response. The sheet should also show whether each response was correct, incorrect, or absent. An example of a recording sheet that can be modified by individual clinicians is given in Figure 5.1.

The recording sheet illustrated in Figure 5.1 shows how the production of the plural morpheme /s/ was baserated in the context of 20 words. Each of 20 target responses was presented on two discrete trials, as described shortly. The clinician then recorded correct, incorrect, and no responses. Finally, the percentage of correct response rate was calculated.

When evoked, this client produced the plural morpheme in single words with 20% accuracy and, when modeled, with 45% accuracy. Statements based on such baserates are stronger than those based on standardized tests of language performance, which often do not yield percentages of correct responses.

The recording sheet could just as easily illustrate a baseline of an articulatory behavior. A client's production of /z/, for example, can be baserated in the context of single words by use of the same two-trial procedure. Each production would be judged as correct or incorrect and marked accordingly. The clinician can then calculate the percentage of correct responses for the production of /z/.

Similarly, vocal characteristics such as hypernasality or hoarseness observed while the client produced selected utterances can be recorded on the sheet when each of the client's attempts is treated as a discrete trial. Under the heading "target behaviors," the clinician may write words, phrases, sentences, manual signs, gestures, or other nonverbal communicative responses.

The format illustrated in Figure 5.1 is most suitable for discrete-trial procedure, not for recording the baselines of target behaviors in conversational speech. Conversational speech is typically audio- or video-recorded for later analysis.

BASELINE RECORDING SHEET

Client:	Clinician:
Age:	Date:
Disorder: Language	Session No.: 2
Target Behavior: Plural /s/	Reinforcement: Noncontingent

	TRIALS	
TARGET BEHAVIORS	**EVOKED**	**MODELED**
1. Cups	–	+
2. Boots	–	–
3. Hats	–	+
4. Plates	–	–
5. Bats	+	+
6. Ducks	–	–
7. Ships	–	+
8. Cats	+	+
9. Boats	–	–
10. Rabbits	–	–
11. Coats	–	+
12. Nuts	0	–
13. Goats	–	–
14. Plants	–	–
15. Blocks	+	+
16. Lamps	0	0
17. Rats	–	–
18. Ants	–	+
19. Trucks	+	+
20. Pots	–	–

Note: + = correct; – = incorrect; 0 = no response.

Correct production of the plural morpheme:

Evoked: 20%   Modeled: 45%

Specified target behaviors can be any measurable behavior at any topography (words, phrases, sentences).

FIGURE 5.1.   Illustration of a two-trial baseline recording sheet.

TREATMENT PROCEDURES IN COMMUNICATIVE DISORDERS

Step 4: Administer the Baseline Trials

As noted before, stimulus items are administered on discrete trials. Figure 5.1 shows that each target response was administered on one evoked and one modeled trial. The difference between these two kinds of trials is the presence or absence of modeling by the clinician. On an evoked trial, the clinician asks a question to evoke a response and records whether the response was correct, incorrect, or absent. For example, in baserating the regular plural /s/, the clinician might show the client selected pictures of plural objects. Immediately, the clinician might ask such questions as "What do you see?" or "What are these?" The client might say "cup" (or "cups"), "book" (or "books"), and so forth.

A modeled trial is designed to find out if a response not typically produced by the client can be imitated. Soon after asking a question, the clinician models the response. For example, the clinician might ask, "What are these?" and add, "Say 'two cups.'" The clinician should probably add the client's name to the modeled response ("John, say 'two cups'"). If the client then says, "two cups," the response is scored as correctly imitated. It is useful to know if the client can imitate the target responses. If the client does not automatically imitate, then he or she must be taught to imitate. If the client can imitate, this step can be skipped. In addition, when multiple responses are baserated, those that are imitated correctly (but not produced on evoked trials) may be trained first.

A third sequence of evoked trial (not illustrated in Figure 5.1) occasionally may be used to informally evaluate the effects of the previous modeled trial. A client who did not produce a particular response on the first evoked trial, but who did produce it on the modeled trial, may be successful on a subsequent evoked trial. This would provide additional information on the relative ease with which baserated responses can be trained. An additional set of evoked trials would extend the time spent on baselines, and therefore may not be used all the time.

What is a trial? A trial is a structured opportunity to produce a given target response with or without modeling. Trials are discrete when they are temporally separated from one another. A trial consists of a sequence of interdependent events. These events are a part of the behavioral contingency discussed earlier.

The steps involved in administering a **discrete evoked trial** are as follows:

1. Place the stimulus picture in front of the client, or demonstrate the action or event with objects.

2. Ask the relevant predetermined question.

3. Wait a few seconds for the client to respond.

4. Record the response on the recording sheet.

5. Pull the picture toward you, or remove it from the subject's view.

6. Wait for 2 or 3 seconds to mark the end of the trial.

The clinician returns to Step 1 to initiate the next trial.
   A **modeled trial** is administered as follows:

1. Place the stimulus picture in front of the client, or demonstrate the action or event with the help of objects.

2. Ask the predetermined question.

3. Immediately model the correct response ("Johnny, say. . .").

4. Wait a few seconds for the client to respond.

5. Record the response on the recording sheet.

6. Pull the picture toward you, or remove it from the subject's view.

7. Wait for 2 or 3 seconds to mark the end of the trial.

The next trial would soon be initiated by placing the picture in front of the client.
   Note that the evoked and the modeled trials are similar except for the clinician's modeling on the latter. It is helpful to have the picture stimuli neatly stacked so that one picture at a time is pulled out and presented to the client. Scattered stimulus materials tend to evoke competing responses from young children. The children may respond to multiple stimuli simultaneously, making it difficult to measure individual responses.
   To measure responses on discrete trials, it is necessary to move or remove the picture at the end of the trial. This action helps separate each attempt on the part of the client. It also prevents the client from responding before the clinician asks the relevant question, or models the response. The procedure also can help the clinician record individual responses, because it can regulate the clinician's behavior as well.

Reinforcement in a Baseline Sequence

Because baselines are response rates in the absence of treatment, correct responses should not be reinforced. Also, no response reduction procedure is used when incorrect responses are produced. The clinician evokes or models responses without reacting to them. However, most baselines require many responses from a client. Sometimes, three or four target behaviors are base rated. This demand can create a motivational problem for some clients, especially for the young. They may not continue to respond in the absence of reinforcement.

To keep the client responding on baseline trials, the clinician should reinforce noncontingently. Periodically, the client may be reinforced for "Doing a fine job," "Good sitting," "Looking at the picture," "Saying the words," and so forth. Tokens and other kinds of reinforcers may also be used, but no reinforcer should be contingent on correct responses. Therefore, every reinforcer is presented during a brief pause period so that there is no contingency between responses and the consequence. For the young child, these reinforcing occasions may also provide needed breaks from structured trials. Such noncontingent reinforcers also may be given when the target behaviors are baserated in conversational speech or oral reading.

Analysis of Baseline Data

Baseline data are analyzed to calculate the percentage of correct responses. The recording sheet illustrated in Figure 5.1 shows the percent correct response rates for the production of the plural morpheme. The measure may be calculated for the production of various speech sounds. The percentage of syllables or words stuttered may be calculated based on the number of words, phrases, or sentences produced by the client. Vocal qualities also can be analyzed in terms of either the time duration for which a given quality was sustained, or the number of words, phrases, or sentences produced with appropriate vocal target. In turn, a percentage of correct responses can be calculated for these measures.

The percent correct response rate also may be calculated when target behaviors are measured in conversational speech. Frequencies of correct and incorrect productions of phonemes may be counted in conversational speech. The number of times a grammatic feature was used correctly or omitted when required may be counted.

Similarly, frequencies of stuttering behaviors along with the number of words spoken may be observed. The number of words (or syllables) on which pitch breaks occurred can be recorded, as can those on which desirable pitch was sustained. Such measures allow calculations of percent correct response rates.

The frequency with which a given communicative behavior is exhibited is probably the most objective of available measures. Absolute number of responses and percent correct response rates are preferable to subjective statements because they are easily verified by other clinicians.

THE BASIC TREATMENT PROGRAM

In treatment or teaching, the clinician produces changes in clients' communicative behaviors by increasing certain behaviors while decreasing certain other behaviors. The clinician accomplishes these tasks by systematic arrangement of appropriate contingencies.

The treatment procedures described in this chapter are based on the treatment paradigm described in Chapter 1. Much experimental–clinical research has been done on the efficacy of behavioral treatment procedures in communicative disorders. In the treatment of many behavior disorders unrelated to speech and language, the evidence has been replicated many times. Also, these clinical procedures are based upon principles established through replicated laboratory research.

The procedures have been used extensively in the habilitation or rehabilitation of a variety of clinical populations, including the mentally retarded, emotionally disturbed, brain injured, autistic, behaviorally disordered, and hearing impaired. The procedures also have been used successfully in regular and special educational classrooms.

Experimental Foundations of the Treatment Program

A comprehensive analysis of verbal behavior based on experimentally established controlling contingencies was published by Skinner in 1957. Following this, some of the earliest applications of the behavioral methodology in the field of speech were done in the area of infant vocalization (Rheingold, Gewirtz, & Ross, 1959; Todd & Palmer, 1968; Weisberg, 1961). These studies showed (and subsequent studies confirmed) that infant vocalizations can be increased or decreased by appropriate behavioral contingencies (Schumaker & Sherman, 1978).

One of the earliest disorders of communication to be researched with the behavioral methodology was stuttering. In 1958, Flanagan, Goldiamond, and Azrin demonstrated that stuttering could be brought under the influence of reinforcing as well as punishing contingencies. This study stimulated a series of investigations on stuttering within the conditioning and learning framework. Many basic and applied research studies have been published and continue to be published (Hegde, 1985; Hegde & Heidt, 1990; Hegde & Parson, 1990; Ingham, 1984; Martin & Haroldson, 1988; Onslow, Costa, & Rue, 1990; Prins & Hubbard, 1988; Ryan, 1974; Shames & Florence, 1980).

Systematic behavioral treatment of language disorders was initiated during the 1960s and early 1970s, when Chomskyan transformational grammar was popular. During this time, the nativists (Chomsky, 1957, 1965; Lenneberg, 1967; McNeil, 1970) raised serious questions about the possibility of empirical manipulations of language. The claim was that because languages are innately determined, behavioral or other environmental manipulations may not have significant effects on them. However, several early clinical experiments demonstrated that language was susceptible to the influence of the behavioral contingency as stated by Skinner (1957). In most of these pioneering studies, language was taught to children who were mentally retarded or autistic (Guess, 1969; Guess, Sailor, Rutherford, & Baer, 1968; Lovaas, 1966; Sailor, Guess, Rutherford, & Baer, 1968).

In subsequent years, operant methods of teaching language to children and adults with various language disorders became well established. Currently, the treatment of language disorders based on the behavioral principles of instructions, modeling, prompting, differential reinforcement, shaping, fading, and maintenance is the most tested of language training procedures. Numerous studies have produced controlled evidence supporting the efficacy of behavioral treatment techniques. It is not practical to cite all or even most of the studies here, but the results of many older studies continue to be replicated by newer studies. Also, behavioral methods continue to be applied to a wider range of clients who exhibit a variety of associated behavioral and physical problems or disabilities (e.g., Charlop & Milstein, 1989; Cole & Dale, 1986; Ezell & Goldstein, 1989; Foxx, Faw, McMorrow, Kyle, & Bittle, 1988; Garcia & DeHaven, 1974; Goldstein & Mousetis, 1989; Gray & Ryan, 1971, 1973; Guess & Baer, 1973; Harris, Handleman, & Alessandri, 1990; Hegde, 1980; Hegde & Gierut, 1979; Hegde & McConn, 1981; Hegde, Noll, & Pecora, 1979; Koegel & Rincover, 1977; Matson, Sevin, Fridley, & Love, 1990; McDonald & Blott, 1974; McReynolds, 1974; Warren & Bambara, 1989; Warren & Kaiser, 1986; Weismer & Murray-Branch, 1989; Welch, 1981).

Experimental evaluation of treatment methods used in the rehabilitation of adult neurogenic communicative problems has been a more recent phenomenon. In recent years, several studies have documented the effectiveness of behavioral treatment methods in the rehabilitation of adults with aphasia, dysarthria, and other neurogenic communicative disorders (Bourgeois, 1990; Doyle, Goldstein, & Bourgeois, 1987; Doyle, Goldstein, Bourgeois, & Oleyar, 1990; Georges, Bellaire, & Thompson, 1990; Thompson & McReynolds, 1986; Till & Yoye, 1988; Wambaugh & Thompson, 1989; Whitney & Goldstein, 1990).

Behavioral technology also has been demonstrated to be effective in the treatment of articulation disorders (e.g., Bailey, Timbers, Phillips, & Wolf, 1971; Baker & Ryan, 1971; Bennett, 1974; Costello & Onstine, 1976; Elbert, Dinnsen, Swartzlander, & Chin, 1990; Elbert & McReynolds, 1975; Fitch, 1973; Gierut,

1989, 1990; Koegel, Koegel, & Ingham, 1986; Koegel, Koegel, Voy, & Ingham, 1988; McReynolds & Elbert, 1981; Mowrer, 1977; Williams & McReynolds, 1975). Despite different approaches to the study and analysis of speech sounds and their errors, behavioral treatment methods have been found to be effective. Most of the currently practiced treatment approaches, based on sound-by-sound analysis, place–manner–voice analysis, distinctive feature analysis, or phonological process analysis, use behavioral methods of training the production of target phonemes.

Fewer studies have been done on the behavioral treatment of voice disorders, largely because of the general paucity of experimental evaluation of voice treatment techniques. Nevertheless, available studies have demonstrated that voice disorders and normal vocal behaviors can be modified by the same procedures as those used in the behavioral treatment of language, articulation, and fluency disorders (e.g., Blake & Moss, 1967; Fitch, 1973; Fleece et al., 1981; Jackson & Wallace, 1974; Lane, 1964; Moore & Holbrook, 1971; R.L. Patterson, Teigen, Liberman, & Austin, 1975; Roll, 1973; Schwartz & Hawkins, 1970).

Teaching various forms of nonverbal communication (e.g., the American Sign Language, communication board usage, and varieties of symbolic communication) to individuals who are profoundly retarded, autistic, hearing impaired, or multiply handicapped also has been researched within the behavioral paradigm. Many excellent studies are available. In addition to nonverbal communication, investigators have addressed many aspects of habilitation and rehabilitation of such populations (e.g., Angelo & Goldstein, 1990; Barrera & Sulzer-Azaroff, 1983; Berg & Wacker, 1989; Carr, 1979, 1982; Carr, Binkoff, Kologinsky, & Eddy, 1978; Carr & Kologinsky, 1983; Clark, Remington, & Light, 1988; Duker & Morsink, 1984; Faw, Reid, Schepis, Fitzgerald, & Welty, 1981; Hurlbut, Iwata, & Green, 1982; Remington & Clark, 1983; Wacker, Wiggins, Fowler, & Berg, 1988).

The treatment procedure described in this chapter is based on extensive laboratory and clinical research of the kind cited above. The effectiveness of the procedure has been replicated across disorders, with individuals of different ages, and by different clinicians.

THE BASIC TREATMENT PROCEDURE

This section outlines an essential sequence of treatment. The sequence may be altered to suit different stages of treatment or individual clients. The sequence includes various objective criteria by which a client's movement throughout the program and eventual progress can be determined. In Chapter 10, some advanced features of the training program are described.

The discrete-trial procedure, used in establishing baselines, is also used in training target behaviors. The studies cited earlier illustrate many aspects of the procedure described below.

The training sequence is initiated after the target behaviors are baserated. Depending on how a client performs, one or more target behaviors may be trained in single treatment sessions. Training is typically started at the level of a word, phrase, or sentence. In the beginning stages, most clients need modeling. Therefore, the training trial is similar to the modeled baseline trials except that it includes the treatment variable.

The treatment variable is the specific consequence programmed for the target responses. Contingencies that increase behaviors are placed on the production of desirable target responses, whereas contingencies that reduce behaviors are placed on undesirable responses.

A training trial is a sequence of events that includes certain actions on the part of the client and the clinician. In a typical discrete training trial on which modeling is included, the clinician performs the following steps:

1. Place the stimulus item in front of the client, or demonstrate the action or event with the help of objects.

2. Ask the predetermined question.

3. Immediately model the correct response.

4. Wait a few seconds for the client to respond.

5. If the client's response is correct, reinforce it immediately by verbal praise and any other potential reinforcer.

6. If the client's response is incorrect, punish it immediately.

7. Record the response on the recording sheet.

8. Pull the stimulus item toward you, or remove it from the client's view.

9. Wait a few seconds to mark the end of the trial.

The next trial is initiated by placing the same stimulus item in front of the client.

In treating adults who stutter or have voice disorders, the clinician may not need to present pictures and objects. The clinician may begin treatment by modeling or evoking one- or two-word responses. The clinician may ask questions that evoke single responses and, if necessary, model the response immediately. However, each attempt on the part of the client is treated as a discrete trial, and responses are measured accordingly.

Modeling is discontinued when the client begins to consistently imitate the correct response. When to stop modeling is one of the early "choice points" the clinician is likely to face. The clinician needs an objective criterion by which to make this decision (e.g., a criterion of five consecutively correct imitated responses). When the client meets the criterion, modeling is discontinued and evoked trials are initiated. The sequence of events is the same for evoked trials as for modeling except that Step 3 is omitted. The client is given a chance to respond appropriately to the clinician's question.

When evoked trials are first introduced, the client may or may not produce the correct response. If the client gives incorrect responses or no responses, the clinician should reintroduce modeling. To make this decision, the clinician needs another objective criterion. For example, the clinician may decide to reintroduce modeling when the client does not respond correctly on two or three consecutive evoked trials. Modeling can be continued until, for example, the client is correct on five consecutive imitated responses. At this point, evoked trials are reintroduced.

As treatment is continued, the client's correct responses on evoked trials are likely to increase and become more consistent. Soon, the clinician must judge whether the first one or few training items are tentatively trained. A training item may be a word, phrase, or sentence. For instance, it may be a word containing a target phoneme, a phrase containing a grammatic feature, or a sentence containing a target syntactic structure. A training item may also include utterances produced fluently or with certain vocal qualities. Specific manual signs and other nonverbal communicative behaviors also are training items.

The clinician should have an objective training criterion that suggests when training on one or more items may be stopped so that training may be started on new items. A **training criterion** specifies how many correct responses must be recorded consecutively before the response can be considered tentatively learned. A range of 10 to 20 consecutive correct responses (sometimes recorded across two consecutive sessions) is required by most clinicians. Ninety-percent correct response rate on a block of 10 to 20 trials may be an alternative criterion.

When the client reaches the adopted training criterion on the first or any item, it is considered tentatively trained. The clinician then selects the next items for training. The correct response is modeled on the first few trials given on new training items. When the client gives four to five consecutively imitated responses, the clinician introduces evoked trials. If necessary, modeling is reintroduced at any time according to the previously described criterion. Training continues until the client reaches the training criterion on the new item or items.

Management of Treatment Contingencies

The most important factor in administering treatment trials is to manage the reinforcing and response reducing contingencies. The correct response, whether imitated or evoked, must be reinforced immediately. There should be ' no hesitation in the clinician's delivery of reinforcement. Some clinicians hesitate because they have trouble judging whether the response was correct. Sometimes, the clinician might first record the response and then reinforce it. This also causes delayed reinforcement. Such delays are undesirable, especially in the beginning stage of training.

The reinforcers or corrective feedback given to clients must be unambiguous. A clinician unsure of a client's response might say, "Maybe your response was okay; I will let you have this token." Such statements are ambiguous in that they do not suggest to the client that the response was fully correct. The clinician must judge the accuracy of responses instantaneously and reinforce immediately and unambiguously.

The clinician should avoid too soft, unsure, and monotonous delivery of verbal praise. A frequent mistake is to deliver such verbal reinforcers as "Good" and "I like that" without any affect, smile, or appropriate facial expressions. Although there is no controlled evidence on this issue, such mechanical delivery of verbal praise may not be effective. Verbal praise must be strong, natural, and full of affect. It must be accompanied by appropriate facial expressions and other gestures.

The consequences that reduce the frequency of incorrect responses also must be delivered promptly. A hesitant and weak "No" may be as ineffective as a delayed and affectless "Good." The clinician must be quick in identifying wrong and uncooperative responses (see Chapter 8 for details).

The clinician also should remember at all times that the selected consequence may or may not increase or decrease responses. The clinician must measure the response rate continuously so as to monitor the effect of consequent events. When the target responses do not change, the consequences must be changed.

Training of Target Responses Versus Target Behaviors

A distinction between a target behavior and a target response is needed to understand the complete sequence of treatment. A target behavior is an empirical class of many similar responses (see Table 5.1). A target behavior is abstract, whereas a response is concrete. To teach a target behavior, clinicians teach target responses that belong to its class. A target response is an exemplar of a target behavior.

TABLE 5.1

Examples of Target Behaviors and Target Responses

TARGET BEHAVIORS	TARGET RESPONSES
The present progressive *ing*	• The girl is running. • The boy is playing. • The woman is reading. • The man is eating.
Requests or mands	• Water, please. • Can I go? • Tell me. • Help me.
Conversational turn taking	Several instances in which the client takes the role of a speaker and listener. Each instance is a target response, an exemplar of the target behavior.
Production of /s/ in word initial positions	• Soup • Soap • Sail • Sun
Prolonged speech (in stuttering treatment)	Utterances in which the syllables are prolonged. Each prolonged utterance is a target response, an exemplar of the target behavior.
Reduced hoarseness of voice	Utterances judged to have reduced hoarseness of voice. Each utterance is a target response, an exemplar of the target behavior.
Sign language skills	Production of selected and specified signs.

A client who learns to produce a target response may not have mastered the target behavior. Several target responses must be learned before a target behavior is fully mastered, generalized, and maintained in natural settings. For instance, a client who learns to correctly produce the /s/ in the word *soup* has learned a target response, not the target phoneme (behavior). Many words that contain /s/ in different positions must be learned before the clinician can say that the client has mastered the target phoneme. Similarly, the correct production of a grammatic morpheme is a target behavior, but the production of a specific exemplar is a target response. For instance, the correct production of the plural morpheme /s/ is a target behavior, but the production of individual phrases, such as "two books," is a target response. Only when the client has learned to say many such phrases ("two boots," "many hats," "nine cats," etc.) can a clinician assume that the target behavior (production of plural morpheme /s/) has been mastered. Many exemplars of specific grammatic, semantic, pragmatic, or other language structures, or nonverbal communicative skills, must be mastered before each of those target behaviors is learned.

Number of Target Responses to Be Trained

As the initial one or several responses meet the tentative training criterion, the clinician can train additional responses of the first target behavior. Soon, the clinician must find out if enough exemplars (target responses) have been trained on a target behavior so that the behavior may be considered tentatively trained. It is necessary to make this decision so that training on the target behavior may be terminated and training on a new target behavior started. For instance, if the client has mastered the production of the plural morpheme /s/ (a target behavior) by learning several exemplars (target responses), the clinician may start training on preposition *on,* a different target behavior. Several exemplars of this behavior will be taught to teach this new target behavior.

The clinician should have an objective basis to determine that a behavior has been mastered. A target behavior is fully mastered when it is produced by the client in his or her natural environment under normal conditions of stimuli and consequences. For continued responding, there should be no need for pictures, modeling, prompts, and other stimuli. Also, the response rate should be maintained with the types and amounts of reinforcers available in the natural environment. In short, a target response has met the final dismissal criterion when it is maintained in everyday situations. This dismissal criterion might specify a correct response rate of at least 90% in conversational speech in everyday situations. Therefore, as many responses as are needed to achieve this criterion must be trained.

The final dismissal criterion is not realized in the early part of training. It may not be realized until maintenance procedures are implemented. This requires additional time and work. Meanwhile, the clinician has the other selected target behaviors to teach. Therefore, within the treatment sequence, only a limited generalization is assessed to determine the need for additional training on the target behavior being taught. When most of the target behaviors are trained to a certain level of proficiency, a program of response maintenance may be started. In essence, then, the clinician needs a tentative criterion by which to decide to proceed to the next target behavior. This decision is made with the realization that additional training and maintenance strategies must be implemented at a later time.

The decision to proceed to the next target behavior is made on the basis of a tentative probe criterion. To determine if the client meets this criterion, the clinician conducts a **probe**, which is a procedure to assess the generalized production of a trained target behavior. This procedure is described in the next section. There may be different tentative probes implemented at different stages of treatment. For example, after teaching a few exemplars of a target phoneme, the clinician may probe to see if the correct production generalizes to untrained words. After teaching the correct production of the same phoneme in phases, the clinician may probe again to see if the phone is correctly produced in untrained phrases. Similar probes may be conducted after completing training at the sentence level.

An **initial probe criterion** used by many clinicians is a 90% correct production of the behavior being trained in the context of selected *untrained* words, phrases, or sentences. Although this type of generalization is limited, it may be sufficient to temporarily discontinue the training on a given target behavior and initiate training on the next.

The **final probe** assesses the generalized production of the target behaviors in conversational speech produced in the client's natural environments. A commonly used **final probe criterion** is the correct production of target behaviors at 90% or better in natural settings. This criterion may be as high as 98% for treated stutterers. It should be noted that such high probe fluency criterion is required only for the client to be dismissed from treatment. The client is not expected to maintain 98% fluency in natural settings, but he or she should maintain a minimum of 95% fluency. A higher criterion allows some increase in dysfluencies while the client's fluency remains acceptable (at least 95%).

To summarize, when a target behavior meets an initial probe criterion of 90% correct or better, the clinician can start the training on the next target behavior. The 90% accuracy may be measured at the level of words, phrases, or sentences, depending upon the level of training.

Thus far, the training sequence described involved the training of individual stimulus items of the first target behavior(s). Perhaps the clinician has trained three or four exemplars for a given target behavior. At this time, the clinician should probe to see if the initial (tentative) probe criterion can be met. If so, the treatment can be initiated on the next target behavior.

The Initial Probe Procedure

The initial probe procedure is administered as soon as the client has met the training criterion on a certain number of stimulus items. Sometimes, the clinician administers the probe after having taught four responses of a given target behavior. In the case of plural /s/, for example, one might probe after the client has met the training criterion on each of the following four responses: *cups, boots, hats,* and *plates.* At other times, probes may be administered after only two responses are trained. As a general rule, probes should be implemented after four to six items have been trained. There is some evidence that in case of language training, four to six stimulus items may be sufficient to obtain an initial, within-clinic generalization on structured probe trials (Guess & Baer, 1973; Hegde et al., 1979). However, such other behaviors as fluency, voice, or articulation may require additional training before generalization is assessed in the clinic. Clinicians may probe after having trained different numbers of responses to determine the best strategy for each client.

Because probes are designed to assess the production of trained responses given to new stimulus items, stimuli that were not used in training are presented on the probe trials. In the beginning, the clinician may have selected at least 20 stimulus items for each target behavior. Perhaps six of them have been used in training a particular target behavior. The clinician can now use the remaining 14 untrained stimulus items to probe generalization.

Probes also are administered on discrete trials. However, responses given on the probe trials are not reinforced. Thus, the probe trials are similar to the baseline trials. Consequently, it may be difficult to have the child respond for prolonged periods of time in the absence of reinforcers; the trained responses may be extinguished. Therefore, a probe in which the already trained items are also used is preferred. This probe type is called an *interspersed* or *intermixed probe.* Intermixed probes are typically used in the initial and intermediate stages of treatment.

In administering an **intermixed probe**, the clinician keeps the already trained stimulus items in one pile and the untrained stimulus items in another pile. Individual stimulus items from the two sets are alternated. Another method is for the clinician to keep all stimulus items in one pile that contains both the trained and untrained items in an alternating arrangement. On the first trial, a trained stimulus item may be presented, as on any training trial. The clinician consequates the response given to the trained item; that is, the clinician presents a response reinforcing or reducing consequence. On the second trial, the clinician presents an untrained stimulus item and asks the predetermined question, but provides no modeling. A few seconds are allowed for the client to respond, and the response is recorded. The client may give no response to the new (untrained) stimulus, or the response may be correct or incorrect. In any case, there are *no* contingent consequences and the clinician gives no feedback to the client. On the third trial, a trained item is presented and the response is appropriately consequated. Thus, trained and untrained items are presented on alternating trials in an intermixed probe sequence.

A probe in which only the untrained items are presented is called a **pure probe**. Pure probes are appropriate when the client is about to be dismissed from treatment. By this time, the clinician will have implemented several procedures to build up the client's resistance to extinction. The clinician will have gradually reduced the amount of reinforcement by using progressively larger response:reinforcement ratios. Primary reinforcers will have been withdrawn. Family members may have been trained to reinforce target responses at home and in other situations. Due to these and other procedures, the client's response rates will have been maintained in the absence of heavy and continuous reinforcement. Therefore, at the time of dismissal, the client can be expected to sustain the response rate on a pure probe that lacks trained items and, hence, reinforcement.

In later stages of training, when the target behaviors are trained in conversational speech, probes also are conducted in conversational speech. Discrete trials are no longer used. The clinician will analyze a conversational speech sample to find out if target behaviors are produced and sustained in words and phrases not used in training. In Chapter 7, procedures designed to enhance and assess generalization and maintenance are described.

A probe trial is identical to a baseline trial in that there is no modeling or response consequences on intermixed or pure probes. However, a probe trial is not called a baseline trial for two reasons. First, baseline trials help establish the operant level of a response, whereas probe trials help assess generalized production of the trained response. Second, the two sets of trials are administered at different times in the training program. Whereas the baselines are administered before the treatment is started, the probes are administered after the behavior has been trained to a certain extent. In essence, the baselines assess the rate of behavior in the absence of treatment, whereas the probes assess certain effects of treatment. Therefore, it is necessary to keep the two terms separate.

Analysis of Probe Results

The probe results are analyzed to calculate the percentage of correct responses given to untrained stimuli. Because only untrained stimuli are presented on a pure probe, the analysis is straightforward. The number of correct responses and the total number of probe stimuli are used to calculate the percentage of correct probe response rate. However, on intermixed probes that contain both trained and untrained stimuli, the probe analysis should include only the responses given to untrained stimuli, not the responses given to trained stimuli. For instance, if the clinician used 14 untrained items and 6 trained items on an intermixed probe, only the correct responses given to the 14 untrained stimuli are counted. If a client gave 7 correct and 7 incorrect responses on the 14 probe stimuli, the percentage of correct probe responses is 50%. The client's responses to trained stimuli are likely to be much higher than those on the probe trials, but are not of concern in the probe analysis.

Sequence of Treatment

The analysis of probe response rates suggests a sequence of treatment. Therefore, at any stage in treatment, what to do next is decided on the basis of probe results. As mentioned previously, a probe generally is administered when four to six items are trained to the training criterion. The results of this probe determine whether additional training is needed for the same target behavior or whether the next target behavior may be trained. The clinician needs an objective criterion by which to make this decision. In many clinical studies, a criterion of 90% or better correct response rate on probe trials has been used. Most clinicians use the same criterion to proceed to the next stage of training.

Behavior that fails to meet the initial probe response rate should receive more training. This training may be provided in one of two ways. If the probe response rate is somewhat low (70% or less), additional stimulus items can be selected for further training. If the probe response rate exceeds 70%, however, then a series of additional training trials on the already trained items may be sufficient to obtain a 90% correct response rate on the next probe.

If additional trials on the previously trained behavior do not improve the correct response rate on the next probe, it is best to train a few new stimulus items. After training new stimulus items, another probe is conducted. In essence, training and probe procedures are alternated until the 90% correct probe response rate is achieved.

If the initial correct probe response rate is at least 90%, the clinician may do one of two things, or both if time permits. The clinician may either start training on the next target behavior, or train the same target behavior at a higher level of response complexity. In doing both, the clinician starts treatment on a new target behavior while shifting training on the old target behavior to a higher level of response complexity. For example, if the first target behavior—for instance, the correct production of the plural morpheme in single words—has met the 90% correct probe response rate, then the training may involve either a preposition (a new target behavior), or the production of the plural morpheme in two-word phrases (a higher level of response complexity), or both.

There is no fixed number of stimulus items that, when trained, will assure the probe criterion. The amount of training needed will vary greatly across individual clients. The probe criterion enables the clinician to make an objective and flexible decision on the amount of training a client needs. The clinician should perhaps avoid the temptation of probing too soon, because probes consume time that may be better used in training. But the clinician should also avoid excessive training at a single level of response topography. Such training, especially at the single word level, may be inefficient because the training must move on to a more complex level, to the next target behavior, or both. Relatively frequent probes, when successful, can help make transitions in the treatment sequence at appropriate times.

When target behaviors meet the probe criterion at one of the higher levels of response topography (e.g., sentences and conversational speech in the clinic), then a program of maintenance can be started so that the target behaviors may be produced and sustained in the client's natural environment. Maintenance programs may be started on some target behaviors while others are still under training.

Single or Multiple Target Behavior Training

In many cases, multiple target behaviors may be trained in the same treatment session. For example, several phonemes can be simultaneously trained in the initial stage of articulation therapy. When a client's misarticulations show phonological patterns, multiple phonemes may be targeted for intervention. In treating language disorders, two to four response classes can be trained in the same treatment session. In the treatment of stuttering, oral reading and speech (at some level) may be simultaneously targeted for treatment. Similarly, a voice disorder can be treated at the level of oral reading and spontaneous utterances of limited response topography.

Some clinicians focus on a single target behavior in the initial stage of treatment. Teaching a single target instead of multiple targets may result in more rapid progress. With some clients, especially those who are profoundly retarded, simultaneous training of multiple targets may be confusing. An initial target behavior may have had a higher baseline level (more correct responses), making it somewhat easier to teach than the other behaviors with few correct responses. Behaviors having more incorrect baseline responses may be better taught at a later stage. However, when baselines of two or three target behaviors are somewhat high, they can all be selected for initial treatment. The sessions then can have some stimulus and response variety.

AN EXAMPLE OF INITIAL TRAINING AND PROBE SEQUENCE

The training procedure, stages of treatment, probe sequence, and various criteria described above are illustrated in this section. The client, Tommy, is a 6-year-old with a language disorder. After the assessment, the clinician baserated the following four grammatic features: the plural /s/, the auxiliary *is*, the preposition *on*, and the regular past tense ending with /d/. Each behavior was baserated with 20 stimulus items on a set of evoked and modeled trials according to the procedure illustrated in Figure 5.1. The percent correct response rate varied from 0 to 37. Figure 5.2 summarizes the baseline data for this client. Figure 5.3 illustrates the treatment data recording sheet and the data for the first target behavior.

The plural /s/ was trained first. Treatment was started at the level of single words. The first word trained was *cups*. Modeling was used in the beginning. Placing a picture of two cups in front of Tommy, the clinician asked the question,

---

Client: Tommy Logos
Age: 6 years
Disorder: Language
Target Behavior: Plural /s/, aux. *is*, prep. *on*, and (reg) past tense /d/

Clinician: Linda Verbose
Date: 1-15-92
Session No.: 2
Reinforcement: Noncontingent, verbal

TARGET BEHAVIORS	PERCENTAGE OF CORRECT RESPONSES	
	EVOKED	MODELED
1. The plural /s/ (*cups, boots,* etc.)	31	37
2. The auxiliary *is* (boy is running, boy is jumping, etc.)	18	30
3. The preposition *on* (on table, on chair, etc.)	9	10
4. Regular past tense /d/ (she opened, she pulled, etc.)	0	4

Note: All error responses involved omission of the target feature.
Each target behavior was baserated with 20 stimulus items.

FIGURE 5.2. Summary of hypothetical baseline data on a 6-year-old language disordered child.

Client: Tommy Logos
Age: 6 years
Disorder: Language
Target Behavior: Plural /s/
Training Criterion: 10 consecutively correct evoked responses.

Clinician: Linda Verbose
Date: 2-5-92
Session No.: 4
Reinforcement: FR2 verbal

BLOCKS OF 10 TRAINING TRIALS

TARGET RESPONSES	1	2	3	4	5	6	7	8	9	10
1. Cups	m−	+	+	−	+	+	+	−	+	−
	+	+	+	−	+	+	+	+	+	e−
	−	mt	+	+	+	+	e+	−	+	+
	~	+	−	+	+	+	−	+	+	+
	+	+	+	+	+	+	+			
2. Boots	mt	+	+	+	+	e−	+	+	−	+
	−	+	−	+	+	+	+	−	+	+
	+	+	+	+	+	+	+	+		
3. Hats	mt	−	+	+	−	+	+	+	+	+
	e−	+	+	+	~	+	+	+	+	+
	+	+	+	+	+					
4. Plates	m−	+	+	+	+	+	e+	+	~	+
	+	+	−	+	+	+	+	+	+	+
	+	+	+							
5. Bats	mt	−	+	+	+	+	+	e+	+	+
	~	+	+	+	+	+	+	+	+	+
	+									
6. Ducks	mt	+	+	+	+	e+	−	+	+	+
	−	+	+	+	+	+	+	+	+	+
	+									

Note: + = correct response; − = incorrect or no response; m = modeled trial; e = evoked trial, no modeling.

FIGURE 5.3. Treatment recording data sheet for the discrete-trial procedure. The data shown are for six target responses.

"What are these?" and immediately modeled the correct response by saying "Tommy, say 'cups.'" However, Tommy said "cup." The clinician said "No," and recorded the response as incorrect (–) on the recording sheet (see Figure 5.3). The clinician pulled the picture toward herself, and after a few seconds started the next trial.

Often, a vocal emphasis on the target response will help the client imitate it. Therefore, the clinician emphasized the /s/ in the word cups by producing it slightly louder and by slightly prolonging the sound. Tommy imitated the response on the second modeled trial, and the clinician immediately reinforced the response verbally and with a token. For 15 accumulated tokens, Tommy would be allowed 2 minutes of play with a toy of his choice. The clinician recorded the response and pulled the stimulus picture away from the child. After a few seconds, the third trial was initiated. The recording sheet shows that this type of discrete-trial procedure continued until Tommy gave five consecutively correct imitated responses. In the beginning, the numbers of correct and incorrect responses were about equal, but soon Tommy gave more correct than incorrect responses. Tommy needed 14 trials before he imitated the response on five successive trials.

The evoked trial was introduced on Trial 20 by omitting modeling. According to the recording sheet, Tommy's responses on the first two evoked trials (Trials 20 and 21) were wrong. The clinician said "No" to these responses. Modeling was reinstated on Trial 22. The next five responses were correctly imitated (Trials 22–26). Therefore, modeling was again discontinued on the 27th trial. This time, Tommy's response on the evoked trial was correct. Although incorrect responses were occasionally given, they became less frequent. Ten consecutively correct evoked responses (the training criterion) were eventually recorded. The recording sheet shows that Tommy needed a total of 47 trials to reach that training criterion.

The clinician then began to teach the next response ("boots"). Again, modeling was used in the beginning, but this time Tommy readily imitated the response. Because his responses were correct on the first five modeled trials, the sixth was an evoked trial. Tommy's response on this trial was wrong, but it was correct on the next trial. Once again, correct and incorrect responses were interspersed to begin with, but the rate of the correct response gradually increased. Tommy reached the training criterion of 10 consecutively correct responses in 28 trials.

Four more responses—"hats," "plates," "bats," and "ducks"—were trained in the same manner. As the recording sheet shows, the number of incorrect responses progressively decreased as the training continued. Tommy gave correct responses from the beginning on the last two training items, with only two incorrect responses each.

After Tommy achieved the training criterion on the sixth response, the clinician probed for generalization. The remaining 14 baserated stimulus items (not used in training) were presented on an intermixed probe sequence. Starting with a trained item, trained and untrained items were alternated on consecutive trials. Responses given to already trained stimulus items were all correct, and were reinforced. Some of the responses given to the probe (untrained) items were correct and others were incorrect, but the clinician presented no consequences for these responses. The first probe showed a correct response rate of 64%. This generalized response rate did not meet the probe criterion, showing a need for additional training. The probe data recording procedure is illustrated in Figure 5.4.

The clinician trained two more responses ("ships" and "cats"), which required fewer trials than the earlier stimulus items. At this point, the clinician decided to probe again, because the previous probe rate, although below criterion, was quite high. The second probe was also intermixed, and showed a probe response rate of 92%. This meant to the clinician that the target behavior plural /s/ was tentatively trained.

To summarize, Tommy was trained in the correct production of plural /s/ with the help of six individual stimulus items. Each of the six responses was trained to a training criterion of 90% correct. Two structured probes were held, and the probe criterion was met on the second probe. At this point, the clinician decided to (1) initiate training on the second target behavior and (2) shift training on the plural /s/ to the level of two-word phrases.

The second target behavior was the auxiliary *is*. This feature was trained in such utterances as "boy is running," "boy is jumping," and "boy is eating." The first six of the baserated phrases were again selected for the initial block of training. Consistent with the previous pattern of responses, Tommy needed modeling on the initial trials, but when modeling was withdrawn, he gave some wrong responses. Modeling was reinstated twice for the first response, and once each for the next three responses. Once the evoked trials were introduced, modeling was needed for the fourth and the sixth responses. The number of training trials needed to teach the individual responses varied from 23 to 58.

An intermixed probe, conducted after six responses were trained, showed only a 33% correct response rate. Therefore, four more responses with the auxiliary *is* were trained. (Note that for the first target behavior, additional training was given on already trained items at a similar juncture.) Adding several new (untrained) stimulus items to the original probe list, the clinician probed a second time. This probe showed an 87% correct response rate on the untrained items. The clinician next trained two more items, and probed for the third time. This probe showed a correct response rate of 95%. Following this successful probe, the clinician concluded that the auxiliary *is* was tentatively trained at the phrase level.

PROBE RECORDING SHEET

Client: Tommy Logos	Clinician: Linda Verbose
Age: 6 years	Date: 2-15-92
Disorder: Language	Session No.: 4
Target Behavior: Plural /s/	Reinforcement: Continuous/Verbal,
Procedure: Intermixed	FR2 cereal

TARGET RESPONSES	CORRECT (+) / INCORRECT (−)
1. Cups (T)	+
2. Ships (U)	+
3. Boots (T)	+
4. Cats (U)	+
5. Hats (T)	−
6. Boats (U)	+
7. Plates (T)	+
8. Rabbits (U)	−
9. Bats (T)	+
10. Coats (U)	+
11. Ducks (T)	+
12. Nuts (U)	−
13. Cups (T)	+
14. Goats (U)	+
15. Boots (T)	+
16. Plants (U)	−
17. Hats (T)	+
18. Blocks (U)	+
19. Plates (T)	+
20. Lamps (U)	−
21. Bats (T)	+
22. Rats (U)	+
23. Ducks (T)	+
24. Ants (U)	+
25. Cups (T)	+
26. Trucks (U)	+
27. Boots (T)	+
28. Pots (U)	+
29. Hats (T)	+
30. Mats (U)	−

Percent correct probe response rate:

Note: The trained (T) and untrained (U) items were alternated. The trained items were used repeatedly. The responses given only to the trained items were reinforced. The percent correct probe rate is based only on the number of correct and incorrect responses given to the 15 probe items.

FIGURE 5.4. Probe data recording sheet. Hypothetical probe data on the first target behavior described in Chapter 5.

While the auxiliary *is* was being trained at the level of three-word phrases during the first half of each session, the plural /s/ was trained at the level of two-word phrases during the second half. Responses such as "two cups," "four books," and "many cats" were used. Initially, four phrases with the /s/ were trained. Modeling was needed in the beginning; however, the correct response rate showed a more rapid increase at this level. There was no need to reintroduce modeling once the evoked trials were initiated. A probe, after four phrases were trained, showed a 76% response rate. Four more items were then trained, and a second probe showed a response rate of 95%.

In the subsequent sessions, training was initiated on the third target behavior: the preposition *on*. In each session, some time was spent in training the first two behaviors at progressively advanced levels of response complexity. When the plural /s/ met the probe criterion at the level of sentences, training on it was tentatively discontinued so that the fourth behavior—regular past tense ending with /d/—could be trained. In this manner, all four behaviors were trained and probed at successive levels of response topography. Eventually, the behaviors met the probe criterion at the level of simple sentences evoked on discrete trials.

When the discrete-trial–based training was completed, the clinician probed the target behaviors in conversational speech. Tommy's correct production of the four grammatic features varied from 57% to 92% in conversational speech. This suggested a need to reinforce some of the features in conversational speech. Therefore, the clinician arranged conversational speech situations that provided maximum opportunities for the production of the target behaviors. Care was taken to make sure that there were plenty of response opportunities on those behaviors that were below 90% on the conversational probe. In the beginning, all correct productions of target responses were reinforced. In subsequent sessions, these responses were reinforced on a VR10 schedule. Only verbal reinforcers were used. Another conversational probe indicated that no behavior was below 94%. At this time, the in-clinic training of the first four target behaviors—the plural /s/, the auxiliary *is,* the preposition *on,* and the regular past tense ending with /d/—was considered complete.

If Tommy had needed training on additional grammatic features, the clinician would have continued to train those features. Since he did not, the clinician assessed generalization of trained behaviors in extraclinical situations and implemented a maintenance program. The clinician first obtained three (the minimum is two) conversational speech samples recorded at home to assess the extent of generalization. Because Tommy's production of the grammatic features at home did not meet the dismissal criterion of at least 90% correct in conversational speech, the clinician decided to implement a maintenance program. Most clients need such a program. Maintenance programs are described in Chapter 7.

Although hypothetical, Tommy's treatment data are not unlike what is often seen in actual training situations. The treatment procedure, the treatment sequence, and the hypothetical results described here parallel data recorded in some treatment studies (Hegde, 1980; Hegde & Gierut, 1979; Hegde & McConn, 1981; Hegde et al., 1979). Figure 5.5, reproduced from a language study by Hegde et al. (1979), shows the target response rates in the baseline, training, and probe sequence involving four grammatic features.

As shown in Figure 5.5, each subsequent behavior has a longer baseline because of the multiple baseline design used in the study. The treatment segments in the graph show the actual response rates of a 3.9-year-old male on discrete trials. The line graphs do not represent averaged response rates; they show the child's responses on the first phrase trained for each of the four grammatic features. Additional stimulus items that were trained followed a similar trend, although the learning was faster on many occasions.

Application of Sequence to Other Disorders

The procedure and the sequence described above may be applied across communicative disorders. Some modifications may be needed depending upon the disorder, the client, or both. Treatment procedures often need to be modified to suit individual clients within the same type of communicative disorder. Such modifications can be made within the scope of the treatment principles discussed earlier.

In the treatment of **articulation disorders**, the same basic sequence can be used. The selected phonemes are baserated at the levels of single words, phrases, sentences, and conversational speech. The training is started on one or two phonemes at the single-word level. Typically, target phonemes are first trained in the initial position of words. Next, final or medial positions of words may be targeted for training. Each word involving the target phoneme in the initial position is trained to the training criterion of 10 consecutively correct responses. After several words are trained to such a criterion, an intermixed probe may be conducted to see if the trained phoneme would generalize to untrained words. If the probe criterion is met, training may be shifted to the two-word level. Also, training may be started on the same phoneme in the medial position. At each position, treatment shifts to progressively higher levels as and when the probe criteria are met for the lower levels. Should treatment time permit, other phonemes or the same phoneme in other position(s) may be trained.

The same procedure may also be used in treating **phonological disorders**. The clinician groups errors according to phonological patterns or pro-

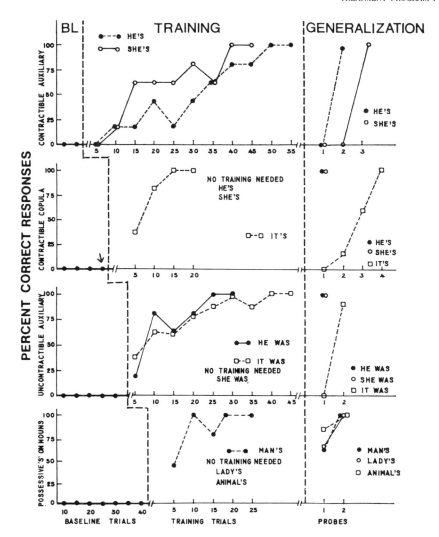

FIGURE 5.5. Percent correct response rates on the baseline, training, and probe trials for the four grammatic features trained in a language delayed child aged 3.9 years. The training segments of the graph represent the actual responses given to the first stimulus item in the case of each target behavior. From "A Study of Some Factors Affecting Generalization of Language Training" by M. N. Hegde, M. J. Noll, and R. Pecora, 1979, *Journal of Speech and Hearing Disorders, 44,* p. 309. Reprinted with permission.

cesses and teaches a few phonemes from a pattern. When these phonemes reach the tentative training criterion, other phonemes within the pattern are probed to see if they are now produced. If the untrained phonemes within a group or pattern meet the probe criterion, phonemes of another pattern, group, or phonological process are selected for training. This procedure continues until all patterns of errors are eliminated. Note that when patterns or processes are identified, the clinician probes all sounds within a pattern or process.

The treatment of **stuttering** also follows the same basic sequence. Target behaviors in the treatment of stuttering typically include an appropriate management of airflow, gentle onset of phonation, reduced speech rate, and prolongation of syllables. Treatment starts at the level of single words or short phrases. The client is asked to inhale, exhale a slight amount, initiate the sound softly, and say the words or phrases with prolonged syllables. Each attempt by the client is a discrete trial, and the target behaviors are scored as correct or incorrect. The training criterion for stuttering may differ somewhat from the one described above. The criterion typically used is 1% or less dysfluency rate. When the client begins to consistently produce words or phrases with the fluency targets, training is shifted to the level of longer utterances with the same targets. Although probes can be held to see if the speech is stutter-free on untrained words or phrases, this is unnecessary because fluency at this level is not of much significance. Next, the client may be asked to speak with target fluency skills in longer utterances and eventually in conversational speech.

The treatment procedure that includes the fluency skills just described results in an unnatural and socially unacceptable speech, although it is free from stuttering. The speech is too slow and monotonous. Therefore, when the client maintains 98% or better fluency (stutter-free conversational speech) with a reduced speech rate and syllable prolongation, the normal prosody must be shaped back to include socially acceptable rate and rhythm. The shaping procedure is described in Chapter 6.

The sequence and the basic procedures involved in the treatment of **voice disorders** are similar to what has been described. For example, in the treatment of pitch disorders, the clinician lowers or raises the vocal pitch of individual clients. After the client's habitual pitch is determined through an assessment procedure, that pitch may be baserated at the level of single words, phrases, and sentences. The clinician may find out that the client uses a certain inappropriate pitch on 80% of utterances, 50% of the time spent in speaking, and so forth. The target may be to have the client use an appropriate pitch on 90% of utterances or 90% of the time spent in speaking. The client may be given a demonstration of the desirable pitch level, and whenever that pitch is sustained on a word (or even a syllable), the clinician may reinforce it. Once again, each of the client's attempts is considered a trial, and the response is scored as correct or incorrect in reference to the targeted pitch.

When the client maintains the desirable pitch at the single-word level with 90% accuracy across a set of 20 trials, treatment may be shifted to the two-word level. Probes are probably better skipped at the early stages of voice therapy. When the training criterion is met at the two-word level, more complex responses, including sentences, may be targeted for treatment. Probes are necessary at this level of treatment. Probes sample vocal behaviors at the level of treatment, but involve untrained productions. Upon reaching the probe criterion for conversational speech in the clinic, generalization to situations outside the clinic is assessed and a maintenance program is implemented.

With suitable modifications, treatment procedures derived from the same principles of contingency management and sequences can be used in the habilitation or rehabilitation of **persons with aphasia, dysarthria, apraxia, laryngectomy, hearing impairment, physical disabilities**, and **developmental disabilities**. In treating such diverse groups, the clinician selects different target behaviors, not different treatment principles. For instance, the target behaviors selected for a patient with aphasia would differ from those selected for a person who is hearing impaired, but the same contingency management procedures and sequence of treatment may be used to teach those target behaviors.

Teaching **nonverbal communicative skills** and **academic skills** also uses the same general principles, most of the same procedures, and the sequences of movement from simpler to more complex levels. For example, in teaching sign language skills to a child who is deaf, the clinician starts with a few, useful, common signs and models them for the client. Modeling is withdrawn as the signs are consistently imitated. Signs that meet the initial training criterion are then trained in phrases and sentences. Additional signs are selected for training as the previous signs meet the training criterion.

The basic sequence presented in this chapter omits certain procedures that are typically a part of most treatment programs. For example, the client is assumed to be able to imitate the target behaviors when modeled by the clinician. However, some clients may not readily imitate target responses. In such cases, the responses have to be shaped. At other stages of treatment, clients need prompting. When these procedures are used to evoke responses, they need to be faded out. These procedures are described in the next chapter. Chapter 10 presents a more advanced sequence of treatment, along with suggestions on modifying planned treatment programs.

SUMMARY

Following an assessment, the clinician selects target behaviors and establishes baselines (i.e., response rates in the absence of treatment). Stable baselines help establish treatment effectiveness and client improvement.

A two-trial (one evoked, one modeled) baseline procedure is recommended. Each behavior is baserated with about 20 stimulus items. A discrete trial is a set of events that includes stimulus manipulations, response requirements, objective recording of responses, and intertrial durations. Baseline data are analyzed in terms of the percent correct response rate of target behaviors.

The basic treatment procedure also includes discrete trials. The target responses are modeled on the initial trials. Modeling is discontinued after five consecutively correct responses are noted. It is reinstated whenever two or more incorrect responses are observed.

A suggested tentative training criterion is 10 consecutively correct evoked responses on a given training item, or 90% accuracy on a block of trials. A 98% fluency may be used in the treatment of stuttering.

The most important aspect of treatment is the prompt and efficient management of reinforcing and response reducing consequences.

All correct and incorrect responses during baseline, treatment, and probe conditions are recorded on separate recording sheets.

The number of stimulus items to be trained depends upon the initial probe criterion. Probes assess generalized production of target responses. The initial probe criterion is 90% correct on untrained stimulus items, the number of which should exceed the number of trained items.

In the intermixed probe, trained and untrained items are alternated. On pure probes, only the untrained items are presented. A probe is administered after four to six items are trained. The results of either procedure are analyzed in terms of percent correct response rates.

The dismissal criterion is 90% or better response rate in conversational speech produced in everyday situations. In case of fluency, the criterion may be 95% or better.

Failure to meet the initial probe criterion results in additional training on new stimulus items or already trained items.

The second and the subsequent target behaviors are selected for training after the first behavior has met the initial probe criterion. Behaviors that meet the initial probe criterion may receive additional training at more complex response topographies.

This basic sequence and procedure can be applied across communicative disorders.

STUDY GUIDE

Answer the following questions. Use technical language. When not sure, re-read the text, and rewrite the answer. Always check your answers against the text.

1. Define baselines.

2. What is an operant level of a response?

3. Why are baselines needed?

4. What is a deteriorating baseline? Is it acceptable or not? Why?

5. Describe a baseline trial.

6. What are the four steps of the baseline procedure?

7. How does a clinician reinforce during probes?

8. How does a clinician determine the percent correct response rate?

9. Describe the discrete-trial procedure.

10. Describe the steps involved in modeled and evoked trials.

11. What is a training trial?

12. When does a clinician stop modeling?

13. When does a clinician reinstate modeling?

14. What is an initial or tentative training criterion?

15. What is a probe? Why is it necessary?

16. What are the two kinds of probes?

17. What is an initial or tentative probe criterion?

18. What is a final probe criterion?

19. When does a clinician start training on the second target behavior?

20. Define an intermixed probe. When is it used?

21. Define a pure probe. When is it used?

22. How does a clinician reinforce during probe sessions?

23. How does a clinician analyze probe results?

24. What are the two ways of providing additional training on already trained items?

25. Describe an initial treatment sequence with four target behaviors.

26. Illustrate, with two separate disorders (e.g., language and articulation), how the sequence can be applied across disorders.

27. What aspects of the treatment of stuttering and voice disorders may differ from that of articulation and language disorders?

28. Can a clinician train more than one behavior in a training session?

29. Specify the importance of managing contingencies during training.

30. Describe the best way of reinforcing correct responses.

6

Stimulus Control in Treatment

- Modeling and imitation
- Shaping
- Instructions
- Prompts
- Fading

The basic sequence of the treatment program described in Chapter 5 did not include details of certain procedures that are used in treatment. In this chapter, some important procedures that are a part of the treatment program are described.

MODELING AND IMITATION

Showing certain pictures and asking relevant questions may be sufficient to evoke responses in some clients. However, many clients, especially young children with articulation and language problems, may not respond appropri-

147

ately to stimuli that are sufficient to evoke speech in most speakers. As noted in the previous chapter, these clients need not only specially prepared stimulus pictures or objects, but also modeling as a special and distinct stimulus. In the treatment of communicative disorders, modeling is frequently used to help teach new responses that were nonexistent in a client's repertoire. Because much of speech–language treatment is designed to bring about new responses, the importance of modeling cannot be overemphasized.

In **modeling**, the clinician produces the target response the client is expected to learn. The client's response that follows modeling is called **imitation**. Because modeling refers to the clinician's behavior, it is a treatment (independent) variable. Imitation is a dependent variable; it is the behavior the client learns. Because imitation is a function of modeling and the reinforcing consequences, it is inappropriate to say that the technique of imitation is used in treatment. The technique used is modeling; the behavior this technique teaches is imitation.

Imitative responses are those that take the same form as their stimuli. When a person imitates a model, the modeling stimulus and the imitative response take the same shape or form. The difference between the two behaviors is in their temporal relation. The modeling stimulus comes first, and the imitative response follows. Thus, whether a behavior is imitative is judged by two criteria: (1) whether it has the same form as the modeled stimulus and (2) whether it follows the stimulus immediately.

The chain of modeling and imitation can be observed frequently in everyday situations. Young babies are often very good at imitation, and give an impression that they learn a lot by imitating events in the environment. The mother claps, and the baby does the same. The mother touches her nose, and the baby gropes for his or her nose. Adults also learn a lot by observing other people perform various activities. A combination of verbal instructions and demonstrations play a large role in learning many complex skills. Most demonstrations include modeling, instructions, and descriptions of target skills. When those who observe respond immediately, a chain of modeling and imitation is demonstrated.

Whether children acquire language by imitating the language they hear was once a subject of debate. Some experts have minimized the importance of imitation in the language acquisition process. Others have thought that, although imitation does not account for everything a child learns to say, it plays an important role. If children did not imitate speech sounds, syllables, and words, then the learning process would probably be prolonged. The child's tendency to imitate speech provides a foundation on which to build a more complex set of verbal skills.

Whether children normally learn language by imitation is not of much clinical significance. Controlled clinical research has repeatedly shown that modeling and imitation are useful techniques in teaching any form of behavior. Therefore, the techniques may be used in treatment regardless of how language is normally acquired. Very little experimental evidence supports the widely held belief that clinical treatment must follow the normal acquisition processes. Certain processes observed in normal acquisition may not be necessary for clinical treatment. For example, behaviors normally mastered earlier need not necessarily be taught before those that are mastered later (Capelli, 1985; De Cesari, 1985; Hegde, 1980). On the other hand, certain other processes, such as modeling, that may or may not play a major role in normal acquisition may be needed in treatment sessions.

Plenty of clinical evidence indicates the usefulness of modeling in the treatment of speech, language, voice, and fluency disorders. Many studies that have successfully used the modeling–imitation–reinforcement sequence in training were cited in Chapter 5. In the early part of treatment, modeling is often essential, although there is no guarantee that the client will be able to imitate the correct response when the clinician models it. When the client does not imitate at all, then the imitative behaviors should be shaped in gradual steps before nonimitative responses can be taught. The shaping procedure is described later in the chapter. When the client can imitate the target behaviors, however, the initial treatment phase can be relatively short and easy.

When to Model

Because modeling is a special stimulus, it is needed whenever typical stimuli such as questions, physical objects, and events do not evoke target behaviors. A language disordered child, for example, may not use the plural inflection when talking about plural objects and events. When asked to, a nonverbal child may not name objects or pictures. In such cases, it is probably of no use telling a client what to do. For instance, telling a child not to distort the /s/ in speech is ineffective. When a stuttering client is told to slow down, the rate may not be reduced. Modeling is needed in such cases.

The need for modeling is the greatest in the initial phase of treatment, when the client has no idea what the clinician wants. Typically, clinicians model on the initial trials until the client meets an objective criterion, such as five consecutively imitated responses. In subsequent stages of treatment, modeling is used when the evoked procedure fails on consecutive trials. Therefore, modeling affords an opportunity to produce an imitated response, thus avoiding repeated failures. When a client gives a few wrong responses on the evoked trials, modeling should be reinstated to make correct (imitated) responses once again likely. This procedure helps prevent a potential extinction schedule or excessive negative feedback because of wrong responses on evoked trials.

Modeling may also be needed every time treatment is shifted to a new phase or level. Although phases of treatment can and often do vary across individuals and disorders, some common phases are relatively constant. Typically, treatment is started at the level of single words or syllables, and progresses through the levels of phrases, sentences, and conversational speech. This is true regardless of the diagnostic category and the client's age. Whether they are asked to produce a phoneme, a grammatical morpheme, a gentle phonatory onset, or a certain vocal pitch, the clients are asked to learn new skills in levels of increasing response complexity.

The clinician may find that each time treatment is shifted to a new phase, the correct response rate is lower than what was recorded in the prior phase. A child who has achieved 90% correct production of /s/ in the initial position of words may drop to 30% correct when moved to the two-word level. A person who stutters may achieve gentle phonatory onset at the level of single words with 99% accuracy, but may revert to abrupt onset when moved to phrases or sentences. Therefore, at each new phase of treatment, modeling may be necessary.

The need for modeling in subsequent phases of treatment should not be as great as in the initial phases. Across treatment phases, there should be a progressive reduction in the amount of modeling needed or used. Marked need for modeling in the later phases of treatment suggests that the evoked trials are not as effective as they should be. In the final stages of treatment, such as those involving conversational speech in and outside the clinic, the need for modeling should be occasional, if at all. Excessive need for modeling in the final phases of treatment means that the target behavior has not been brought under its usual stimulus control. Usual stimuli for speech are natural events including speech, not modeling. Excessive need for modeling in later phases of treatment may also mean that the client was moved too fast from phase to phase, resulting in insufficient amount of treatment at each phase.

How to Model

Models are typically provided by the clinician; however, it is not always necessary or possible for the clinician to model target responses. For example, a clinician of one sex may not be able to model the correct vocal pitch for a client of the opposite sex. A clinician who speaks a dialect that differs from that of the client may not be able to model certain phonemes. These limitations are easily overcome because mechanically produced models can be used.

Mechanical models may actually be preferred to clinicians' live models. Mechanical models, which may be professionally prepared and made available to clinicians, may be more reliable and less variable from trial to trial. Increasing use of computers in treatment can be expected to reduce the need for live models. Sophisticated computer programs may represent various target responses in both visual and auditory modes. Several computer programs already show most target vocal characteristics. Other communicative behaviors may be similarly displayed on a computer monitor and through its audio system for the client to imitate.

In some cases, a client may be able to generate his or her own model. A client who misarticulates certain sounds may correctly produce them in certain contexts. These correct productions, when taped, can serve as modeled stimuli. The voice of many voice clients is not invariably abnormal. A clear voice or a certain desirable pitch may be captured on an audiotape and used as a self-model.

It is necessary for the clinician to provide a good transition from modeled to evoked trials. There is no such transition when the modeled and the evoked trials are not similar except for modeling. The clinician asks questions to evoke responses on most evoked trials on which the target response is not modeled. For instance, the clinician may ask, "What is the boy doing?" to evoke a verb + *ing*. To evoke plural word responses, the clinician might show appropriate pictures and ask, "What do you see?" Such questions are not necessary to have the client imitate on modeled trials. For example, the clinician can show the stimulus picture and state, "Say, 'the Boy is running'" or "Say, 'I see two books.'" The client may imitate the response. However, when modeling is discontinued, the question becomes necessary to evoke the response. If the question had not been asked on the modeled trial, its addition on the evoked trial may fail to provoke the response. Therefore, although questions are not necessary to have the client imitate correct responses, appropriate questions must precede modeling. For example, in modeling the verb + *ing*, the clinician first should ask the question and then immediately model the correct response: "What is the boy doing? Say, 'the boy is running.'" Similarly, in modeling the plural morpheme, the clinician should ask a question first: "What do you see? Say, 'two books.'" Later, the question is retained, but modeling is dropped or faded.

In the treatment of language disorders, a target response or responses may be a part of an utterance that contains nontarget responses. One example just given is a case in point. The target response being taught may be merely the *ing*; the child may be able to produce the main verb. Or the target response may be *is* and *ing* (the auxiliary and the present progressive). In either case, the sentence used on the training trials contains nontarget responses (*The, boy, run*). When the response to be taught is thus embedded in a phrase or sentence, it may be necessary to highlight it. Otherwise, the client may not imitate it.

An effective way of highlighting an embedded target response is to put **vocal emphasis** on it. When the clinician increases the vocal intensity on the specific target responses ("Say, 'the boy *is* running'"), the client may be more likely to imitate the target. Sometimes this procedure is described as a prompt, but prompts also can be a part of modeling. Other ways of prompting responses are described later in this chapter.

In the treatment of stuttering, the clinician may model the reduced rate of speaking, the gentle onset of phonation, or the prolongation of the initial sylla-ble of words. Even with adult speakers, it is often insufficient to tell them that they should reduce the rate of speech or prolong the initial syllable of words. The clinician must demonstrate a rate that is judged to be adequate to eliminate stutterings. Often, the rate at which stutterings decrease in a given client must be determined empirically. This means that a suitable rate must be found for each client through informal experimentation.

In the rate control treatment of stuttering, it is useful if the clinician also speaks at a noticeably slower rate. In this case, the clinician models a certain rate and expects it to be imitated, but the client does not imitate what the clinician said. If the questions are asked at a very fast rate, it may be difficult for the client to answer at a slow rate. A question asked at a slower rate has a better chance of being answered at a slower rate.

Live or mechanical models are frequently used in the treatment of voice disorders. In treating a vocal intensity disorder, for example, the clinician may have to model the louder or softer level that is being targeted for a given client. Modeling techniques may be equally necessary in the treatment of resonance disorders. Reduced or increased nasality on appropriate target sounds (and words) may have to be modeled before the client can imitatively produce responses with appropriate resonance.

Correct production of speech sounds in the treatment of articulation disor-ders is almost invariably modeled, although the clients are not often able to imitate the sounds in the initial stages of treatment. Modeling in the treatment of articulation can take different forms. Most modeled responses have the appro-priate acoustic (audible) properties of the target sounds. This is the typical "Say, 'sun'" variety of modeling. But modeling can also be nonacoustic, and purely topographic. This type of modeling involves a demonstration of the correct placement of articulators in the production of target phonemes. The clinician might silently demonstrate the position of the tongue for the production of /l/, or the relationship between the upper dental arch and the lower lip in the production of /f/. A distorted /s/ can sometimes be modified by modeling a very soft /s/ produced with minimum articulatory effort.

Reinforcing Imitative Behaviors

The clinician should immediately reinforce only correctly imitated responses. Sometimes, the client may not imitate the response fully. For example, a clinician might model the correct production of an /s/ in the initial position of words, but the child's response may not be an accurate imitation. Another clinician might model a word response in teaching a core vocabulary to a nonverbal child, but the child's response might at best be a partial imitation. Technically, imitative behaviors must resemble the modeled stimulus very closely. If not, they are not imitative behaviors, and therefore they may not be reinforced.

In clinical practice, insistence upon technically defined imitative behaviors can create problems in the initial stages of treatment. The client simply may not be able to imitate the modeled response fully, and therefore may never receive reinforcers. This will extinguish even partially correct imitative responses. To avoid this problem, clinicians can reinforce a response if it shows some improvement or movement in the right direction. The clinician judges whether the attempted imitation is better than the responses typically given by the client on the baseline trials. If it is, the response may be accepted as imitative, and reinforced accordingly.

When less than full imitations are accepted, the clinician should gradually raise the performance accuracy required for the client to receive reinforcers. Therefore, what was accepted on the initial trials are not accepted on subsequent trials. Progressively better imitations must be required to earn reinforcers. Eventually, the client's responses should match the modeled stimuli as fully as possible.

The procedure in which less than desirable responses are accepted initially, and the criterion of performance is raised gradually as the client's level of mastery increases is known as shaping or successive approximations. The procedure, which is not limited to modeling–imitation sequences, is described later in this chapter.

How to Withdraw or Fade Modeling

As noted earlier, modeling is an additional stimulus, and explicit modeling is typically not one of natural stimuli. Therefore, modeling must be used only when necessary and must be discontinued as soon as possible. However, it is always possible that, when modeling is discontinued, the client may not give the correct response. Thus, the clinician should give some thought to the manner in which modeling is discontinued.

Modeling can be either withdrawn all at once or faded gradually. In **withdrawal of modeling**, the clinician simply stops modeling as soon as a criterion of imitative responses has been met. Evoked trials are then introduced. In **fading the modeled stimulus**, the clinician progressively reduces the length of the modeled utterance. The longer the modeled utterance, the more steps involved in fading it. When the modeled stimulus is faded, the correct response is better maintained than when the modeled stimulus is suddenly withdrawn.

In fading the modeled stimulus, the clinician first drops the last word of the utterance with a rising intonational pattern. Sometimes, what is dropped may be a morphologic component of the last word. The resulting modeled utterance may sound like a sentence completion task. For example, a clinician is training a child in the production of the present progressive (*ing*). The clinician models the sentence, "The boy is running," and the client meets the initial criterion of five consecutively correct imitated responses. When the clinician discontinues modeling, the child does not produce the correct response. This suggests that the behavior is under the control of the modeled stimulus, and this control must be faded, not abruptly eliminated.

In this case, the clinician can model the response without the *ing*. After having asked the relevant question, the clinician models, "Tommy, say, 'The boy is run . . . ,'" with a rising intonational pattern, which resembles a question and suggests that the utterance is incomplete. If the response is only "running" and is not acceptable, the client can be instructed to "start with 'The boy.'" If the client produces the correct response, the clinician can drop the word *run*. The modeled stimulus would then be "Tommy, say, 'The boy is. . . .'" In subsequent steps, the words *is, boy,* and *the* are dropped one at a time. Eventually, only the question is asked. If fading is done in small and carefully planned steps, the correct response is likely to be produced on the evoked trials.

The procedure of fading the modeled stimulus control can also be called **partial modeling** or **verbal prompts**. In the earlier example of fading, the clinician modeled parts of the correct response that may have prompted the full correct response. All partial models may work as prompts, but not all prompts are partial models. Partial models contain some part or parts of the correct responses. Some prompts contain no part of target responses, and therefore are not partial models. For instance, a hand gesture may prompt the client to lower his or her pitch. This gesture is unlike a partial model in which the clinician displays some part of the target behavior for the client. Many prompts are used in shaping a new response, and these are described in a later section.

SHAPING

As noted in the previous section, modeling is a technique to teach new responses as long as the client can imitate, even if imperfectly. However, some clients cannot imitate a modeled stimulus unless special procedures are used. Such clients cannot be taught new behaviors with the straightforward modeling–imitation–reinforcement sequence. This sequence can only increase the frequency of already existing behaviors. Also, certain target behaviors are complex, and unless they are broken into smaller components, the client may not learn them. In sequential steps, the client learns the smaller components, which are later put together to achieve the final, complex, integrated behavior.

When a client cannot imitate a response that is not in his or her repertoire, or when the response is complex and needs to be broken into smaller components, the clinician can use the shaping procedure. This procedure is also known as **successive approximation**. It has been used widely in the treatment of speech–language disorders. **Shaping** is the technique used to teach new behaviors in small, sequenced steps. New behaviors must be created in many clients who are nonverbal, who cannot imitate the target behaviors, or who find the final target behavior too complex to master in total.

How to Shape a Response

Shaping, like any other treatment procedure, starts with the selection and definition of a target behavior according to the procedures described in Chapter 3. Once the target behavior has been selected, the clinician baserates the response. When both modeled and evoked trials are used in baserating the behavior, the clinician learns whether the client can imitate the responses. If the rate of imitative behavior is close to zero, then there probably is a need for shaping. Also, the need for shaping may become evident at any stage of treatment. When the treatment moves to a more complex level, the client may be unable to imitate the more complex responses.

As noted in earlier chapters, a final or dismissal criterion is the production of clinically taught behaviors in conversational speech emitted in everyday situations. In most cases, this final target behavior is too complex to be attempted in the initial treatment phases. Therefore, the treatment almost always starts at a certain lower level at which the client can perform the required response with the help of modeling. Hence, the shaping procedure is a part of most treatment programs, and the specific steps of the shaping procedure described below apply to most programs.

Step 1: Describe the Terminal Response

In the shaping procedure, the final target is called the **terminal response**. For example, with a nonverbal child, a terminal target might be the production of specified words in conversational speech emitted in the child's home and other situations. However, the child is unable to imitate the words. Because the treatment would not be started at the conversational speech level, a starting point must be identified. This is done in Step 2.

Step 2: Describe the Initial Response

The initial response must fulfill two basic criteria: (1) the client should be able at least to imitate it, and (2) it must bear a relation to the terminal response. Perhaps the first target word to be taught to the nonverbal child is "mommy." The initial response in this case may be putting the upper and lower lips together so that the initial articulatory posture for the production of /m/ is achieved. The child can probably imitate it with the help of some additional procedures that are described shortly. The articulatory posture bears a systematic relation to the response "mommy."

Step 3: Describe the Intermediate Responses

Intermediate responses bridge the gap between initial and terminal responses. These responses form a chain so that, when trained systematically and in sequence, the end result is the production of the terminal response. It is difficult to specify ahead of time all the intermediate responses needed to achieve a terminal response.

To learn the same response, one client may need more intermediate responses than another client. The target response must be broken into more and smaller components for a client who needs to learn additional intermediate responses. Therefore, the clinician must be able to identify smaller components of terminal responses.

In the example just given, some intermediate responses may include the following: vocalization while the lips are in the articulatory posture for the production of /m/, which might result in a nasal resonance; opening of the mouth when this vocal response is still being made; closing of the mouth again; and opening the mouth while adding an /i/ sound. These intermediate responses should be taught in that order. The resulting response will be an approximation of "mommy," which needs to be "put together" and practiced further.

Step 4: Model the Specific Response Under Training

The specific response under training may be the initial, the terminal, or one of the intermediate responses. Each response is modeled in its initial stage of training. The criteria for modeling, evoking, and reintroducing modeling can be the same as described in Chapter 5. The nonvocal (or nonverbal) responses should be modeled nevertheless. In our example, the clinician models the articulatory posture for the initial /m/.

Step 5: Use Manual Guidance When Necessary

When the child does not imitate the modeled response, manual guidance is needed. **Manual guidance** is physical assistance provided to shape a response. Typically, the clinician first models the needed response and immediately manually guides the response. For example, in teaching the initial articulatory response for the production of /m/, the clinician models the posture, and then manually "shapes" the client's lips. In teaching appropriate pointing responses, a clinician may say "Show me the cup," and immediately take the client's hand and point to the appropriate picture placed among alternatives. This is another example of manual guidance. Such guidance is more frequently used with nonverbal or minimally verbal clients. It is needed whenever clients fail to imitate a target response.

Step 6: Reinforce the Correct Responses

Correctly imitated responses are immediately reinforced on a continuous schedule. Subsequently, when the responses are evoked, an intermittent schedule of reinforcement is used. However, any of the intermediate responses should *not* be excessively reinforced. If they are, it would be difficult to proceed to the next response in the hierarchy. Sometimes clinicians talk about clients who "get stuck" or "perseverate" during treatment; this may be a consequence of the clinician's overly reinforcing an intermediate response in a shaping program.

Move Swiftly Through the Sequence of Responses. As soon as an initial or an intermediate response shows a consistent increase over the initial level, the clinician must proceed to the next response. In this way, the sequence of responses is taught as quickly as possible. The terminal response, however, should be strengthened so that it is maintained. Therefore, it should receive more training than the initial and the intermediate responses. The training and probe criteria for the terminal response are the same as those discussed in Chapter 5.

Shaping in the Treatment of Communicative Disorders

The six steps described above are effective in teaching many kinds of new responses. Shaping is a valuable tool in treating children who are **autistic** or **mentally retarded**. These children may not readily imitate target behaviors. In teaching syntactic structures, shaping is useful with most clients. For example, a target behavior such as "The boy is running" may not be fully imitated by the client. The clinician then asks the client to imitate "The boy," and subsequently "is running," and finally "The boy is running."

The rehabilitation of persons with **aphasia** typically requires the shaping procedure. The more severe the aphasia and associated neurological problems, the greater the need for the shaping procedure. In many cases, manual guidance, extensive prompts, frequent modeling, and simple response topographies that are changed in small increments are all a part of treatment programs designed for persons with severe aphasia.

In the treatment of **articulation disorders**, the terminal response is the production of target sounds in conversational speech in extraclinical situations. This target is achieved in small steps, starting with the production of a given sound in isolation, syllables, words, phrases, and sentences. When the client cannot produce a target sound in isolation, the clinician might ask the child to move an articulator in a certain direction. For example, the child trying to learn the production of /l/ may be asked to lift the tip of the tongue and touch the alveolar ridge. When this response is performed reliably, the clinician might ask the child to vocalize while the tongue tip is in contact with the alveolar ridge. Next, the child might be asked to release the air stream by lowering the tongue tip. The resulting sound would resemble an /l/. Additional intermediate responses would be trained at the level of syllables, words, phrases, and sentences.

The sequence of responses involved in the treatment of **voice disorders** is similar to that described above. A client with excessive nasality may be asked to say /a/ without nasal resonance (initial response). Non-nasal productions of /a/ are immediately reinforced. When the client has done this a few times, the /a/ may be shaped into a simple word such as *all*. Additional syllables and words may be added to expand the utterance length, reinforcing each intermediate response until all are produced consistently.

Shaping plays a major role in the treatment of **fluency disorders**. In achieving such targets as reduced speech rate, gentle onset of phonation, prolongation of syllables of words, or airstream management, the treatment starts at a simple level of response topography. The initial response is usually one or two words spoken at a time while the new skills are practiced. Intermediate responses include progressively longer utterances produced with the specific target topography. Each increment in the length of an utterance is an intermediate response in the overall treatment program.

In the treatment of adults who stutter, there is a different kind of need for the shaping procedure. Many of the target responses specified in such cases, especially the explicit management of airflow and rate reduction, result in a socially unacceptable speech pattern. Unusually slow speech does not "sound" normal, even though it is free from stuttering. Speech is similarly altered when clients are taught to initiate each sound gently and softly. Under each of these treatment targets, the resulting speech does not have some aspects of normal prosody. Consequently, in the final phases of treatment, normal prosodic features must be shaped. A more natural sounding rate, subtle management of airstream during speech production, normal phonatory onset, appropriate rhythm and intonation must be shaped in gradual steps. Thus, in the treatment of stuttering, shaping is needed first to teach skills of fluent speech and then to shape normal prosodic features.

In the case of young children who stutter, a straightforward technique of reinforcing fluent utterances may be effective. In this technique, young clients are not taught a particular skill, such as gentle phonatory onset. The treatment starts with an initial response (e.g., single-word utterances) which is reinforced when spoken fluently. Intermediate responses once again include utterances of increased lengths. The terminal response is conversational speech produced fluently in everyday situations. Because this type of treatment does not alter the pattern of speech, there is no need to shape the prosodic features of speech.

INSTRUCTIONS

Although our profession is concerned mainly with speech and language, the role of verbal instructions and prompts remains a little researched technique of behavior change. Yet, in everyday situations, verbal instructions (and prompts, to a lesser extent) play a major role in controlling human actions. Many skills, including washing a dish, learning the alphabet, playing a piano, and ballet dancing, are taught through verbal instructions combined with modeling. The pupil listens to the instructions, watches demonstrations, and then tries to duplicate the action. Many do-it-like-this demonstrations are a combination of modeling and verbal instructions. After some learning has taken place, prompts ("hints") can increase the probability of the skill's being performed. Prompts are then gradually removed so that responses are maintained without these additional stimuli.

Instructions are verbal stimuli that gain control over another person's actions. They illustrate a special kind of stimulus control of behavior. For the most part, subhuman behaviors are under the control of chemical and physical stimuli. Many human behaviors are also under the control of those kinds of stimuli. However, one distinct aspect of human behavior is the verbal stimulus control, which makes the process of learning adaptive and creative behaviors economical and efficient. Instructions combined with modeling spare the learner of tedious and slow workings of natural contingencies. Instead of fumbling through the sequence of actions, making many mistakes, and thus learning the hard way, one can listen, watch, perform, and learn new skills with fewer mistakes and in less time.

TREATMENT PROCEDURES IN COMMUNICATIVE DISORDERS

Although modeling is the actual demonstration of a response, it is mostly preceded or accompanied by verbal instructions. Before modeling the tongue placement for the correct production of a speech sound, the clinician describes the sequence of actions necessary for the production. Descriptions of the following kind may be given: "See the tip of my tongue? I am going to make it real small like this. Then I am going to lift it up. See? Then the tip of my tongue is going to touch this part of my mouth. Did you see that? Can you do it?" Also, just before modeling, do-as-I-do types of instructions are given. Without these additional stimuli, the client may or may not imitate the modeled response. Therefore, the initial treatment sequence involves an instructions–modeling–imitation–reinforcement sequence. However, instructions are also useful in the subsequent phases of treatment. Instructions given during later stages of treatment may be more complex.

With some clients who seem to learn the target behaviors quickly, the clinician need not model frequently. In treating such clients, instructions may play an even more important role. Specific instructions, minimum amount of modeling, and reinforcement contingencies may be effective in treating such clients.

Much research work regarding the effects of instructions on target behaviors remains to be done. It must be recognized that instructions alone may not be effective in many cases. They are effective, however, when combined with modeling, shaping, and reinforcement.

PROMPTS

Prompts are also special stimuli that increase the probability of response productions (Kazdin, 1984). Prompts are like "hints" in everyday life. A question is asked, and when the response is not forthcoming readily, an additional stimulus is given. This stimulus may draw the response from an unsure person.

Prompts can be verbal or nonverbal. **Verbal prompts** are special verbal stimuli that help trigger a response. Some verbal prompts are similar to partial modeling, which was described earlier. After having asked the question, "What is the boy doing?" the clinician might say "The boy is . . ." and wait for an answer. This partial modeling works as a prompt because it suggests the answer. As suggested in an earlier section, this type of prompt is an effective way of fading the stimulus control exerted by modeling. In gradual steps, more of the modeled response is omitted. It was also noted earlier that this type of prompt contains parts of the answer for the target behavior under training.

Vocal emphasis is a special kind of verbal prompt. In modeling various grammatic features, the clinician might place additional emphasis on the target behavior under training. For example, the clinician might state, "Say, 'the boy is runn*ing*,'" placing greater vocal emphasis on the *ing*. Similarly, in treating children with articulation disorders, the clinician may vocally emphasize the missing speech sounds that are targeted for treatment.

Some verbal prompts need not contain any part of the response expected. The clinician might ask, "What do you say?" or "Do you remember?" after having asked the question designed to evoke the answer. Such prompts may lead to correct responses.

Nonverbal or **physical prompts** are various signs and gestures that suggest the target behavior to the client. After having asked the question, "What is the boy doing?" the clinician might gesture a motion. The client then might immediately say "running." While training the correct production of /l/ in the initial position of words, the clinician might show the picture of an /l/ word and ask the client to name it. Before the client makes an attempt, the clinician might demonstrate the tongue-tip position needed for the production of /l/. The clinician does not produce the sound or the word itself. Such physical prompts may be given when the client begins to imitate the modeled response.

In the treatment of fluency and voice disorders, certain gestures can be used to prompt the target behaviors. If the treatment target is a lower pitch level, the clinician can hand-gesture a lower level during conversational speech. A gesture at a higher level may suggest to the client that the pitch is too high. While reducing a stutterer's speech rate, the clinician may show a slower hand movement as a prompt for reduced speech rate.

Prompts should not be confused with manual guidance. In manual guidance, the required response is physically shaped by the clinician. When the clinician moves the client's lips or takes the client's hand and makes it point to an appropriate picture, the entire response is being physically guided. Prompts, on the other hand, contain at best only a part of the response required of the client, and there is no physical contact with the client. Many physical prompts contain no part of the target response.

By and large, the need for prompts should be minimal. A few prompts should lead to evoked trials so that there is no need for either modeling or prompts. If the clinician must prompt constantly, more modeled trials were needed.

FADING

Treatment of people with communicative disorders, especially people with language delays or disorders, involves extensive manipulation of special stimuli. Clients seek clinical services because natural stimuli encountered in everyday situations have not entered into a contingency. Objects, events, and persons are not meaningful stimuli that evoke appropriate communicative behaviors. Normally speaking persons find "many things to talk about," but language delayed children and adults may not. Technically, objects and events surrounding persons with language problems have not acquired the discriminative stimulus value (see Chapter 7). Therefore, the clinician arranges a variety of special stimulus conditions, including pictures, modeling, instructions, manual guidance, and prompts, so that the client will learn to respond verbally and appropriately to stimulus conditions encountered in everyday life.

Although they are necessary to establish certain target behaviors, the special clinical stimuli are not a part of the client's typical environment. The parents of a language handicapped child do not systematically arrange pictorial stimuli, followed by explicit questions, modeling, prompting, and so on. Therefore, even when correct responses are reliably given in treatment sessions, the client may fail to respond appropriately in everyday situations that lack the special stimulus support. This means that the two situations are *discriminated:* Because the home situation differs from the clinical situation, the responses produced in the clinic may not be produced at home.

The client may respond reliably in extraclinical situations when the clinical and nonclinical situations are not discriminated. If the two situations contain similar stimuli and consequences, then the responses learned in one situation may be produced in the other. Because the special stimulus conditions associated with treatment create a difference between clinical and nonclinical situations, steps should be taken to minimize or eliminate this difference. Fading is the technique designed to make the treatment conditions more like everyday situations.

Fading is a technique in which the special stimulus control of target behaviors created and exerted by the clinician is reduced gradually. While the same responses are evoked, the special stimuli are gradually withdrawn. Various aspects of fading were described in the section on modeling. The procedure is summarized below.

As pointed out previously, one method of fading is **partial modeling**. Another method of fading a modeled stimulus is to change its **acoustic properties**. For example, the vocal intensity (loudness) of the modeled stimulus may be faded. Initially, the clinician models the response with normal loudness. As soon as the client begins to imitate the response reliably, the clinician reduces the loudness of modeling. The clinician models in a softer voice on successive trials until his or her voice is completely faded out.

Sometimes, when the voice is faded out, the client may stop responding correctly. In such situations, additional fading steps can be introduced. The clinician can simply "mouth" the target response without vocalization. These articulatory movements can also be faded. On successive trials, fewer and fewer movements can be modeled, or the movements can become less conspicuous.

Physical stimuli are **faded physically**. For instance, pictures and objects used on discrete treatment trials should be faded physically. These stimuli are initially placed directly in front of the client. The clinician can begin to move them around on the table such that they eventually are no longer in front of the client. Finally, the physical stimuli are removed from the client's sight.

Manual guidance is also physically faded. The extent of guidance can be reduced gradually. To begin with, the clinician may take the child's hand and point to the correct picture while making a "Show me . . ." type of request. Soon, the clinician may move the child's hand close to the relevant picture and let the child actually touch it. Then, only the initial movement of the hand may be guided by the clinician. Next, a gentle touch on the hand may be sufficient to evoke the response. In this manner, the entire manual guidance may be faded out, so that the correct pointing response is given as soon as the clinician makes a request.

Nonverbal prompts may be similarly faded. The hand gestures suggesting a certain pitch level or speech rate can be made less and less conspicuous, or maintained for progressively shorter time durations. The gesture is eventually eliminated. The position or movement of articulators used to prompt the correct production of speech sounds can be similarly faded.

As noted before, fading is necessary to promote generalization and maintenance of target behaviors. The potential for generalization is enhanced when modeling, prompts, and other such stimulus manipulations are faded. However, other kinds of special stimuli associated with treatment must also be faded. The entire physical setup of treatment and the clinician who provides the treatment also become special discriminative stimuli for target responses. Natural settings and audiences other than the clinician may lead to discrimination rather than generalization. In many cases, therefore, the stimulus control exerted by the physical setup and the clinician also must be faded out. To do this, the clinician holds informal treatment sessions in nonclinical settings so that such settings also become discriminative stimuli for target responses. The clinician also trains the family members and others in prompting and reinforcing target behaviors in natural settings. These and other methods of fading the special stimulus control to promote generalization and maintenance are described in the next chapter.

SUMMARY

Many clients need special stimuli, without which they do not produce the target responses. A significant part of treatment is to create stimulus control for nonexistent communicative behaviors.

Modeling is the clinician's response that the client imitates. The clinician produces the target behavior and asks the client to reproduce it. It is a frequently used technique.

Imitation is the client response that reproduces its own stimulus. Clinically, approximations of stimuli are often accepted and reinforced.

Shaping is a technique designed to teach nonexistent target behaviors. In this procedure, a terminal target behavior is broken down into an initial response and several intermediate responses. All responses are modeled and reinforced. In successive stages, more complex response topographies are trained.

Manual guidance is a procedure in which the response is physically shaped or directed by the clinician.

Prompts and instructions also are important aspects of special stimulus control used in treatment. Verbal instructions often are accompanied by demonstrations. Prompts can be verbal or nonverbal.

Special stimulus control procedures, such as modeling, prompts, manual guidance, and instructions, must be faded in gradual steps. If not, the target behaviors may not generalize to natural environments.

STUDY GUIDE

Answer the following questions in technical language. Verify your answers against the text. Rewrite inadequate answers.

1. What is stimulus control?

2. Define modeling.

3. Define imitation.

4. Are modeling and imitation dependent or independent variables?

5. State the two criteria for judging whether a response is imitative.

6. Do you think the modeling–imitation–reinforcement sequence should be used in clinical language training if it is demonstrated that children do not normally learn language in that manner?

7. What kinds of evidence would be required to determine whether the modeling–imitation–reinforcement sequence should be used clinically?

8. Why is modeling needed?

9. When should the clinician model?

10. Should the clinician require perfect stimulus–response matching for reinforcement in initial stages of training? Justify your answer.

11. What are the two methods of discontinuing modeling?

12. What is partial modeling?

13. Define shaping

14. When is shaping used?

15. What is another name for shaping?

16. Describe the six steps of shaping.

17. What two kinds of shaping are needed in some stuttering treatment programs?

18. Define verbal instructions.

19. Describe the importance of verbal instructions.

20. Describe a prompt.

21. What are verbal prompts?

22. What are nonverbal prompts?

23. As described in the text, what is vocal emphasis?

24. Describe fading.

25. Specify the need for fading.

26. What is "fading in terms of acoustic properties"?

27. How are nonverbal prompts faded?

28. Why is fading helpful for generalization?

29. What is manual guidance?

30. Describe the variables that need to be faded out.

7

Discrimination, Generalization, and Maintenance

- Discrimination

- Generalization

- Generalization: Intermediate or final clinical target?

- Maintenance strategies

After establishing the target behaviors in the clinical setting with the procedures described in the previous chapters, the clinician should implement additional procedures for two main reasons. First, established behaviors may be used inappropriately. Second, established behaviors may not be produced and maintained in nonclinical settings. The client is ready to be dismissed from clinical services only when the target behaviors are produced appropriately and maintained in home, school, playground, workplace, supermarket, and other settings. In this chapter, how to prevent inappropriate generalization by training discrimination and how to promote maintenance of target behaviors across situations and over time are addressed.

DISCRIMINATION

Discrimination is a common behavioral process in which different responses are given to different stimuli. Apples and oranges are discriminated through their different names, appearances, flavors, and so on. We do not confuse tables with chairs. We react differently to attractive and repulsive stimuli. We stop when we see the red traffic signal and proceed when the signal is green.

Discriminated responses may be verbal or nonverbal. When we call some objects "edible" and others "inedible," we give verbal responses. When we move *away* from the burning sun and *toward* the cool shade, we exhibit discriminated nonverbal response. Obviously, speech–language pathologists are concerned with discriminated verbal responses.

In everyday language, lack of discrimination results in confusion. When there is no discrimination, events and stimuli that should be kept separate get mixed up. A driver who does not stop for a red light does not show discrimination between red and green signals. A baby girl who puts everything she can grasp into her mouth does not discriminate between edible and inedible objects.

Technically, lack of discrimination is generalization, another behavioral process. The two behavioral processes are opposite. When there is discrimination, there is no generalization. When there is generalization, there is no discrimination. In an advanced stage of clinical training, discrimination and generalization are important. The client's response rates must show appropriate discrimination and generalization.

In **discrimination**, different responses are given to different stimuli. In generalization, the same response is given to different stimuli. Responses generalize because different stimuli share certain common properties. Sometimes, however, a person may inappropriately generalize when he or she should be making a discrimination (different, not the same, response). For example, a young child who is learning words and their meanings may call all adult females "Mommy." This child has inappropriately generalized the word "Mommy" to all women because of their similarities. Such an inappropriate generalization illustrates lack of discrimination. When the child is eventually able to call only his or her mother "Mommy" and other females with different and appropriate names, we say the child has learned discrimination.

Studies of language acquisition have documented many instances of failure to discriminate (inappropriate generalization). Words and morphologic features learned initially tend to generalize inappropriately (Gleason, 1989; Owens, 1988). A child may use the word "truck" to describe all vehicles, or the word "doggie" to name all four-legged animals. Any circular stimulus may be called "moon," and any colored drink "juice." A child who learns to produce the regular plural morpheme /s/ (e.g., *cups, boots*) may overgeneralize it to irregular plural words (e.g., *mans, womans*). Eventually, children begin to discriminate and produce labels that are specific to stimulus classes.

Whereas responses generalize because of stimulus similarities, they are discriminated because of stimulus differences. In formal and informal teaching, discrimination is the result of a procedure called **differential reinforcement**. In this procedure, a response in the presence of a stimulus is reinforced and the same response in the presence of other stimuli is extinguished (not reinforced). As a result, the response is more likely in the presence of the stimulus associated with reinforcement and less likely in the presence of all other stimuli. In the previous example, the child may be reinforced for calling the mother "Mommy," but not for calling other women by the same name. The child may also be told "No, she is not your mommy," when that word is used for other women. Such differential reinforcement (and corrective feedback) is responsible for the eventual discrimination between the mother and other women.

A stimulus in the presence of which a response is reinforced is called a discriminative stimulus. It is abbreviated S^D (pronounced ess-dee). The response becomes more probable in the presence of its S^D, presumably because the stimulus signals reinforcement. For instance, in the presence of the mother, the child is more likely to say "mommy" because that response is typically reinforced in her presence. The child's mother is the S^D for the word "mommy." The stimulus in the presence of which a response is not reinforced is known as S^Δ (pronounced ess-delta). For instance, the child's aunt is an S^Δ for the word "mommy" because the response is not reinforced in her presence. Similarly, the green traffic light is an S^D for proceeding and an S^Δ for stopping, and the red light is an S^Δ for proceeding and an S^D for stopping. These stimuli evoke such discriminated responses because of past reinforcement history.

People need to learn both discrimination and generalization, which are the bases for learning concepts. Without discrimination and generalization, people do not learn abstract concepts. Generalization within a class of stimuli and discrimination across classes are the bases of concept formation. People learn one concept when they generalize; they learn multiple concepts when they discriminate. For example, a speaker who could say only "flower" to all kinds of flowers has learned only one concept. This speaker has overgeneralized the word "flower" to all kinds of flowers because he or she has not been taught to discriminate among different kinds of flowers. But another speaker who could produce different names for different kinds of flowers has learned many concepts because he or she has learned to discriminate among different kinds of flowers and not to overgeneralize the same label "flower" to all kinds of flowers.

The fact that stimuli belong to different classes is the basis of concept formation. Society accepts generalization within a class of stimuli; it is appropriate to call all kinds of roses "roses." But generalization across classes of stimuli is not acceptable. It is not appropriate to call chairs "tables." Because chairs and tables belong to different classes of stimuli, responses given to them must be discriminated.

In addition to generalization and discrimination, a process known as abstraction is involved in the formation of complex conceptual behaviors. For generalization to occur across members of a class of stimuli that may differ in many ways, the response should come under the control of a single or very few properties shared by those stimuli. For instance, the single word "flowers" applies to flowers of varied color, shape, texture, and fragrance. Although the different kinds of flowers are very different, the same word is used. This means that the response could not be controlled by the differences between flowers; it could be controlled only by the similarities between them.

To take another example, when a mother says that her child "knows the colors," what she means technically is that different color naming responses are controlled by their respective single (or unique) properties of the wavelengths of stimuli. When a child has learned to say "red" appropriately, then the actual stimulus events for which the term is a response may be infinitely varied in terms of shape, size, texture, use, and so forth. The following stimulus events may be called "red": chair, brick, dress, sky, book, lipstick, telephone, car, carpet, Jupiter, blood. Unless a single property (wavelength) of these varied stimulus events comes to control the response "red," the child can neither generalize nor discriminate red from other colors. In the behavioral analysis, control over a response exerted by a single or unique property of stimuli is called abstraction. Abstract stimulus control will result in appropriate generalization and discrimination.

Discrimination Training in Clinical Work

After certain behaviors have been established in the clinic, there are times when discrimination training is needed. Whenever there is unacceptable generalization (overgeneralization), discrimination training is necessary. Overgeneralization is common both to children who acquire language normally and to those who receive clinical language training. For example, a child who has just been taught to produce the plural /s/ correctly may overgeneralize it to nouns that take plural /z/. Any of the trained plural morphemes may also overgeneralize to singular stimulus conditions or irregular plural forms. The trained singular verbal auxiliary (*is*) may be produced in contexts where the plural form (*are*) is appropriate. When the regular past tense is trained, it might overgeneralize to irregular past tense. In situations such as these, discrimination training is needed so that different and appropriate responses are produced in relation to different stimulus classes.

The procedure to eliminate such overgeneralization is the same that produces discrimination: differential reinforcement. A response in the presence of one stimulus is reinforced, whereas the same response in the presence of another stimulus is not reinforced. In training discrimination between singular and plural noun labels, the clinician has two sets of stimuli: singular and plural objects. When singular objects are presented, a singular label is reinforced, whereas when plural objects are presented, a plural form is reinforced. In this procedure, each stimulus has an S^D and an S^Δ. For instance, the picture of a single book is an S^D for "book" (reinforced) but an S^Δ for "books" (not reinforced and corrective feedback given). A picture of two or more books, on the other hand, is an S^D for "books" but an S^Δ for "book." Through such differential programming of consequences that match the stimulus conditions with expected responses, appropriately discriminated response classes can be generated. The same discrete-trial procedure described in Chapter 5 can be used in discrimination training.

GENERALIZATION

Most clinicians believe that generalization is the final goal of treatment, and that behaviors trained in clinical settings should generalize to natural environments. I believe, however, that generalization should not be the final goal of treatment, but that response maintenance should be. Although generalization is not useful as a final target, it is useful as in intermediate target of clinical intervention. When clinically taught responses generalize, it is easy to implement maintenance procedures. Therefore, it is helpful to understand different types of generalization.

Generalization has a stimulus dimension and a response dimension. It is the basis upon which some new learning is demonstrated without additional conditioning. Generalization refers to an extension of learning to new situations and stimuli, or to new responses based upon old learning.

Stimulus Generalization

Stimulus generalization occurs when a response learned in relation to one stimulus is evoked by stimuli that were not used in teaching that response. In stimulus generalization, new stimuli (those that were not used in teaching) evoke a response. Most of the basic research information on stimulus generalization can be summarized as follows:

1. All learning necessarily takes place in a certain situational context, which is a bundle of stimuli. When a response is taught in a context, all stimuli in that context acquire some power to evoke that response because of reinforcement.

2. No stimulus is a discrete entity. All stimuli are generic in that they are members of larger classes. A large number of stimuli may fall into a class because they share certain properties, such as size, color, shape, or texture. Stimuli may also form classes on the basis of use, which means that people act upon them in similar manners. Different items of furniture, for example, may fall into a class on this basis.

3. Initial learning takes place in relation to one or a few stimuli. The clinician teaching the word *ball* to a child uses a specific ball or a few pictures of balls. When the client later comes in contact with other (novel) balls, the response may be likely. The greater the similarity between the training and the novel stimuli, the higher the chances of stimulus generalization.

4. As the difference between the training and the novel stimuli increases, the response rate decreases. In the example above, if the clinician were to present progressively different balls to the client, the response "ball" would eventually diminish because of an increasing (and eventually extreme) difference between the training stimulus and the new stimulus. This phenomenon is known as the *generalization gradient*. In laboratory situations, researchers measure generalization in the absence of reinforcement while presenting stimuli that are progressively different from the training stimulus. Therefore, measures of generalization are similar to measures of extinction.

5. Although people (and animals) show stimulus generalization, it is not an activity of the subject. Clients do not generalize, but untrained stimuli evoke responses from them. However, generalization is dependent upon a number of manipulable variables, such as stimulus variety and reinforcement schedule.

6. Although the clinician programs initial learning in relation to specific stimuli, the actual learning takes place in a larger stimulus context, which includes the entire physical setting, the therapy room, the verbal antecedents of responses, the clinician, and so forth. These different kinds of stimuli lead to different types of stimulus generalization.

Types of Stimulus Generalization

Physical Stimulus Generalization. This type of generalization takes place because of stimulus similarity. Physical stimulus generalization occurs when a learned response is evoked by standard stimuli that were not used in teaching the response. Although responses are typically controlled by a bundle of discriminative stimuli, there are standard stimuli for most responses. For example, "ball" may be the verbal response to a variety of standard physical stimuli, such as actual balls, pictures of balls, or the printed word "ball." In clinical training, certain pictures or actual balls may be used. Should there be any generalization, the word "ball" may be evoked by pictures of balls or actual balls that were not used in training.

If a client were to generalize the target behaviors to most of the standard stimuli, training time and effort would be minimized. Then a maintenance program can be started.

Verbal Stimulus Generalization. In the treatment of communicative disorders, verbal stimuli provided by the clinician play a major role. In most language treatment programs, the clinician asks questions such as "What is this?" and "What do you see?" or makes requests such as "Tell me about this" and "Say what I say." As a function of training, these questions, requests, and other verbal devices may come to evoke the target responses from the client. Such verbal devices are antecedents because they become a part of the S^Ds evoking target behaviors.

Typically, the same verbal behaviors have multiple antecedents. A target behavior such as "The boy is running" may be evoked by "What is the boy doing?" or "What is happening in the picture?" or "Tell me about the boy," or so on. In treatment, a particular antecedent may be used consistently. **Verbal stimulus generalization** is evident when target behaviors are evoked by verbal antecedents that were not used in training.

Verbal antecedent generalization is important for clinical speech–language training. Speech itself is probably the most pervasive stimulus for speech. Unless natural speech stimuli become S^Ds for clinically taught speech, the success of the treatment program remains questionable. The child who sees a ball or wants a ball or has something to say about a ball in the natural environment should not need the same triggering stimuli that were used in clinical training.

Physical Setting Generalization. All treatment takes place in a certain physical setting. Most treatment occurs in small, isolated rooms with minimum furnishings and equipment arranged in a relatively constant fashion. Most therapeutic settings are discriminated because they are unlike the client's natural environment. Discriminated therapeutic settings are desirable, and sometimes even necessary, for initial learning because they minimize distracting stimuli. However, when responses are reinforced in discriminated settings, they become "attached" to those settings. In other settings, the target behaviors may not be produced.

Physical setting generalization occurs when responses trained in one physical setting are produced in other settings in which training is not done. For example, after having taught the correct production of /r/ in the context of 10 single words, the clinician might take the client to another room, the outdoors, or the client's home. In these settings, the clinician might try to evoke the same 10 words using the same pictures presented during training. If the client uses the target phoneme, physical setting generalization has been demonstrated.

Audience Generalization. One of the most powerful discriminative stimuli for speech is the presence of other people. In behavioral analysis, people are called the audience when they serve as discriminative stimuli for speech (Winokur, 1976). Speech is reinforced by other people; thus, people are discriminative stimuli for speech.

Audience generalization takes place when responses taught or typically evoked by a given audience are evoked by audiences not involved in training. The clinician who reinforces a target behavior quickly becomes the audience for that behavior. Family members and other people who have not reinforced the behavior may not serve the role of audience. These other people become audience for speech when they reinforce the client's speech, at which time audience generalization is evident.

Factorial Stimulus Generalization. The four types of stimulus generalization—physical stimulus, verbal stimulus, physical setting, and audience—may not always be independent of each other. In most cases, different types of stimulus generalizations are concurrently active, although they can be separately manipulated. This combination of different types of stimulus generalization, called **factorial stimulus generalization**, is the most complex form of stimulus generalization.

When the correct production of a grammatic feature—for example, a plural morpheme—generalizes to the home situation, this may be factorial stimulus generalization. It is likely that the client responds at home to plural objects that differ from any encountered in the treatment sessions. At home, the client responds to family members and not the clinician. Possibly, the verbal antecedents of those target responses are different from those in the clinical setting. Therefore, the client's correct production of the plural morpheme at home is a product of all types of stimulus generalization. The responses may be the same (e.g., "books" and "cups"), but they are emitted in a new setting, given in relation to stimuli not used in treatment, evoked by people other than the clinician, and triggered by verbal stimuli that were not a part of treatment. In essence, this generalization is a combination of physical setting, standard physical stimulus, audience, and verbal stimulus generalization.

Response Generalization

Stimulus generalization involves untrained or novel stimuli, but the same (trained) response form. Response generalization, on the other hand, involves new (untrained) responses.

A newly learned response can be a basis for new responses. A child who has been taught to cooperate with other children in play situations may smile more often. A child who receives language training and thus becomes verbally more proficient may also show increased social activity. A man who gets his high vocal pitch treated successfully may speak more in conversational situations. A stuttering woman who becomes more fluent because of treatment may begin to seek the company of men. Each of these examples has a response trained by the clinician and a new (untrained) response based upon that learning. **Response generalization** is evident when new (untrained) responses are produced because of prior teaching.

Typically, response generalization is defined as the production of new and, therefore, unreinforced responses that are similar to those that have been reinforced. In its purest form, response generalization is evident when new responses are evoked by the same stimuli that were used in the original teaching. In stimulus generalization, new stimuli evoke the old response, whereas in response generalization, old stimuli evoke new responses. Therefore, in stimulus generalization, stimuli change, and in response generalization, responses change.

In language learning, response generalization rarely occurs in its purest form. Most clinical studies in which verbal response generalization has been documented involved changes in both stimulus and response variables. Take, for instance, the earlier example of a client trained to produce the plural morpheme in such words as *cups* and *books*. To assess generalization of this target behavior, the clinician might present a variety of untrained stimulus items, such as *hats* and *plates*. A correct production of the responses would mean there was some generalization. But what kind of generalization is this?

Consider another example from treatment of articulation disorders. Suppose the clinician teaches a child to correctly produce /f/ in the context of a few single words. The clinician then tries to evoke some untrained words to assess generalization. If the child were to produce such untrained resposes as "fire," "fish," and "foot," the child would have demonstrated generalization. But again, what kind of generalization?

In the two examples, when the untrained pictures or words were presented, the stimuli changed. But in both instances, one feature of the stimulus complex (which is supposed to evoke the target response) was common to the trained and untrained stimuli. The response also changed, for the particular words containing the plural morpheme or the target phoneme were not involved in training. Nevertheless, the generalized response was not entirely new; it contained either the trained plural /s/ or the target phoneme /f/. This means that it was not a pure form of either stimulus or response generalization. It was actually both. For this reason, the term *intraverbal generalization* is suggested here to describe the kinds of posttreatment changes that may take place in verbal behaviors.

Intraverbal Generalization

Posttreatment changes in verbal behaviors include either a substitution of old responses by new responses of the same class, or an expansion of the entire response topography. **Intraverbal generalization** involves stimulus and response generalization *within* forms of verbal behaviors. The term refers to generalized verbal response substitutions, topographic expansions, and some new stimuli.

A client who learns to produce such sentences as "The boy is running" and "The boy is walking" may generalize the target *is* not only to sentences such as "The boy is eating," but also to sentences such as "The girl is writing," "The man is washing," and "The rabbit is hopping." Each generalized response illustrates the substitution process: New nouns and verbs are substituted for trained nouns and verbs. This type of generalization is characterized by some constant responses, one or more substituted responses, many new stimulus elements, and one constant property of the stimulus complex. The stimulus property that is constant is discriminative of the auxiliary *is*. The property discriminative of the definite article is also constant, but that is beside the point.

The process of generalized expansion of trained verbal responses can be illustrated as follows. Suppose the client who has learned to use the plural /s/ in the context of single words produces untrained responses such as "I see two books," "Books are here," "Look at the cups," and "Where are the cups?" These are generalized verbal expansions. Similarly, if the phoneme /f/ trained only in the context of single words were to generalize to appropriate phrases and sentences, this would be another instance of generalized expansion of response topography. It is important to note that intraverbal generalization necessarily includes new discriminative stimulus control.

Many language training studies have demonstrated that it is possible to induce intraverbal generalization. It is known that clients are typically able to use trained grammatic features in the context of untrained responses. This might result in either substituted or expanded verbal responses.

Intraverbal generalization, like stimulus generalization, can help minimize training time and effort. When it does occur, it may be one of the best forms of generalization because it includes new and expanded responses as well as additional discriminative stimulus control.

Response Mode Generalization

A debated issue in speech and language training is whether clients should necessarily imitate or produce the target behaviors they are taught. Some clinicians believe that clients may learn from either listening to the target behaviors the clinician repeatedly produces or from giving a nonverbal response to verbal stimuli. For example, a child may learn to produce sentences containing the present progressive *ing* by simply watching and listening to a clinician who repeatedly models such sentences. The child in this case is not asked to imitate the clinician or produce the sentence forms during auditory stimulation. Some children may learn to produce sentence forms when they are frequently stimulated auditorily.

Some clinicians also believe that clients who are trained to "comprehend" a target speech or language response or are taught to auditorily discriminate between two similar sounding responses, will begin to produce those responses. In both comprehension training and auditory discrimination training, the client may be asked to nonverbally respond to verbal stimuli. For example, a client in articulation training may be asked to distinguish the target phoneme from the nontarget phoneme when the phonemes are produced by the clinician. In this procedure, the client may raise the right hand when the target sound ("radio") is heard, and the left hand when the nontarget sound ("wadio") is heard.

In language training, the client may be trained to respond nonverbally when verbal signals are given. For example, in teaching possessive morphemes in such phrases as "Mommy's hat" and "Daddy's coat," a child may be trained to differentially point to appropriate pictures. In a more complex example, instead of teaching a client to say "Please open the door," the clinician may train the client to actually open the door when that request is made. While saying nothing, the client performs an appropriate action. From this action, the clinician infers that the client comprehended the verbal statement. Some clinicians believe that a client who comprehends an utterance will soon produce it without production training. Others believe that production training is necessary, but becomes easier if comprehension training precedes it.

A client who begins to produce an utterance because he or she has heard it many times, but did not produce it during training, shows response mode generalization. A child who begins to distinguish the clinician's productions of "radio" and "wadio" may begin to correctly produce the /r/ in words, demonstrating a response mode generalization. In both the cases, there is generalization from the auditory mode to the production mode. If clients who have learned to respond appropriately to verbal commands also begin to produce the commands without training, they show response mode generalization from comprehension to production. For example, the child who learns to correctly point to pictures of "Mommy's hat" and "Daddy's coat" may begin to produce those responses.

Whether such response mode generalizations take place has been a controversial issue. Available evidence suggests that response mode generalization from comprehension or auditory stimulation to production is limited, unstable, and unreliable. Therefore, the best strategy is to train production. When production of responses is trained, both comprehension and auditory discrimination are achieved without much extensive training, whereas when only comprehension or auditory discrimination is trained, production may not follow (Connell, 1987; Connell & McReynolds, 1981; Ezell & Goldstein, 1989; Guess & Baer, 1973; Keller & Bucher, 1979; Thompson & McReynolds, 1986; Weismer & Murray-Branch, 1989; Williams & McReynolds, 1975). When only production is trained, the clinician should probe for comprehension. If comprehension is absent, it should be trained as well.

Concurrent Stimulus–Response Generalization

The final form of generalization to be described is probably the most complex, and it includes all the forms of generalization discussed previously. Factorial stimulus generalization, which is a combination of multiple types of stimulus generalization, was discussed earlier. Factorial stimulus generalization combined with response generalization results in concurrent stimulus–response generalization.

Concurrent stimulus–response generalization is evident when both the stimulus and the response variables change subsequent to original learning. The change may be sudden, simultaneous, or achieved over a period of time, but the end result is a complex form of stimulus and response generalization in which a variety of new stimuli control forms of responses that were not trained.

Suppose a clinician teaches a child to produce the possessive /s/ in the context of short phrases (e.g., "Cat's tail," "Pat's coat"). The child then goes home and begins to produce untrained sentences such as "Here is cat's food," "These are rabbit's ears," and "I see the parrot's cage." Assume that the child's productions of these verbal responses were preceded by various questions and comments from the mother. In this case, the child has shown a complex combination of stimulus and response generalization of the possessive morpheme. The responses produced at home may show concurrent stimulus–response generalization of the following kinds: (1) setting generalization, because they were produced in a nontraining situation; (2) verbal stimulus generalization, because the verbal antecedents may not have been a part of training; (3) physical stimulus generalization, because the stimuli that triggered the responses may not have been involved in training; (4) audience generalization, because the mother was a new audience for those responses; and (5) response generalization of the intraverbal variety, because of additions to and expansions of the response topography.

If the concurrent stimulus–response generalization occurs, it is beneficial from the clinical standpoint. Clinically trained responses must be triggered by natural physical stimuli, in various nontreatment settings, in response to everyday verbal antecedents, in the presence of people with whom the client would come in contact, and in expanded and novel forms. When this happens, it is concurrent stimulus–response generalization.

GENERALIZATION: INTERMEDIATE OR FINAL CLINICAL TARGET?

Generalization has been described at some length because it is an important phenomenon of learning and teaching. More research is necessary to fully explain the complex changes that take place after learning new verbal behaviors. Unfortunately, the nature of generalization is not researched much because the past and current research focus has been on promoting generalization of clinically established behaviors.

The popular idea that generalization is the final goal of intervention poses many serious problems. The essence of the argument presented in this section is that generalization has been conceptually and methodologically distorted in clinical research. When generalization does occur, it can serve as a basis for further clinical programming, but it cannot be the final, programmed goal.

In the laboratory, **generalization** is a measure of a declining rate of response under conditions of changing stimuli and absence of reinforcement. The eventual course of a generalized response is extinction. How long the generalized response rate continues depends upon many factors. The most important are the schedule, the amount, and the quality of reinforcement received during training, and the length and amount of training. Also, how different the novel stimuli are from the training stimuli affect generalized responding. Stimuli that are very different from the training stimuli may not produce generalized responding. As a function of these variables, generalized responding may be high or low, and may continue for relatively long or short durations, but in the end there is extinction.

One of the basic tenets of behaviorism is that all responses are maintained by their consequences. Generalization, however, is a short-term phenomenon of response rate in the absence of consequences. It lasts as long as it does only because of the discriminative stimulus value. This means that new stimuli evoke generalized (unreinforced) responses only because they signal reinforcement. If reinforcement does not occur, the generalized responses do not continue.

In clinical settings, generalization has been considered the final goal because it has seemed to be what is needed. The clinician cannot continue to reinforce the target behaviors because he or she will not be present in the client's natural environment. It has been thought that the solution is generalization, because generalized responses (as long as they last) do not require reinforcement. In the clinical contexts, this amounts to a presumption that response rates will be maintained indefinitely in the absence of reinforcement contingencies. Obviously, this is impossible from the standpoint of behaviorism. Therefore, generalization cannot be the ultimate goal of clinical intervention programs. Whenever it has been treated as such, two major problems have emerged.

First, this highly desirable final goal of clinical treatment has been elusive. Clinical studies have observed some stimulus and response generalization, but often the extent is negligible. Some trained behaviors are produced some of the time in certain naturalistic situations. More typically, however, behaviors that are produced reliably in the clinic are not generalized to nonclinical settings.

Second, and more important, generalized responses may not last in the natural environment. That is, even when responses do generalize, they may not be maintained over time. This is not surprising, because generalization is not an indefinite process. Generalized but not maintained responses show that generalization can lead only to extinction.

Because of these two problems, the clinical researchers have suggested that generalization should be programmed to promote its occurrence. Many tactics have been suggested to promote generalization. For instance, it has been suggested that the clinician should use common stimuli to train responses, use intermittent reinforcement schedules, and train parents and others to reinforce generalized responses produced in natural settings.

The so-called generalization strategies are useful but, ironically, not for promoting generalization. When they are thought of as strategies to promote generalization, several conceptual problems arise. First, the very idea of programming generalization is conceptually confusing. When generalization is programmed, a temporary and declining rate of response without reinforcement is being programmed. However, no researcher who recommends programming generalization believes that the goal of clinical intervention is a declining rate of response. Nonetheless, many researchers recommend that clinicians promote generalization.

Second, programming generalization means that lasting response rates in the absence of reinforcement contingencies are expected. Such an expectation violates one of the most important principles of behaviorism (Ferster, Culbertson, & Boren, 1975; Kalish, 1981; Skinner, 1953, 1969, 1974): Any behavior lasts only because of the lasting contingencies. If behaviors are to be maintained, they should be reinforced. Therefore, generalization (as a decreasing response rate in the absence of reinforcement) should not be the goal of clinical intervention.

Third, some tactics of generalization offer a de facto definition of that phenomenon as response rates reinforced in other situations, or by other persons. For instance, one of the previously noted tactics of generalization is to have parents and others reinforce generalized responses. Another strategy is to treat generalized response as the target and reinforce its occurrence. Such strategies confuse generalization with treatment done outside the clinical settings. It is not clear why reinforcement of responses in clinical settings is treatment, whereas the same thing done outside the clinic is generalization. Both are treatment. The pill a patient takes is medicine when given by the physician in his or her office; the same pill taken at home by the patient is also medicine.

Fourth, the concept of programmed generalization seems to be based on the questionable assumption that the only contingencies of importance are the ones administered by the clinician. When the clinician withdraws the contingencies, the response is supposedly maintained because of generalization. Behaviorism asserts that response maintenance is also due to operant conditioning (Skinner, 1953), which means that the initial learning and eventual maintenance of behaviors are both due to the same reinforcement contingencies. Whether the reinforcing agent is the clinician or another person is irrelevant.

These four problems suggest that to conceptualize the final target of clinical treatment in terms of generalization is inconsistent with behaviorism. As Drabman, Hammer, and Rosenbaum (1979) pointed out, "the current practice of subjective reference to a variety of phenomena as generalization is unacceptable" (p. 204). Scott, Himadi, and Keane (1983) stated that many techniques that seek to extend the treatment effects to nontreatment conditions are "not always consistent with the process of generalization. Using a single experimental term to describe a number of different clinical phenomena can only invite confusion and imprecision" (p. 118). There is no compelling reason why the term generalization should not be restored to its original meaning: a declining rate of response in the absence of reinforcement. When behaviors are reinforced, it is not generalization. It is conditioning. Maintenance requires not tactics of generalization, but a continued process of conditioning.

Although it is not a final goal, generalization can be an intermediate goal of clinical intervention. When the transition from the clinic to natural environments is being made, generalization can help. When generalization does take place, it can serve as a basis for maintenance strategies that help strengthen the responses in natural environments. Obviously, those strategies must be instituted before generalized responses are extinguished.

The final target of clinical intervention is not generalization, but response maintenance in natural environments. After the treatment contingencies are terminated, contingencies of everyday life should sustain behaviors. If natural contingencies are defective, as they may often be, then steps must be taken to ensure that they become effective. According to this view, there will be no attempt to have the target behaviors produced in the absence of reinforcement (generalization). Instead, the clinician will focus upon the problems involved in contingency management in nonclinical settings.

Why Newly Learned Behaviors Are Not Maintained

Responses often are not maintained after the termination of treatment, possibly for two reasons. First, the clinician and the clinical setting are the only discriminative stimuli for the target behaviors. Other persons and natural settings are not discriminative stimuli for those behaviors because only the clinician has reinforced them in the clinical setting. Therefore, the target behaviors are likely to be exhibited only in the treatment setting. Second, the natural environment might still contain S^Ds for undesirable behaviors, and no S^Ds for desirable ones. The undesirable behaviors may receive reinforcement while the desirable behaviors are extinguished. The clinician's task in promoting response maintenance is to reverse the process: The natural environment should become discriminative of the target behaviors and should not support the undesirable behaviors.

MAINTENANCE STRATEGIES

A **maintenance strategy** is an extension of treatment to the client's natural environment. Behaviors are maintained when persons in the client's life sustain those behaviors by reinforcement. Contingency management is the key to reinforcement. Therefore, a maintenance strategy is not unlike treatment offered by the clinician. The single most important difference between treatment and maintenance is the locus of response control. During treatment, responses are controlled in the treatment setting by the clinician. During maintenance, the same responses are controlled by people in a client's everyday situations. Thus, a shift in the locus of response control is the heart of maintenance strategies.

Behavioral maintenance strategies must be planned even before treatment is started, not after the behaviors have been established. Contingency management for the sake of maintenance involves manipulation of all three aspects of that contingency: stimuli, responses, and consequences. Many issues related to stimulus, response, and contingency deserve consideration *before, during,* and *after* treatment. Maintenance strategy is described below in terms of (1) stimulus manipulations, (2) response considerations, and (3) contingency manipulations.

Stimulus Manipulations

The kinds of stimuli used in training target responses may promote or retard the initial generalization and subsequent maintenance of those responses. Neutral stimuli used in training eventually become discriminative stimuli capable of evoking target responses. This training stimulus control should be extended to stimuli in the natural environment. The suggestions mentioned in the following subsections help achieve such a transfer of stimulus control from the clinic to the natural environment.

Select Standard Stimuli from Natural Environments

Typically, stimuli for target behaviors are selected somewhat arbitrarily. Most stimulus materials used in training happen to be present in the clinic. Often, commercially prepared stimulus materials may be used. These materials may or may not be particularly relevant to individual clients. Response maintenance may be enhanced when stimuli used in training are present in the client's environment. When stimuli selected from natural environment are used in training, they acquire discriminative stimulus value. Later, when the client faces those stimuli at home, the production of target behaviors is more likely.

Clinicians often use pictures in teaching speech–language behaviors. Even a cursory glance at commercially available stimulus pictures suggest that their quality and the extent to which they represent true objects vary tremendously. Pictures selected from popular magazines may be more representative of the real objects than some of the commercially available materials. Whenever practical, it is better to use real objects, which tend to promote generalization. Another advantage of real objects is that they can be used to represent events because they are more manipulable than pictures. In teaching verb + *ing*, for example, toy trucks, cars, and several other objects can be used to demonstrate movement. Whether selected stimuli are pictures or objects, they should be a part of the client's environment.

Careful selection of stimulus materials that are present in the client's environment is probably more crucial in treating articulation and language disorders than in treating voice or fluency disorders. The ideal strategy may be to ask parents to bring in selected stimulus materials from home. The child may bring to the therapy session his or her own toys and other belongings, which may then serve as stimuli for the target behaviors under training. When this is done, the discriminative stimuli used in training are carried back to the home situation.

Select Common Verbal Antecedents

In addition to real objects and events, communicative behaviors have unique verbal stimuli. In many cases, verbal antecedents may be the sole triggering stimuli of language behaviors. Questions, requests, comments, suggestions, hints, prompts, modeling, and so on, are potentially effective verbal antecedents of target behaviors.

Some verbal antecedents may be more frequently encountered in everyday situations than some of the antecedents used in clinical situations. For example, modeling, leading to imitative responses, is not as frequently associated with verbal responses as are questions and requests. Therefore, when modeling is used, the clinician must fade it out as soon as possible and use the kinds of antecedents that may be found more frequently in natural settings. Questions and requests, such as "What is happening?" "What is the girl doing?" "Tell me about this," are more natural than the clinician's formal models, hints, and prompts.

Vary Audience–Antecedent Controls

Because the clinician initially reinforces correct responses, he or she quickly becomes the discriminative audience for those responses. As a result, the correct responses are more likely in the presence of the clinician, and less likely in the presence of other people, including family members. Because the clinician is not the typical audience of verbal responses, family members and other persons should eventually be involved in the training sessions so that they can also become a discriminative audience. Parents and siblings should take part in training sessions. Initially, they may simply observe the clinician and the training procedure being implemented. Soon, they may be asked to administer some stimulus items. Eventually, they may be trained to reinforce correct responses, in which case they also may be expected to acquire discriminative stimulus value. The correct responses may then be more likely in their presence.

Student observers, other student clinicians, or colleagues of the clinician also may serve as audience. When this is done systematically, the exclusive control exerted by a clinician on target behaviors is reduced, and a broader control by people other than the clinician is achieved.

Vary Physical Setting Controls

The physical setting in which the target behaviors are taught also can quickly acquire discriminative stimulus value. In more natural settings, such as home, school, or office, however, the target behaviors may be absent. To overcome this problem, the clinician should vary the physical setting of treatment so that multiple settings come to control target responses.

A desirable strategy is to hold training sessions in different rooms that vary in size and setup. As target behaviors become more stable, training can be less formal and may be conducted in more naturalistic settings. When different physical settings are used, an important aspect of stimulus control of responses will have been broadened. Contingency management in more naturalistic settings must be subtle, however. This point is discussed again in a later section.

In some clinical populations, such as children who are autistic, the physical setting and other stimulus conditions used in training seem to exert unusually circumscribed control on target behaviors. This means that the target behaviors are not produced outside the training setting. Stutterers also tend to exhibit tight stimulus control of fluent and dysfluent behaviors. Compared with nonclinical populations, clinical populations that need explicit management of reinforcement contingencies to learn behaviors are likely to come under relatively strict stimulus controls. Thus, varying physical setting controls is an important aspect of stimulus manipulations designed to promote generalization and maintenance.

Response Considerations

Several maintenance strategies relate to certain characteristics of target responses. Some responses may have a better chance of being reinforced and thus maintained in natural environments than some others a clinician might arbitrarily select for training. This suggests that maintenance should not be considered only after target behaviors are established; it should be considered even at the stage of target behavior selection.

Select Client-Specific Responses

Target behaviors often are selected because developmental norms suggest them, or because most clients seem to need them to be able to interact socially. However, such responses may or may not have special relevance to individual clients. It may be more meaningful to select target responses specific to the individual client's needs as assessed by an examination of that client's environment. For instance, children who are nonverbal may be taught labels of colors or furniture items, but such responses may not have pragmatic relevance. Instead, children can be taught labels of toys, food items, or clothing articles. Useful responses generalize more readily than labels of furniture items or body parts. Useful responses help the client gain better control over the environment. Once generalized, those responses are likely to be reinforced at home and in other natural settings.

This approach of selecting client-specific target behaviors was described in Chapter 3. Consult that chapter for additional information.

Select Multiple Exemplars

A target behavior is a collection of multiple responses, all being controlled by the same or similar contingency. Each response is an example of a given response class. For a class of target responses to be produced and reinforced in everyday situations, an adequate number of responses from that class must be sampled and taught.

The number of responses that must be trained to achieve an initial generalization and eventual maintenance varies with clients and types of behaviors under training. Most often, the number of exemplars to be taught to a client is determined empirically. A clinician teaches a few exemplars and probes for generalization, which can serve as a basis for maintenance strategies. If there is no generalization, then additional exemplars are taught.

Traditionally, generalization of some sort has been the basis to judge the necessary number of exemplars to be taught in a given case. Several studies have shown that some language behaviors can generalize only after training a few exemplars. When sufficient numbers of exemplars are trained, the resulting generalization can provide a basis for a contingency-based maintenance strategy.

Reinforce Complex Response Topographies

Typically, responses are initially trained at simple topographic levels, such as single words or short phrases. Responses may not be produced or maintained in everyday situations simply because naturally occurring topography— conversational speech—was not reinforced by the clinician. Both in the clinic and at home, target behaviors produced in conversational speech must be reinforced.

In some cases, clinicians simply continue to train target behaviors at simpler, more manageable topographic levels. Training may not proceed to more complex levels of sentence productions and conversational speech. Monitoring and reinforcing speech and language target responses in conversational speech are difficult and require sharp observational skills. This difficult task must be accomplished if responses are to be generalized and maintained.

Contingency Manipulations

Contingency manipulation is the most important element in maintenance strategies. Although this form of management should eventually occur in natural settings, there are some techniques that, when used during training sessions, can also promote generalization and maintenance. These techniques are discussed in this section.

Use Intermittent Reinforcement Schedules

Intermittent reinforcement schedules help generate target responses that may be maintained over longer periods of time than those that are reinforced continuously. When target behaviors have increased notably above the baseline, the schedule of reinforcement may be shifted from continuous to intermittent. Initially, an intermittent schedule that permits a relatively high level of reinforcement (e.g., an FR2 schedule) may be appropriate. The schedule may be gradually stretched so that progressively greater numbers of responses are unreinforced.

Whenever possible, variable ratio schedules must be used during the latter stages of training. In everyday situations, reinforcers are more likely to come on a variable ratio. Sometimes, people get reinforced for few responses; other times, many responses may go unreinforced. Variable ratios might help minimize discrimination between treatment and nontreatment conditions.

During the final phases of treatment, the client must be able to tolerate a fairly large response:reinforcement ratio. Occasional reinforcers should be sufficient to maintain target responses.

Use Conditioned Reinforcers

As discussed in Chapter 4, it is sometimes necessary to use primary reinforcers (food and other consumables) for clients who have not had a history of successful language use. Also, primary reinforcers may not support generalization or maintenance. Because most classes of verbal behaviors are reinforced by social reinforcers, it is most appropriate to use attention, approval, and praise to strengthen communicative behaviors.

Even when primary reinforcers are necessary, conditioned reinforcers must always be used. This will help fade out primary reinforcers while maintaining responses on social and other conditioned reinforcers. The best strategy is to use conditioned generalized reinforcers (tokens) that are backed up by a variety of reinforcers.

Delay Reinforcement

In teaching behaviors, the importance of immediate reinforcement usually is emphasized. On the other hand, in everyday situations, reinforcers often are delayed. Prompt reinforcement in the clinic and delayed reinforcement in nonclinical settings can encourage discrimination between clinical and everyday situations. Therefore, delayed reinforcement in clinical settings may be a useful maintenance strategy. If reinforcers are delayed in both clinical and nonclinical settings, the discrimination between the two situations will be less sharp. Consequently, target behaviors may be more readily produced in nonclinical settings.

Delayed reinforcement should not be used during the early stages of training when target responses are shaped or increased from a low operant level. Immediate reinforcement is necessary at this stage of treatment. Once the responses have been established, the delivery of reinforcers may be delayed. When this is done, the durations of delay should be increased gradually. In the beginning, the responses must be reinforced only with a slight delay. Progressively longer delays may be implemented as the response rate is maintained.

Train Significant Others in Contingency Management

Perhaps the most important element of behavior maintenance strategy is to have the people associated with a client manage the reinforcement contingency at home and in other nonclinical settings. When other persons begin to reinforce the target responses in natural settings, the response control is shifted from the clinical to the extraclinical situations, and the behaviors are more likely to be produced and maintained in natural settings.

Who should be trained in contingency management is determined on an individual basis. The people with whom the client spends the most time (his or her significant others) are the primary targets for training. These people include parents, caretakers, spouses, siblings, teachers, friends, colleagues, relatives, and others who are in regular contact with the client. In the case of child clients, parents, siblings, babysitters, and grandparents may be the primary people to be trained. With school-age children, it is often useful to train the classroom teacher and close friends. In the case of adult clients, spouses, friends, and some colleagues may be the primary people. Training caretakers and other staff is important in the case of institutionalized clients.

Initially, the clinician may ask the family members to attend the treatment sessions to observe how the clinician evokes and reinforces target responses and how he or she stops the client at the earliest sign of a wrong response. Through discussion and observation, the significant others learn to clearly describe the target responses. They can then expect the same behaviors at home. The family members should understand how to evoke responses in natural settings. They should be able to model and prompt the responses. If necessary, they should know how to manipulate concrete stimuli (pictures and objects) to evoke the responses learned in the clinic. Most importantly, they should learn to promptly reinforce the target responses and prevent the occurrence of wrong responses.

After a few sessions of observation, the clinician might ask the significant others to administer treatment trials in the clinic under his or her supervision. These people should be especially involved in later stages of treatment when the client reliably produces the target responses in conversational speech. It is important for the parents to learn to reinforce target responses produced in conversational speech. For instance, they should know how to monitor fluency, desirable vocal qualities, correct production of phonemes, and morphological and other features of language. They should also learn to promptly stop the client when he or she produces dysfluencies, undesirable vocal qualities, misarticulated phonemes, and inappropriate language structures. The significant others should learn to prompt the correct responses in a subtle and objective manner.

Significant others should not only reinforce desirable target behaviors, but also withhold reinforcers for undesirable behaviors. In some cases, appropriate communicative behaviors taught in the clinic may not be maintained in natural environments because the incompatible, undesirable behaviors are still being reinforced in those environments. For example, if a nonverbal child continues to receive reinforcement for gestures at home, the verbal responses trained in the clinic may not be produced at home. When the child has learned an alternative verbal response, the incompatible nonverbal response should not be reinforced at home and in other situations.

In addition to training others in contingency management, the clinician should develop methods to determine whether other persons are indeed managing the contingencies. This is a difficult task. The clinician needs some evidence that the others are efficient in managing the treatment contingencies at home. The clinician may ask the parents and others to tape-record some formal and informal treatment sessions held at home. The clinician may visit the client's home, office, classroom, and other relevant settings to see if the target behaviors are being reinforced. A limitation of these strategies is that other persons may act as expected during taping or while the clinician is present, but not at other times. However, if significant others are asked to tape verbal interactions frequently, the chances of home management of contingencies might increase simply due to this requirement.

Teaching contingency management to significant others is an important clinical task. However, the clinician should work with significant others to achieve other targets as well. Chapter 9 is devoted to a more comprehensive discussion of working with families and others.

Reinforce Generalized Responses

Traditionally, generalized responses are not systematically reinforced. This is partly because, by definition, generalization is an unreinforced (albeit declining) rate of responses. In describing training and probe sequences in Chapter 5, it was suggested that responses given to probe items should not be reinforced. That suggestion was made because the clinician wishes initially to *assess* generalization. Because a probe is designed to find out the extent of generalization, if any, correct responses given to probe items should not be reinforced. However, while promoting maintenance, generalized responses, first documented through unreinforced probes, should be reinforced.

When a target behavior generalizes to home and other settings, the family members do not have to work on establishing the behavior. They can then promptly reinforce the initially generalized responses to prevent its extinction. In this sense, when stimulus and/or response generalization does take place, it is not the end of programming efforts. It is the beginning of a maintenance strategy in natural environments. Note that generalized responses are not reinforced to promote generalization, which has already taken place; they are reinforced so that generalized responses are maintained because of maintained contingencies.

The clinician can also reinforce generalized responses while not assessing them. When the clinician takes the client into nonclinical situations, such as stores and other public places, appropriate responses should be reinforced on a relatively large ratio. Even in clinical situations, novel (untrained) responses may be required and reinforced.

Hold Informal Training Sessions in Natural Environments

Even before parents or others are asked to manage contingencies at home and in other situations, it may be worthwhile to hold some informal training sessions outside the clinic. If possible, the clinician should hold informal sessions at the client's home.

Training sessions held in the home and other nonclinical situations can use "incidental" or naturalistic teaching procedures (Hart, 1985; Warren & Kaiser, 1986). These procedures are less formal than the discrete-trial–based technique described in earlier chapters. In incidental teaching, stimuli and responses are allowed to vary as they do in real-life situations. The clinician and the client might interact in typical manners in the client's home, stores, restaurants, playgrounds, and other places. Whenever the client produces a target response, the clinician might reinforce it, but the clinician does not strictly control the opportunities for such productions. In essence, naturally occurring responses in real-life situations may be reinforced. For example, a clinician may reinforce a stutterer's fluent speech while ordering in a restaurant, a child's correct production of targeted speech sounds or grammatic features in natural conversational speech at home, and a deaf individual's correct sign language in a store.

It is important to hold informal training sessions in those situations where trained responses are not produced on the basis of generalization. It is also important that parents or other family members be present during such training so that they can eventually take over the response control function. Holding informal training sessions in situations that do not show generalization has been called sequential modification (Stokes & Baer, 1977).

Contingency management in all natural settings, especially in public places such as stores and restaurants, must be as subtle as possible. A subtle signal, such as a hand or finger movement, may suggest to the client that the response was correct. A different signal might suggest that the target response was missed. The clinician and the client should agree beforehand on the meaning of such gestures. See Chapter 9 for additional information on this matter.

Teach Self-Control Procedures

Probably one of the most effective maintenance strategies is to make the client his or her own therapist. Self-control is evident when a client is able to monitor his or her behaviors in such a way as to decrease or increase them. A client who can do this can more readily begin to produce them in natural settings and maintain therapeutic gains with sporadic reinforcement from other persons (Koegel et al., 1986; Koegel et al., 1988).

Self-control refers to certain kinds of behaviors that can be taught and learned. A person who hides cookies so that they are not readily available for indiscriminate consumption is showing self-control. A student who habitually reads a certain number of pages in textbooks before going to a movie also exhibits self-control. Similarly, a teenage girl who monitors the number of cigarettes smoked per day to reduce smoking is modifying her behavior through self-control. The man who stutters may learn to measure his dysfluencies; in turn, this measurement will help him control his dysfluencies. Clients who can plot their own incorrect phoneme productions may be better able to monitor their correct and incorrect productions of phonemes.

To teach self-control, the clinician should reinforce clients for accurately discriminating their correct and incorrect responses. Whenever clients tell the clinician that their responses were not correct, they should be reinforced for their self-monitoring skills. Clients may be asked to mark their correct and incorrect responses on a separate recording sheet. They may also be taught to pause as soon as they exhibit a wrong response. This is self-administered time-out, which also is useful in teaching self-control.

Teach Contingency Priming

Despite a clinician's best efforts to teach contingency management to significant others, the other people sometimes may fail to notice the production of target behaviors. In that case, the client would not be reinforced. This problem can be handled by teaching the client to prime others to reinforce when he or she produces the newly learned target behaviors. In **contingency priming**, the client is taught certain actions that prompt other persons to reinforce him or her.

Everyday examples of contingency priming are numerous. A child who writes something, shows it to the mother, and says, "See Mom, how nice is my handwriting," is priming reinforcement. Adults who draw attention to their good work and then ask questions such as, "How about this now?" are also priming reinforcement. Clients may be taught to draw other persons' attention to their own target responses in an effort to obtain reinforcers that may not otherwise be forthcoming. A person who stutters may draw his or her recently acquired fluency to the attention of his ignoring family members or colleagues. A child who has been taught to produce certain grammatic features may also be taught to draw the teacher's attention whenever those features are produced.

Make Sure the Duration of Treatment Is Adequate

Sometimes the behaviors may not be maintained simply because of insufficient treatment (Kazdin, 1984). Unless target behaviors are well established and stabilized, they may not be produced often enough in natural environments to get reinforced. As a result, target behaviors may not come under the influence of maintaining contingencies.

The clinician must make sure that the trained behaviors are occurring reliably in extraclinical situations before considering dismissal from treatment. Periodic probes in extraclinical situations will help determine whether target behaviors are produced in those situations and, if so, to what extent. An extremely low or fluctuating response rate in everyday situations might suggest that more treatment is needed. Either a premature termination of the treatment program or a premature introduction of a maintenance strategy may be detrimental to response maintenance.

Follow Up and Arrange for Booster Treatment

Treatment given some time after the client is dismissed from the original program is called **booster treatment**. Many clients can benefit from a booster treatment. Although there is little empirical evidence regarding the need for booster treatment across different disorders, clinical impressions suggest that the need for booster treatment probably varies from disorder to disorder. For example, most stutterers and many voice clients need booster treatment.

The need for booster treatment is typically established through follow-up procedures. Unfortunately, follow-up procedures are among the most neglected aspects of treatment in communicative disorders, and very few follow-up studies are published in journals. The clinician must establish a regular follow-up procedure in which dismissed clients are periodically recalled to the clinic so that response maintenance can be measured over time.

A **follow-up** is a probe of previously trained target behaviors. These behaviors are sampled at the level of conversational speech. After taking a conversational speech sample, the clinician calculates the percent correct response rate. When appropriate, oral reading samples, telephone conversations, and conversations with unfamiliar people may also be sampled. These latter procedures are especially important in a follow-up of treated stutterers. In addition, clients, parents, or both may be asked to tape conversational speech samples at home and send them to the clinician periodically. Clients or family members may be requested to bring two or more recorded samples to the clinic when they come for a follow-up.

To establish reliability, the clinician needs a minimum of two samples of each speech task. The results are analyzed the same way as any assessment or probe data. The most important factor is the measured rate of target responses across samples. Booster treatment is needed when the measures show that, since the client's dismissal, the response rate has fallen below the desirable level.

Typically, booster treatment is not as extensive or intensive as the original treatment. Often, a session or two may be sufficient to reestablish the high rate of target response recorded at the time of the original dismissal. A greater number of treatment sessions may be needed if deterioration in response rate has been severe. Even then, in booster treatment sessions, most clients recover their target behaviors fairly rapidly.

Booster treatment may be the same as the original treatment or a variation of it. A new treatment, found to be more effective than the original, may also be used. In all booster treatments, the clinician may focus on specific problems of maintenance identified for given clients. For instance, a client may have maintained fluency in most situations, but not while talking on the telephone. In this case, the clinician must spend extra time on stabilizing fluency skills in telephone conversations.

The first follow-up after a client's initial dismissal may be scheduled after 3 months. If the target behaviors are maintained, the next follow-up may be scheduled after 6 months. Subsequent follow-ups may be done annually. Any time a follow-up measure shows a deterioration in response rate, booster treatment is arranged. After a booster treatment, more frequent follow-ups may be required until the target behaviors are again maintained.

At the time of dismissal, clients or parents must be informed of the need for future treatment. Clients and their family members who do not understand that fluency and other target behaviors may deteriorate and that additional treatment may be needed may think that treatment has failed and that nothing more can be done. However, those who understand that brief periods of booster treatment will help maintain target behaviors may be more willing to return for follow-up and booster treatment. The clinician should tell clients and their families that they should get in touch with the clinic any time they detect a change for the worse in treated behaviors. This can help initiate needed booster treatment before a scheduled follow-up takes place.

SUMMARY

Discrimination and generalization are two concepts that are especially relevant to an analysis and training of speech–language behaviors. Discrimination, which involves different responses to different stimuli, is achieved through a process called differential reinforcement. Whenever there is unacceptable generalization, discrimination training is needed.

Most clinicians believe that generalization is the final goal of clinical intervention. However, generalization is a declining response rate under changing stimulus and response properties in the absence of reinforcement. Therefore, it should not be the final goal of clinical intervention. Stimulus and response generalization are the two major types of generalization, and each has a variety of subtypes. Because generalized responses may be reinforced, it is desirable to promote their occurrence.

The final criterion of treatment success is response maintenance in everyday situations. Response maintenance refers to durability of treated behaviors across situations, across persons, and over time. Responses are maintained not because they show an initial (and temporary) generalization, but because they come under natural maintaining contingencies.

To achieve the final goal of treatment, the clinician must implement a maintenance strategy, which is defined as the extension of treatment to a client's natural environment. Maintenance strategy includes stimulus manipulations, response considerations, and contingency manipulations.

Stimulus manipulations include (1) selecting standard stimuli from the client's natural environment, (2) selecting common verbal antecedents, (3) varying audience antecedents, and (4) varying physical setting controls.

Response considerations include (1) selecting client-specific target behaviors, (2) selecting multiple exemplars of each of the target behaviors, and (3) reinforcing complex response topographies.

Contingency manipulations include (1) using intermittent reinforcement schedules, (2) using conditioned reinforcers, (3) delaying reinforcement, (4) training significant others in contingency management, (5) reinforcing generalized responses, (6) holding informal training sessions in natural settings, (7) teaching the client self-control procedures, (8) teaching the client contingency priming, (9) providing treatment for an appropriate duration, and (10) arranging for follow-up and booster treatment.

More research is needed to experimentally demonstrate the effectiveness of these and other maintenance strategies. It is hoped that because clinicians are now more concerned than ever about maintenance, systematic research information on effective maintenance techniques will become available in the near future.

STUDY GUIDE

Answer the following questions in technical language. Check your answers with the text. When necessary, rewrite your answers.

1. Define discrimination.

2. State the clinical need for discrimination training.

3. What is differential reinforcement?

4. What is the basis of concept formation?

5. What is abstraction in behavioral analysis?

6. Compare and contrast generalization and discrimination.

7. Define generalization.

8. Define stimulus generalization.

9. What is a generalization gradient?

10. Summarize the basic research information on stimulus generalization.

11. Define the following types of stimulus generalization:

    - Physical stimulus generalization.
    - Verbal stimulus generalization.
    - Physical setting generalization.
    - Audience generalization.
    - Factorial stimulus generalization.

12. Write your own examples of each type of stimulus generalization.

13. Define and describe response generalization.

14. Write your own examples of response generalization.

15. What is intraverbal generalization? Give examples.

16. Describe response mode generalization.

17. How is "comprehension" treated in behavioral analysis?

18. Describe concurrent stimulus–response generalization.

19. State precisely why generalization should not be the final goal of clinical intervention programs.

20. State the two problems that emerge when generalization is treated as the final goal of treatment.

21. State why the concept of "programming generalization" is confusing.

22. What is the final goal of clinical treatment?

23. How are responses maintained?

24. What are the three sets of maintenance strategies?

25. Define and describe each of the specific maintenance strategies. Give examples.

26. What are the four stimulus manipulations related to response maintenance strategies?

27. How are physical setting controls varied?

28. Why should complex response topographies be reinforced?

29. How does a clinician determine how many exemplars should be trained?

30. When and why are intermittent reinforcement schedules used?

31. What additional steps should be taken while using primary reinforcers?

32. What is meant by "train significant others"?

33. What is meant by "shift the locus of control"?

34. As a maintenance strategy, can generalized responses be reinforced?

35. Is reinforcing generalized responses a "strategy to promote generalization"? Justify your answer.

36. How are contingencies managed while holding informal training sessions in naturalistic settings?

37. Define self-control.

38. What are some of the self-control procedures that can be taught?

39. What is contingency priming?

40. How is treatment duration related to maintenance?

41. What is the purpose of a follow-up?

42. How are behaviors measured during a follow-up?

43. What is booster treatment?

44. When is booster treatment appropriate?

45. Can you give a new treatment during booster?

8

Decreasing Undesirable Behaviors

- More or less aversive methods of response reduction

- Assessment of undesirable behaviors

- Direct methods of response reduction

- Indirect methods of response reduction

- Negative side effects of aversive methods

- Positive side effects of aversive methods

- Implementing a least aversive response reduction strategy

As described in Chapter 4, speech–language pathologists have two major clinical tasks: to increase desirable communicative behaviors in their clients and to decrease undesirable behaviors. The procedures described in the previous chapters—positive and negative reinforcement, shaping, modeling, and differential reinforcement—help achieve the first task. This chapter describes procedures to achieve the second task. In many cases, the two kinds of tasks must be accomplished simultaneously. By using carefully selected procedures, the clinician increases certain behaviors while decreasing certain other behaviors.

Clients typically exhibit two sets of behaviors that need to be decreased: (1) *inappropriate* communicative behaviors and (2) behaviors that *interfere* with the training process. **Inappropriate communicative behaviors** are the typical undesirable behaviors clients give in place of desirable or appropriate speech–language behaviors. These inappropriate behaviors include misarticulated sounds; stutterings; improper or undesirable pitch, loudness, or other vocal qualities; wrong usage of grammatic features; and unacceptable use of language in social situations. While teaching appropriate behaviors, the clinician must decrease these inappropriate behaviors.

Interfering behaviors are extraneous nonspeech behaviors that interrupt the treatment process. A client who does not pay attention to the stimulus, a child who cries and whines during sessions, a teenage stutterer who yawns incessantly during treatment, or children who try to play with whatever material is on hand, all illustrate interfering behaviors.

Also, most uncooperative behaviors, including wiggling in the chair, offseat behaviors, interruptive talking, lying under the table, and constantly paying attention to irrelevant stimuli are interfering behaviors.

It is rarely necessary to concentrate on the inappropriate behaviors at the expense of teaching the desirable communicative behaviors. For instance, a clinician can continue to reinforce correct production of speech sounds while withholding reinforcing consequences for incorrect productions. Desirable vocal qualities may be reinforced while undesirable qualities are ignored.

Sometimes, however, it is necessary to concentrate on the interfering behaviors because they can make it difficult if not impossible to teach the desirable behaviors. Therefore, control of these behaviors becomes a priority. For example, it is difficult to teach anything to a crying child. The crying must be stopped first.

Throughout this chapter, the term undesirable behaviors is used to include both types of responses—inappropriate and interfering—that need to be reduced. Whenever greater specificity is needed, the specific term, inappropriate or interfering, is used.

MORE OR LESS AVERSIVE METHODS OF RESPONSE REDUCTION

Educators and clinicians would like their methods to be attractive to their pupils and clients. Historically, however, educational practices have never been totally free from methods that the recipients find unattractive or aversive. An event (or a procedure) is **aversive** if persons work hard to avoid it or move away from it; in this case, aversive events increase response frequency because the response is successful in terminating or avoiding the event. This is *negative reinforcement.* An event is aversive also when persons **respond less frequently** if responding is followed by the aversive event; in this case, aversive events decrease the response frequency because the event follows the response. This is *punishment.* An event is **nonaversive** if persons work hard to obtain it, or frequently move toward it. Such an event is a positive reinforcer because, when it follows a response, the response increases in frequency.

In recent years, research on various behavioral treatment programs has been concerned with developing nonaversive methods of reducing behaviors. A major debate is on the most desirable method of reducing undesirable behaviors (Carr, Robinson, Taylor, & Carlson, 1990; Repp & Singh, 1990). Some behavioral specialists believe that, among response reduction strategies, operant punishment procedures are aversive, unethical, inappropriate, and socially unacceptable and, therefore, should not be used in reducing any behavior. The proponents of this view also believe that totally nonaversive methods of reducing behaviors are now available and should be used.

Other specialists believe that at least some aversive response reduction procedures are necessary to control very serious inappropriate behaviors, including the self-injurious and aggressive behaviors of some clients. These specialists also believe that totally nonaversive methods of controlling all kinds of serious inappropriate behaviors are not yet available, and that the available nonaversive methods have not been proven to produce lasting effects.

Most clients of speech–language pathologists do not exhibit extremely serious inappropriate behaviors, such as head banging, self-mutilation, and physical assault. These behaviors are most frequently exhibited by persons who have multiple handicaps, profound retardation, and autism. However, speech–language pathologists who work in psychiatric institutions and rehabilitation facilities for the profoundly retarded are likely to face the same challenges as other health care and rehabilitative professionals. If they are otherwise acceptable, procedures that reduce serious inappropriate behaviors may be used in reducing the less serious but equally undesirable behaviors seen in routine speech, language, and hearing treatment sessions. Therefore, speech–language clinicians who work in any setting need to be aware of developments in response reduction strategies. The clinicians can then critically analyze the data and make judgments about accepting or rejecting certain procedures.

The debate on the use of aversive and intrusive methods is intense in relation to such procedures as electric shock, loud noise, water mist sprayed in the face, lemon juice squirted into the mouth, and so forth. Such procedures are used only when the client's or other person's life or safety is threatened by outbursts of powerful, serious, repetitive, and dangerous behaviors. Clinicians who use such procedures contend that they are used only after less aversive procedures have failed to stop the behavior. The advocates also claim that the aversive procedures may be more humane than the less aversive but ineffective procedures that condemn the individual to endless unhappiness. Another justification offered by many is that, without such aversive methods, some individuals will hurt or kill others, destroy property, or hurt themselves so badly that they are a threat to their own lives.

The dichotomy of aversive and nonaversive methods is somewhat artificial. It is doubtful that any of the direct response reduction procedures is totally nonaversive. As described in a later section, the direct response reduction procedures place a contingency on the undesirable behavior itself. The indirect strategy does nothing directly to the undesirable behavior, but does increase, by reinforcement, desirable behaviors. This increase in desirable behaviors may have an indirect effect of decreasing undesirable behaviors.

The indirect strategy of doing nothing to an undesirable behavior while reinforcing a desirable behavior comes close to being a nonaversive strategy; however, it still may be aversive to some extent. All indirect strategies involve ignoring or not reinforcing the undesirable behavior when it occurs. Can it be assumed, then, that not getting reinforced in the way someone was accustomed to is nonaversive? Probably not. All response reduction strategies force the person to unlearn. Most if not all unlearning may be aversive to some extent; if so, most if not all response reduction strategies are aversive to varying degrees. Therefore, it is best to describe methods of response reduction as *more or less aversive.*

All clinicians prefer totally nonaversive methods to those that are aversive to any extent. Clinicians who are not convinced that totally nonaversive methods are available will use the least aversive methods in conjunction with positive methods that shape and maintain desirable behaviors. Even those clinicians will always emphasize positive methods that teach the desirable communicative behaviors.

ASSESSMENT OF UNDESIRABLE BEHAVIORS

Most undesirable behaviors are somehow reinforced. Otherwise, they would not be maintained. An undesirable behavior whose reinforcer is known may be reduced efficiently and with fewer aversive consequences. Therefore, in recent years, many behavioral research efforts have been made to understand how undesirable behaviors are maintained (Carr et al., 1990; Repp & Singh, 1990).

The method of finding causes of behaviors is called **functional analysis**. In a laboratory, functional analysis may discover the original causes of behaviors, but this is possible mostly with animal subjects. With human subjects, functional analysis mainly discovers the maintaining causes of behaviors. This is fine, because in most cases, controlling maintaining causes will reduce unwanted behaviors. The original cause of many behaviors may or may not be working at a time when clinicians try to reduce them.

The causes of already established behaviors are a combination of antecedent stimuli and consequent events: Certain stimuli trigger undesirable behaviors, and certain consequences maintain them. By manipulating stimuli and consequences of undesirable behaviors, researchers have discovered that most undesirable behaviors are learned and maintained by positive, negative, or automatic reinforcement.

Positively Reinforced Undesirable Behaviors

As mentioned, events that increase the frequency of a behavior because they followed that behavior are positive reinforcers. Positive reinforcers make no distinction between good and bad behaviors; they increase the probability of any behavior that preceded them. Society makes the social or ethical judgment about the nature of the behavior. Thus, it is up to society to reinforce certain behaviors and not reinforce other behaviors.

An important point to remember is that one person's actions may reinforce another person's undesirable behavior even though there was no intention to increase such a behavior. Often, intentions do not matter; consequences do. Although most people do not want to reinforce undesirable behaviors, people may reinforce behaviors they do not wish to see in others.

The fact that some undesirable behaviors are maintained by positive reinforcement has been known for a long time. Recently, functional analysis has confirmed this (Iwata, Vollmer, & Zarcone, 1990; Repp & Karsh, 1990). A teacher or parent, for example, may pay attention to a disruptive child who is otherwise ignored. The attention need not be "positive" in the everyday sense of that term. Disapproval and reprimand also may reinforce and maintain the disruptive behavior. It has been shown that some autistic children's head banging and other self-injurious behaviors may be maintained by social attention. An autistic boy who bangs his head may be immediately picked up by a staff member, or reprimanded for that action, or taken out for a walk, or given something to do to keep himself busy. Each of these and many similar staff actions may be sufficient to increase the future probability of head banging. When the boy is not banging his head, he may simply sit in a corner with no attention paid to him.

Behaviors maintained by positive reinforcement increase when attended to and decrease when ignored. Therefore, in assessing the maintaining cause of positively reinforced behaviors, the clinician may reinforce for a brief duration to see if the behavior increases. Subsequently, the clinician should withdraw reinforcers to see if the behavior decreases. For example, if the child frequently interrupts treatment trials with distracting questions, the clinician may first attend to those interruptions and later withdraw all attention to see if the frequency of interruptions increases and then decreases.

A clinician may inadvertently strengthen undesirable behaviors with positive reinforcers. Hoping to stop a child's crying behavior by reasoning, the clinician may talk to the child. However, this may reinforce the crying behavior. Other things clinicians do include dangling toys before fussing or uncooperative children or showing them pictures or other interesting but nontherapeutic materials. All such actions may positively reinforce the child's undesirable behaviors.

Established undesirable behaviors may be under **stimulus control**; that is, the mere presence of a person or a setting may trigger the behavior. For example, a clinician who typically reinforces undesirable behaviors may become a discriminative stimulus for such behaviors. The clinician is likely to complain that the child is more disruptive in his or her presence than in the presence of other clinicians. Likewise, a child may be more disruptive at home than at school because the undesirable behavior is reinforced at home. These examples show that disruptive behaviors may be controlled by antecedent stimuli as well as by consequences (reinforcers).

Negatively Reinforced Undesirable Behaviors

Some undesirable behaviors may be maintained by negative reinforcement because the behaviors provide escapes from aversive situations or stimuli. People can turn off aversive events or escape from them by exhibiting desirable or undesirable behaviors. The behaviors become problematic only when socially unacceptable behaviors are learned to terminate aversive events.

For instance, a student who is studying for an examination may find the roommate's music loud and aversive. The student can seek termination of this aversive event by several means. The student can politely request the roommate not to play music or to play it softly. If the roommate complies immediately, the student's polite request has been **negatively reinforced** because the request terminated the aversive music. In the future, when the roommate turns on loud music, the student who is studying is more likely to request that it be stopped or its volume reduced. This is what is meant by negative reinforcement: A behavior that is successful in terminating an aversive event is more likely in the future. In this case, the student learned a socially acceptable behavior to terminate an aversive event. It is fine to request people not to disturb.

Unfortunately, and just as effectively, a person can learn a socially unacceptable or undesirable behavior to eliminate aversive stimulation. For example, the student could terminate the loud music by shouting at the roommate, pulling the plug, or destroying the roommate's boom box. Each of these undesirable behaviors may immediately terminate the aversive music. The worst of the three actions (destroying the stereo) is guaranteed to eliminate the aversive event; however, the roommate may buy another, bigger stereo financed generously by the student's insurance company. Nevertheless, the student's destructive behavior will have been strongly and negatively reinforced by the immediate result it produced: cessation of music. Next time, the student is more likely to exhibit destructive behavior to eliminate music or other aversive stimulation. The student will have learned to exhibit undesirable behaviors by negative reinforcement.

For many children in therapy, the task demanded of them may be difficult to perform. Repeated trials are aversive to the child who cannot imitate or produce the target phoneme or grammatic morpheme demanded by the clinician. If some behavior may terminate or postpone such unpleasant treatment trials, the child is likely to exhibit it. Suppose that the child leaves the chair and crawls under the table during the treatment session. If this action was a response to repeated trials on which the child failed to imitate or produce the correct responses, the action successfully terminated aversive treatment trials. While under the table, the child cannot be presented with the difficult treatment task. This termination of treatment trials may negatively reinforce the undesirable behavior of crawling under the table. Similarly, a child who begins to cry and thus shortens an aversive treatment session may also be negatively reinforced.

Several research studies have documented negative reinforcement of undesirable behaviors. Most of these studies were made with developmentally disabled or autistic children with a history of serious undesirable behaviors, including head banging and other forms of self-injury. To show that these behaviors were negatively reinforced, the researchers terminated difficult educational demands whenever the children they were treating exhibited some undesirable behavior. The result was an increase in those undesirable behaviors. Because the undesirable behavior was negatively reinforced by task termination, the children showed that behavior more frequently to escape from the aversive task. On the other hand, when the researchers continued to present the difficult task demands, the undesirable behavior decreased in frequency. In this case, the child's undesirable behavior did not provide an escape from the aversive task; that is, there was no negative reinforcement for the undesirable behavior (Iwata, 1987; Iwata, Pace, Cowdery, Kalsher, & Cataldo, 1990; Iwata, Vollmer, & Zarcone, 1990; Pyles & Bailey, 1990; Repp & Karsh, 1990).

To find out if a client's undesirable behavior is negatively reinforced, the clinician *removes* the suspected aversive stimulus contingent on the occurrence of that behavior. Recall that in finding out if a behavior is positively reinforced, the clinician *presents* the suspected positive reinforcer immediately after the behavior is exhibited. In both cases, the behavior increases in frequency.

To prevent negative reinforcement for an undesirable escape behavior, the clinician must block escape. This is done, however, only when the escape attempted is from such harmless aversive stimulation as a difficult educational or therapeutic task. The procedure extinguishes the escape response by not (negatively) reinforcing it. Therefore, the procedure is called **escape extinction**. The procedure of decreasing undesirable behaviors through escape extinction has three components: continued presentation of treatment trials; prevention of the escape response; and, thus, elimination of negative reinforcement.

As noted before, stimuli associated with aversive events may also acquire the power to evoke the undesirable behavior. For example, the sight of the therapist may be sufficient for a child to start crying. The parent then stays with the child to console. The result is that the aversive treatment is postponed and the crying behavior is negatively reinforced. The longer the child cries, the longer the duration of escape from treatment. Eventually, the child may begin to cry or fuss when approaching the clinic. Later, the child may refuse to get into the car when it is time to go to the clinic. Finally, the child may fuss when it is about time to leave the house for the clinic. These are examples of various environmental stimuli that become associated with the aversive event (therapy) and that evoke the undesirable (escape) behavior.

Automatically Reinforced Undesirable Behaviors

It is difficult to identify environmental events that reinforce certain undesirable behaviors. Some undesirable behaviors of developmentally disabled and autistic children are hard to explain on the basis of observable positively or negatively reinforcing events. The reinforcers in such cases may be the stimulation derived from the behaviors themselves. When this is the case, the behaviors are said to be automatically reinforced. **Automatic reinforcers** are also described as sensory reinforcers because the reinforcing events are sensory consequences of undesirable actions.

Research has shown that rocking and other kinds of self-stimulatory behaviors—often described as stereotypic behaviors—are more likely when developmentally disabled children experience a general lack of stimulation. Absence of play and other forms of activities and social interactions deprive children of reinforcing stimulation. Conversely, research has shown that children are less likely to indulge in stereotypic behaviors when environmental stimulation is increased (Iwata, Vollmer, & Zarcone, 1990). These data suggest that certain undesirable behaviors provide stimulation that the environment does not.

To find out if an undesirable behavior is maintained by automatic reinforcement, the clinician may manipulate the amount of stimulation to determine if the behavior changes accordingly. If the behavior increases when the amount of available environmental stimulation is decreased (deprivation of stimulation) and the behavior decreases when *noncontingent* stimulation is provided, then the behavior is likely reinforced automatically. The clinician must make sure that the stimulation provided *does not follow* the occurrence of the undesirable behavior. This is the meaning of noncontingent stimulation. The undesirable behavior is reinforced if stimulation is made contingent on it. Although this method will show that external stimulation reinforced the undesirable behavior, it will not show that the behavior was reinforced by sensory stimulation in the first place.

Summary of Assessment of Undesirable Behaviors

Undesirable behaviors may be maintained by positive, negative, or automatic reinforcement. By programming the consequence thought to be reinforcing a behavior for a short duration, the clinician can determine the potential source of reinforcement for most undesirable behaviors. Following this assessment, the clinician may develop a behavior reduction program.

DIRECT METHODS OF RESPONSE REDUCTION

In **direct** methods of response reduction, a contingency is placed on the undesirable behavior itself. This contingency reduces the behavior. The direct strategy is contrasted later in this chapter with the indirect strategy in which no contingency is placed on the behavior to be reduced.

There are four direct behavior reduction procedures: extinction, stimulus presentation, stimulus withdrawal, and imposition of work. The latter three are traditionally described as operant punishment. In extinction and punishment, the clinician's attention is focused on the undesirable behavior. The clinician stops reinforcement (extinction), presents a stimulus, withdraws a reinforcer, or imposes effort (work) when an undesirable behavior occurs. Therefore, they are all direct methods.

Extinction

The behavioral process of extinction was originally discovered by Pavlov in classical conditioning and Skinner in operant conditioning. These two scientists found that if the response is continuously evoked without reinforcement, the response rate eventually decreases, and may even reach zero. Therefore, extinction is common to both classical and operant responses. The Pavlovian dog will stop salivating if the experimenter continues to present the tone (conditioned stimulus) without food (unconditioned stimulus or the reinforcer). The Skinnerian pigeon will stop pecking the button when that response no longer produces food (reinforcer).

A general rule is that behavioral procedures are defined in terms of their effects on the rate of behaviors. Recall that a reinforcer is an event that increases the rate of a response it follows. *But extinction is an exception to this rule.* It is not defined in terms of its effects on the behavior. Instead, **extinction** is defined as a procedure of terminating the reinforcer for a response (Ferster et al., 1975; Holland & Skinner, 1961; Kazdin, 1984). This definition simply points out the procedure of extinction: A reinforcer is terminated, and the response is allowed to be made. Extinction is so defined because it does not have an invariable, single effect. Its initial and subsequent effects may be different. That is why it is sensible to describe it only procedurally.

When a previously reinforced response no longer produces reinforcers, the person does not stop responding abruptly. In fact, the person may redouble the efforts and increase the rate of response, presumably to produce the reinforcer. But if the responses continue to go unreinforced, the rate eventually decreases to its prereinforcement level. Thus, the clinician who stops reinforcing a response may see first an increase and then a decrease in the rate of that response. This increase in the response rate is called an **extinction burst**. Because of extinction burst, it is not appropriate to define extinction as a decrease in the rate of response under no reinforcement. Extinction is similar to what people call ignoring. When an action is consistently ignored by a person, that action becomes less likely in the presence of that person.

Factors that Affect Extinction

Typically, extinction is a gradual process. Responses under extinction decrease slowly, often over a period of time. The time needed to extinguish a response depends upon several factors.

Reinforcement Schedule. Extensive laboratory research has shown that behaviors maintained on an intermittent reinforcement schedule are more difficult to extinguish than those maintained on a continuous schedule (Ferster et al.,

1975; Ferster & Skinner, 1957). Intermittently reinforced behaviors persist even when the reinforcer is withdrawn. Most undesirable behaviors are probably reinforced intermittently. It is unlikely, for example, that each time a child fusses, the parents pay attention. Sometimes they do and sometimes they do not. But this is precisely the kind of schedule that creates a very strong behavior that resists extinction.

The somewhat long duration it takes to extinguish such behaviors may afford opportunities for unplanned reinforcement. For example, if the child's crying has been intermittently reinforced at home, it is likely to take a long duration to extinguish it in the clinic. If it takes very long, the clinician may accidentally look at the child and reinforce the crying in some other fashion. This will prolong the extinction process even more.

Amount of Past Reinforcement.   A response that is heavily reinforced is more difficult to extinguish than the one reinforced not so heavily. Note that an intermittent schedule may involve a high or low density of reinforcement. If the amount or the magnitude of reinforcement is high when it does come, it creates a strong response that resists extinction.

Duration for Which the Response Has Been Reinforced.   A response reinforced over a long period of time is more difficult to extinguish than the one reinforced for a shorter duration. Crying, fussing, or other undesirable behaviors clinicians try to extinguish in the clinic may have been reinforced at home over months or even years.

Previous Exposure to Extinction.   If the behavior is being extinguished for the first time, it takes longer than if the behavior has been previously exposed to extinction. Extinction is somewhat fast if the behavior has been extinguished several times before. The clinicians are often the first persons to apply extinction correctly and systematically. Many parents may have *attempted* extinction in the past, but may not have carried it through.

In essence, the most difficult response to extinguish is the one that has been reinforced intermittently, with large amounts of reinforcement, over a long period of time, and with no prior history of extinction.

Effective Use of Extinction

Before extinction can be initiated, the reinforcer that is maintaining the behavior must be identified. This is not a major problem in laboratory research. The experimenter conditions the response with a specific reinforcer, which is then withheld, and the subject is allowed to respond.

Clinicians typically do not know the conditioning history of a given client's undesirable behaviors. Nevertheless, to extinguish a behavior, the clinician should remove the reinforcer that maintains it. Therefore, clinicians often guess at the possible reinforcers maintaining given undesirable behaviors and then withhold them. This is why extinction is less efficient in clinical situations than in laboratory experiments. However, the efficacy of extinction can be greatly improved if the clinician makes a functional analysis of the undesirable behavior. As described before, this analysis may show that the behavior is maintained either by positive, negative, or automatic reinforcement.

How the clinician extinguishes a behavior depends on how it is reinforced. The following are suggestions to extinguish behaviors depending on how they are reinforced.

Extinction of Positively Reinforced Behaviors. Although reinforcers maintaining responses are difficult to identify without functional analysis, many interfering behaviors children show in clinical situations can be effectively controlled by a systematic use of attention. A child's interfering responses, such as "Is it time to go yet?" "We are all done for today," and "You know what?" are best ignored. If the child begins to play with stimulus materials or reinforcers, they should be promptly removed from the subject's reach. If the child looks at the mirror and makes faces, the seating arrangement can be changed. If a picture on the wall is a distracting and reinforcing stimulus, it must be removed. These examples illustrate how reinforcers can be withdrawn to extinguish inappropriate responses.

In extinguishing a positively reinforced undesirable behavior, the following steps are necessary. First, the behavior to be extinguished must be clearly defined. If the child exhibits multiple undesirable behaviors, only one behavior may be extinguished at a time.

Second, at the earliest sign of the target behavior, the clinician should tell the child in simple language what is going to happen. For instance, the clinician may tell a crying child that "You may get these tokens if you stop crying. We will not work together as long as you are crying." This sort of explanation should be brief.

Third, the clinician should turn away from the child and sit motionless. The clinician should not do anything (e.g., reorganize the stimulus material) that might be reinforcing to the child. A child lying under the table in a treatment session may be looking at a comic book or playing with a small toy. In this case, although the clinician has withdrawn attention, the response is still being reinforced. As suggested earlier, all reinforcing stimulus material must be out of the child's reach. A frequent mistake of beginning clinicians is to reinforce the undesirable behavior by talking to the child. Some clinicians think they can reason with the child who is crying, whining, or lying under the table to convince him or her that the behavior is bad. Other clinicians think that when the child interrupts the training trials by asking irrelevant questions or by narrating "you know what" types of stories, a quick approval or a response will stop the interfering behavior. However, paying attention in any form reinforces the behavior to be extinguished.

Fourth, the clinician should not give in when there is an initial increase in the response rate. Sometimes, the clinician might think that extinction is not working because the behavior has intensified and, therefore, does something that actually reinforces the response. For example, when the intensity of the crying behavior increases, the clinician might pick up the child or bring the mother into the therapy room. These actions may stop the crying behavior, but the clinician will have reinforced the crying behavior so that it is more likely in the next session. Also, the clinician will have reinforced a more intense crying behavior! Once extinction is initiated, the clinician should resist the temptation to stop that behavior by other means.

Extinction of Negatively Reinforced Behaviors.
Recall that escape from aversive treatment provides negative reinforcement for some undesirable behaviors exhibited in treatment sessions. If the treatment trials involve difficult tasks, the child may try to terminate or postpone treatment in many ways.

One example given earlier is that the child crawls under the table to escape aversive trials of therapy. Other examples of escape include frequent and abrupt verbal interruptions ("You know what I ate for breakfast?"), inattention, leaving the seat, and grabbing the clinician's pen to scribble on paper.

To extinguish negatively reinforced behaviors, the clinician must prevent escape. As mentioned before, this is **escape extinction**. Any behavior is extinguished only by removing the reinforcer. In case of positive reinforcers, undesirable behaviors may be allowed to be exhibited while withholding the reinforcers. However, negatively reinforced behaviors cannot be extinguished in this manner, because the behavior terminates the aversive event and thus gets immediately reinforced. Therefore, to prevent negative reinforcement, the clinician must prevent the behavior itself.

Escape may be prevented physically or by changing the treatment procedure. Physical prevention of escape involves restricting the client's movements. For example, if the clinician sat right in front of a child with the child's chair between his or her legs, escape may be physically prevented. The clinician may also hold the child's face and make sure the child attends. Every time the child tries to leave the seat, the clinician may physically restrain the movement. How an escape behavior is prevented depends on its form.

As the examples show, a negatively reinforced behavior must be prevented so it will not be reinforced (extinguished). For example, when crawling under the table is prevented and the treatment trials continue to be presented, the clinician will have done two things: maintained aversive trials and prevented escape behavior. Consequently, the negative reinforcement was terminated. This is escape extinction.

An important point to remember is that the traditional extinction procedure in which the behavior is simply ignored is not effective in reducing negatively reinforced behaviors. Ignoring the behavior means allowing it to happen without offering reinforcement. But the clinician does not have to present anything to reinforce many negatively reinforced behaviors; behaviors instantaneously earn their own reinforcers. Therefore, if a negatively reinforced behavior is allowed to occur, the behavior is reinforced without the clinician's help. Although a clinician may ignore temper tantrums, the behavior was reinforced because it terminated aversive treatment.

Preventing an escape response while continuing to make difficult task demands probably has a high level of aversiveness. A preferred method is to reduce the aversiveness of therapy. The escape extinction procedure should be used only when serious and systematic attempts at reducing the aversiveness of the therapeutic task has failed. Because reducing aversiveness of therapeutic tasks is not an extinction procedure, it is described in a later section.

Extinction of Automatically Reinforced Behaviors. While working with clients who are emotionally disturbed, profoundly retarded, and brain injured, the speech–language pathologist may encounter undesirable behaviors that are automatically reinforced. One form of automatic reinforcement that may maintain these behaviors is sensory reinforcement, which may be extinguished. For example, if the child begins to bang on the table during therapy, reinforcement for this behavior may be the auditory feedback (noise) generated by the response.

To reduce this behavior, the table may be covered with a soft material that eliminates the auditory stimulation. A child who inappropriately claps his or her hands during treatment sessions may be made to wear thick, soft gloves that reduce or eliminate the sound that might reinforce the response. If the clinician's charting of the target behaviors seems to distract the child constantly, the clinician can hold the writing pad such that the child is unable to see the charting. This will eliminate the reinforcing visual feedback.

Some self-injurious behaviors also may be automatically reinforced. Researchers have reduced such behaviors as head banging by placing on the children padded helmets that reduced sensory feedback for the children (see Iwata, Vollmer, & Zarcone, 1990, for a review of studies).

Combination of Extinction and Reinforcement

To make extinction work faster, and hence make it less aversive, it should be combined with other procedures. The best procedure to be combined with extinction is positive reinforcement for desirable behaviors.

As stated before, the clinical goals are to reduce undesirable behaviors *and* to replace them with desirable behaviors. Extinction (and other procedures to be described) helps reduce undesirable behaviors, and positive reinforcement helps increase desirable behaviors that will replace the undesirable behaviors; while a competing response is weakened, an alternative response is strengthened. Extinction of a response is faster when an alternative response is positively reinforced.

For each undesirable behavior to be extinguished, the clinician must have a clearly identified desirable behavior to be reinforced. For example, when extinguishing a child's crying behavior, the clinician should be ready to promptly reinforce the child if crying were to stop. Even a brief period of no crying should be immediately reinforced. While ignoring nonattending behaviors, the clinician must positively reinforce attending behavior. Sometimes clinicians make the mistake of not taking note of the alternative behavior quickly enough, with the result that the undesirable behavior picks up speed again.

In teaching parents to use extinction, clinicians must emphasize that reinforcers must be removed promptly and consistently. If the behavior is likely to be reinforced by different members of a family, each should be trained in the correct use of extinction. The procedure will fail if only one person occasionally reinforces the behavior. The clinician should take extra time in training parents and others in extinguishing negatively reinforced behaviors.

Limitations of Extinction

Extinction has certain limitations. In using extinction, the clinician should make efforts to overcome its limitations.

First, some experiments have shown that extinction may have certain negative side effects. When the reinforcer is withheld, the client may react with anger, frustration, and even aggression. I once observed a child whose crying behavior under extinction was interrupted by such shouts as "I don't like you" and "You are not nice." In everyday situations, adults also show emotional reactions when the reinforcer is not forthcoming. A flat tire might prompt the driver to curse and kick the car, and a losing tennis star might throw his or her racket on the ground.

The frequency or intensity of such emotional reactions is minimized when the clinician clearly defines an alternative, desirable behavior and reinforces even the earliest signs of that behavior. The actual extinction and reinforcement contingency must be made clear to the client. For example, the clinician might tell a crying child that as soon as he or she stops crying, they can go out to see the mother. Otherwise, the clinician should not interact with a child whose behavior is being extinguished.

Second, an extinguished response may recover sooner or later. If the response is reinforced at this time, it might rebound with alarming force. However, if the clinician were to put that behavior back on extinction, the process would be quicker than originally. With succeeding cycles of extinction, the behavior is eliminated sooner and with more lasting effects.

Third, an extinction procedure can be uncomfortable to the clinician. When a child begins to cry in a session, the clinician must cease all forms of attention and turn away from the child. The crying behavior may not subside immediately. Only when the clinician persists with the extinction procedure is there a decrease in crying behavior.

Fourth, extinction should not be used to reduce aggressive, self-destructive, or highly disruptive behaviors. Before the slow process of extinction works, aggressive behaviors might result in damage to other persons or property or harm to the person. Extremely disruptive behaviors in clinic and classroom situations may have to be controlled by other means that produce faster results.

Carefully planned extinction procedures combined with positive reinforcement can be effective in controlling undesirable behaviors while encouraging desirable alternative behaviors. Once extinction is initiated, the clinician should not reinforce the client until signs of desirable behaviors occur.

Stimulus Presentation

Although extinction is a "do-nothing" procedure, in other direct methods of response reduction, the clinician either presents a stimulus immediately after a response is made or withdraws a stimulus promptly. If the response rate decreases because of the stimulus presentation or withdrawal, the stimulus is traditionally described as punishing. **Punishment** in operant conditioning is a procedure of reducing behaviors either by presenting certain stimuli or by withdrawing certain others immediately after the behaviors occur. Technically, the procedure of reducing behaviors by presenting stimuli is Type I punishment, and the procedure of reducing behaviors by withdrawing stimuli is Type II punishment.

Presentation of any stimuli, including shock, noise, distasteful material, reprimands, and so forth, are included in direct procedures or Type I punishment. In most speech–language treatment sessions, the stimulus presentation used is corrective feedback. Many clinicians do not and would not use other types of stimuli that are more aversive, invasive, and socially and personally unacceptable.

Some clinicians are alarmed at the term punishment, but it is not used in the popular sense here. In everyday use, the term is emotionally charged. The popular use of punishment is often questionable. Nonetheless, many popular and scientific connotations of the term make it a difficult and confusing concept. Both the educated and lay persons constantly confuse the word's use as a scientific term and its use in everyday and legal language. Therefore, I limit use of the term in this book. Still, it should be clear that, except for extinction, other direct methods of response reduction may be described as punishment procedures.

Some people confuse negative reinforcement with punishment. When they mean punishment, they use the term negative reinforcement. Recall, however, that negative reinforcement increases response rates, whereas punishment decreases response rates. Because the two procedures have opposite effects on behavior, they should not be confused.

Corrective Feedback

The direct response reduction procedure of corrective feedback is frequently used in speech–language treatment sessions. It is described as *corrective feedback* because, immediately after a response is made, a stimulus is presented to suggest the acceptability of the response. The feedback may be verbal, nonverbal, or mechanical. Feedback of this nature, especially verbal and nonverbal, is most frequently used in treatment sessions.

Corrective Verbal Feedback.   Clinicians constantly and instantaneously evaluate the appropriateness of each response given by a client. If a response is judged to be inadequate, inappropriate, or unacceptable for any reason, clinicians tell the client about this evaluation. Clinicians may say words such as "no," "wrong," and "not correct." These verbal stimuli, presented contingent on an inappropriate response, may decrease the response. Traditionally, these stimuli are classified as punishing stimuli.

Some clinicians may be reluctant to give corrective feedback. However, there is little justification for withholding minimally aversive verbal, nonverbal, or mechanical stimuli that tell the client in unmistakable terms whether the response was acceptable. Because many clients may not be able to make that judgment, they need feedback from the clinician. One 7-year-old girl who received training for correct articulation of phonemes brought this idea home to a clinician who was reluctant to say "no" or "not correct." After wondering for a while whether the clinician's silence meant good or bad, the girl told the clinician, "You know, if you don't tell me if I am correct or not, I can't learn!" The clinician immediately began to provide feedback.

Corrective Nonverbal Feedback. Gestures and other nonverbal signals presented response contingently may reduce the frequency of undesirable behaviors. For example, the clinician may raise a finger when the production of a target phoneme is unacceptable. Eyebrows may be raised when the child wiggles in the chair. A hand signal may be given to slow the rate of speech in a stuttering person under a rate reduction treatment. Hand signals also may suggest to a voice client that the pitch is too low.

Most gestures and other nonverbal signals work only when paired with verbal instructions and verbal corrective feedback. For instance, the clinician may say "slow down" and simultaneously give a hand signal to suggest a lower rate. In articulation therapy, while saying "no" to incorrect sound productions, the clinician may raise the index finger. Later, the hand signal or raised index finger alone may give the client the necessary corrective feedback.

Mechanical Feedback. Biofeedback has been the most researched of the mechanical feedback forms used in reducing undesirable behaviors. Small electronic electromyographic units that monitor muscle action potential, for example, are used to reduce muscular tension and anxiety. Both visual and auditory feedback may be provided. For instance, a red light or a high-frequency tone may suggest an unacceptable level of muscular tension. Most biofeedback units give dual feedback, signaling both acceptable and unacceptable responses. A green light or a low-frequency tone, for example, may signal acceptable (lower) levels of tension.

Recent developments in computer technology have vastly expanded the range of mechanical feedback that can be provided to clients. Many computer programs used in treatment provide immediate, animated, colorful feedback that signal correct and incorrect responses. Colorful graphics on the computer monitor may represent correct sound production; acceptable pitch, loudness, and voice quality; appropriate rhythm of speech; and many other speech and voice characteristics. These representations provide an immediate evaluation of the response and signal both appropriate and inappropriate behaviors.

Stimulus Withdrawal

Another direct procedure to reduce behaviors is withdrawal of certain stimuli. This is also a response-contingent procedure in that a stimulus (or an event) is withdrawn immediately after an undesirable response is made. It is presumed that what is withdrawn reinforces the undesirable behavior. Therefore, the stimulus or event withdrawal procedure removes a potential reinforcer, and thus reduces the behavior.

There are two kinds of stimulus withdrawal procedures: time-out and response cost. Both are frequently used in educational and clinical work with children and adults.

Time-out

Time-out (TO), which means time-out from positive reinforcement, is a period of nonreinforcement imposed response contingently, resulting in a decreased rate of that response. This period of time may be imposed in different ways, giving rise to variations in TO procedures. There are three major types of TO (Brantner & Doherty, 1983).

The first and the most extreme form is called **isolation TO** in which a person is removed from the environment and placed in a specially designed situation with few, if any, reinforcers. For instance, parents of misbehaving children may send them to a barren room for a few minutes. Time-out booths also illustrate this procedure. When a person is placed in a barren room, or a TO booth, naturally occurring reinforcers are denied during the TO period. Prison terms are intended to be isolation TO, but they may not have the expected effects. An important reason for this failure is that prison terms are rarely response contingent: In most cases, criminals are sent to prison months or years after they commit criminal acts. The isolation TO is controversial and is used mostly in institutional settings with appropriate legal and ethical safeguards.

The second type of time-out is called **exclusion TO**, which is common in educational settings. A teacher might ask a misbehaving child to sit outside the classroom, in a corner, or facing the wall. The child is not physically isolated, but is excluded from the normal activities of the classroom. Exclusion TO is rarely used in clinical speech–language services. When the sessions are as brief as they are in the treatment of communicative disorders, the response reduction procedures must also be brief.

The third type is **nonexclusion TO**. In its most common form, the clinician gives the client a response-contingent signal to start a brief period of TO, during which (1) the clinician does not interact with the client, (2) the client is prohibited from responding, and hence, (3) no reinforcers are forthcoming. This form of TO can be described as a "frozen moment" of no interaction. For example, any time a client gives a wrong response, the clinician might say "stop," and avoid eye contact for a brief period, such as 5 seconds.

Nonexclusion TO is more acceptable socially than the other forms because it does not involve physical removal, isolation, or exclusion. This technique is effective in reducing many forms of incorrect and interfering behaviors (Brantner & Doherty, 1983). In speech–language treatment sessions, nonexclusion TO has been frequently used. Several studies have demonstrated the effectiveness of nonexclusion TO in the treatment of stuttering (Costello, 1975; Hegde & Parson,

1990; James, 1981; Martin, Kuhl, & Haroldson, 1972). Typically, the clinician gives a signal such as a verbal "stop" or a red light that is turned on contingent upon stuttering and imposes a brief TO period during which the client is not allowed to talk. The clinician avoids eye contact. As long as the stutterer sustains fluent speech, the clinician continues to reinforce with eye contact, smile, and attention.

To make TO more effective, verbal stimulus presentation may be combined with nonexclusion TO. For example, whenever a child yawns or looks away from the stimulus item, the clinician might say "no," and then avoid eye contact for a few seconds.

Ineffective Use of Time-Out.

In some cases, the clinician may be dismayed to find an increase in a behavior subjected to time-out. This paradoxical effect is typically due to two reasons. First, TO may negatively reinforce an undesirable behavior. Suppose the child finds the treatment trials aversive because either the target behaviors are too difficult or the reinforcers are not effective. The child then begins to look away from the treatment stimuli, and the clinician asks the child to sit in a corner for a few seconds. This is what the child wanted: relief from aversive treatment trials. After the TO period, the child returns to the boring treatment trials, but knows precisely what to do to escape. The child's inattentive behavior is thus negatively reinforced instead of being reduced by TO.

Second, TO may provide opportunities for positive reinforcement. For example, the child sitting in a corner may begin to scribble on the wall, play with a toy, or do other things that are more reinforcing than the treatment trials. Therefore, the child may seek TO by exhibiting the undesirable behavior with increasing frequency.

Effective Use of Time-Out.

To use TO effectively, the clinician must make sure that TO is not an opportunity for either negative or positive reinforcement. If it appears that the child is escaping from aversive treatment trials, the aversiveness must be reduced by simplifying the target behavior and a more effective reinforcer should be used. During the TO, the child should not have access to reinforcers. For instance, the child should not be sent to a place where play and other reinforcing activities are possible. The child should not be released from exclusion TO if undesirable behavior does not cease. As soon as it does, however, the child should be promptly released from TO. To control opportunities for reinforcement, the duration of TO should be brief. Less aversive nonexclusion TO should be preferred over exclusion TO. Invariably, a desirable behavior should be positively reinforced.

Response Cost

In **response cost**, reinforcers are withdrawn response contingently so that the rate of response decreases (Pazulinec, Meyerrose, & Sajwaj, 1983). Each incorrect response results in the loss of a reinforcer to which the person has access. In other words, each wrong response *costs* the client a reinforcer.

The distinction between TO and response cost is that opportunities to earn reinforcers are terminated in TO, whereas the client's reinforcers are taken away in response cost. In TO, the person may be removed from a reinforcing state of affairs or denied the opportunity to respond. In TO, a specific reinforcer is not taken away from the person in a response-contingent manner. In response cost, each response results in the loss of a reinforcer, but the person is neither removed from the scene nor prevented from responding. The difference between TO and response cost is similar to the difference between a prison term and legal fines. Whereas the prison term is similar to TO, the fines are similar to response cost. However, note that neither the prison term nor the fines may be effective because of a lack of response contingency.

Response cost is somewhat easy to use and is effective in controlling many forms of interfering and inappropriate behaviors in clinical, educational, and home settings. It is not as restrictive as some forms of TO, and may generate much less emotional resistance.

To use response cost, the client must have accumulated a certain number of reinforcers, or must have access to some reinforcers. Also, some reinforcers can be withdrawn, but others cannot be. For instance, the clinician can take away tokens, but cannot withdraw verbal praise. Many clinicians reinforce the correct production of target behaviors by giving points, stickers, stars, tokens, and edible items that the client can collect. When the client accumulates these reinforcers, the clinician can begin to use response cost. This may speed up the reduction of still-troublesome incorrect responses. Reinforcers earned for correct responses may be lost for incorrect ones. For example, a child may receive a token for every correct production of a phoneme, but lose one for every incorrect production. This procedure of losing only those reinforcers the client has earned is called the **earn-and-lose** variety of response cost.

In the other variety, the client does not earn reinforcers that are lost. In this **lose-only** type of response cost, the clinician gives the client a certain number of tokens at the beginning of the session. The clinician then takes them away as the client exhibits inappropriate behaviors. In the lose-only procedure, the tokens are given noncontingently, but are withdrawn response contingently.

In general or special classrooms, response cost can be used as a group contingency. In this procedure, the educator gives a certain number of points to an entire class. When any student exhibits an inappropriate behavior, the educator withdraws a point. Undesirable behaviors within groups are known to decrease under this arrangement.

Few studies have been reported on the effects of response cost in the treatment of communicative disorders. In one study, stuttering frequency decreased when subjects lost points on a counter every time they stuttered (Halvorson, 1971). In other treatment programs, persons who stutter may lose tokens for increased rate of speech, abrupt onset of phonation, inappropriate use of airflow, and other behaviors to be reduced.

Response cost may be readily applied to other communication disorders. For example, every incorrect production of a phoneme or a grammatic morpheme may result in the loss of a reinforcer. Clinicians may withdraw tokens contingent on pitch breaks, brief episodes of hoarseness or hypernasality, and other voice characteristics targeted for reduction. Similarly, every time a client exhibits an interfering or uncooperative behavior, the clinician can withdraw a reinforcer.

Ineffective Use of Response Cost.   When used inappropriately, response cost may be ineffective or may even increase the undesirable behavior. The clinician who promptly takes away a token from a child also pays attention to the undesirable response. This attention (a positive reinforcer) may increase the response rate. If this happens, the clinician should use some other method of response reduction.

Response cost may be ineffective when the clinician begins by taking more tokens per responses, and then takes fewer. If there is a change in the number of tokens taken away, it should be an increase, never a decrease. Also, when the clinician takes away multiple tokens, the client may run out of tokens. Some children react emotionally when tokens are withdrawn. Generally, this response subsides.

Effective Use of Response Cost.   To use the technique effectively, the clinician should generously reinforce the desirable target behaviors so that the client earns many tokens, ensuring that the client does not run out of tokens. To begin with, only one token should be taken away. If this does not work, two or more tokens may be withdrawn in an ascending series. But there should be no descending series. If the client's strong emotional responses to token loss persist, the clinician should discontinue the use of response cost and find another method of response reduction.

Distinctions Between Response Cost, Time-Out, and Extinction

Time-out and response cost must be distinguished from extinction. The three procedures share one common feature: Behaviors are reduced by manipulating reinforcement. The difference between extinction on the one hand and time-out and response cost on the other lies in how the manipulation is done. In extinction, the reinforcer is simply suspended; otherwise, the clinician does nothing specific each time the behavior occurs. The undesirable behavior runs its course and runs dry. In both time-out and response cost, however, the clinician does something each time the behavior occurs.

In time-out, a brief duration of no reinforcement is arranged after the response is made. The person exhibiting the undesirable behavior may be put into a less reinforcing situation. No action of this sort is taken in extinction. In response cost, a reinforcer to which the client has access is taken away. In time-out and extinction, reinforcers are terminated. In response cost, it is taken away from the person. In extinction and time-out, the person exhibiting an undesirable behavior sees a potential reinforcer suddenly suspended. In response cost, the person exhibiting a similar behavior loses what he or she was already given.

Imposition of Work

The final direct method of response reduction is imposition of work contingent on a behavior to be reduced. This method, called **overcorrection**, requires the person to eliminate the effects of misbehavior *and* practice its counterpart, an appropriate behavior (Foxx & Bechtel, 1983).

Overcorrection was originally developed for the treatment of mental patients and has been used mainly in institutional settings. The method has three components: (1) the person who misbehaves must eliminate the immediate effects of that behavior; (2) the person must vastly improve the environment; and (3) the person must practice an incompatible, appropriate behavior repeatedly without reinforcement. For example, a patient in a mental hospital who has kicked a bucket of water and made a mess is first asked to straighten up the bucket and mop the floor. Next, the patient is required to mop and polish the floor of the entire ward. Finally, the patient is asked to walk appropriately around the bucket several times (Matson & DiLorenzo, 1984).

The first two components are called **restitution**, and the last component is called **positive practice**. Restitution requires not only that the effects of misbehavior are corrected, but that the situation be improved beyond its original state. Positive practice may appear to be a method of encouraging alternative, desirable behaviors, but it still is a response reduction procedure because heavy work is made contingent upon misbehavior and there is no positive reinforcement.

Overcorrection has been used extensively in many settings to control a wide range of problem behaviors. In special educational settings, the technique is applicable in controlling disruptive and aggressive behaviors, and to encourage more appropriate social behaviors. A study by Barton and Osborne (1978) provided an interesting example of the positive practice component of the overcorrection method. The authors increased the verbal sharing behavior, which was defined as either a verbal request to share another child's toys or an invitation to share one's own toys, in five kindergarten-age children who were hard of hearing. In a play situation, any occurrence of nonsharing behavior led to a required positive practice of one of two roles: the initiator who invited another to share, and the acceptor who agreed to share. This type of positive practice led to decreases in the nonsharing behaviors, with concomitant increases in sharing behaviors.

Overcorrection has also been used in teaching correct spelling to children in elementary and junior high schools (Foxx & Jones, 1978). The children were required to correctly spell the misspelled words and to give a dictionary definition of those words in five sentences. Studies of this kind have shown that spelling errors can be decreased dramatically.

Overcorrection or its components have rarely been used in clinical speech–language work. A study by Matson, Esveldt-Dawson, and O'Donnell (1979) illustrated the potential of this technique in treating certain language disorders. When an elective mute boy was required to write the words he refused to speak 10 times each, his speaking behavior was reinstated. Children who exhibit unruly behaviors that disrupt and alter the classroom arrangement may be asked first to restore the original arrangement, and then to vastly improve it. A desirable behavior may be overpracticed.

Summary of Direct Methods of Response Reduction

In the direct methods of response reduction, a contingency that reduces the behavior is placed on an undesirable behavior. In these methods, the clinician focuses on the behavior to be reduced. The direct methods include extinction, stimulus presentation, reinforcement withdrawal, and imposition of work. In extinction, the reinforcer is withheld, and the response is allowed to occur until it is extinguished. In stimulus presentation, corrective feedback is given for inappropriate behaviors. The most frequently used feedback is verbal ("no," "wrong," etc.). Reinforcement withdrawal includes time-out and response cost. In time-out, a brief period of no reinforcement follows an inappropriate response; the person may also be removed from the reinforcing situation. In response cost, each undesirable response costs the person one or more reinforcers.

INDIRECT METHODS OF RESPONSE REDUCTION

In **indirect methods** of response reduction, the clinician places no contingencies on the behavior to be reduced. Instead, positive contingencies are placed on desirable behaviors. By increasing certain desirable behaviors, the clinician replaces undesirable behaviors. Because no aversive contingency is placed on the behavior to be reduced, indirect strategies are the least aversive of the behavior reduction strategies.

When a desirable behavior is reinforced, the undesirable behavior to be replaced is ignored. Therefore, in using indirect methods, the clinician uses a combination of extinction and positive reinforcement. This method of simultaneously increasing one behavior and decreasing another is called **differential reinforcement**.

Four differential reinforcement techniques have been extensively researched and found to be effective in replacing undesirable behaviors with desirable ones (Repp & Karsh, 1990; Rolider & Van Houten, 1990): (1) differential reinforcement of other behavior, (2) differential reinforcement of incompatible behavior, (3) differential reinforcement of alternative behavior, and (4) differential reinforcement of low rate of responding.

Differential Reinforcement of Other Behavior

Previously described as a *schedule* of reinforcement, differential reinforcement of other behavior (DRO) is one of the oldest reinforcement methods for replacing undesirable behaviors. Most reinforcement schedules specify which responses and how many of them will be reinforced, but the DRO schedule specifies which behavior will *not* be reinforced. This widely used technique has been effective in reducing a variety of undesirable behaviors in both clinical and educational settings (Carr, Robinson, Taylor, & Carlson, 1990; Rolider & Van Houten, 1990).

The behavior selected for nonreinforcement is the one to be reduced. In its place, the client may exhibit any of the many unspecified desirable behaviors to receive reinforcers. For instance, during treatment sessions, a young boy may persistently chew on his shirt collar. Under the DRO schedule, the clinician reinforces the child as long as the collar chewing behavior is not exhibited. Desirable behaviors to be reinforced are not specified, but they can include looking at pictures, sitting in a certain posture, and responding to the clinician's modeling. The essential feature of the schedule is that behaviors to be reinforced may be many, varied, and left unspecified, whereas the behavior that will not be reinforced is clearly specified.

Many clinicians probably routinely use the DRO schedule in controlling uncooperative behaviors by reinforcing a variety of cooperative behaviors. Possibly, the schedule is used most frequently with young children. Whenever the clinician tells the child, "If you *don't* do this, you will get this" (and follows through with expected results), the clinician is using the DRO schedule. A child may be given a token for not yawning during 10 training trials, or for not wiggling in the chair during the previous few minutes, or for not looking into the observational mirror while the clinician is trying to have the child's attention focused upon a stimulus picture. Because the client is reinforced for omitting a certain behavior, the procedure is sometimes called **omission training**. When a client omits a specified action and exhibits another, appropriate behavior, an undesirable behavior is replaced with a desirable one.

The method may be used in replacing disordered communicative behaviors with desirable behaviors. For example, in treating persons who stutter, the clinician may specify behaviors that are stutterings, and ask clients to talk without them. If no specific skills of fluency are targeted for reinforcement, the procedure would be DRO.

Similar strategies can be used in the treatment of other disorders. For example, in treating voice disorders, a client with an undesirable pitch may be reinforced as long as he or she does not exhibit *that* pitch level while saying words or sentences. Assuming that the new pitch is in the direction of the final target, the clinician may reinforce it because it is not the client's undesirable baseline pitch. In treating clients with articulation disorders, reinforcers may be given as long as the speech is free from misarticulated sounds.

In implementing the DRO schedule, one potential mistake is to inadvertently reinforce a different undesirable behavior the clinician has not specified. For example, an educator may reinforce a child for not walking around in the classroom for 10 minutes. But at the end of 10 minutes, when the reinforcer is to be given, the child may be hitting another child. In such cases, the reinforcer must be withheld and the second undesirable behavior should be added to the contingency (no walking around, no hitting).

Differential Reinforcement of Incompatible Behavior

Some behaviors are incompatible in that they cannot be produced simultaneously. When one behavior is produced, another, which is incompatible with it, is absent. For example, a child cannot simultaneously wiggle in a chair and sit quietly. A client is either looking at the clinician or looking elsewhere. Such incompatible behaviors provide an excellent opportunity to decrease undesirable behaviors. In using **differential reinforcement of incompatible behaviors (DRI)**, the clinician reinforces a desirable behavior that is not compatible with an undesirable behavior. As the desirable behavior increases, the incompatible undesirable behavior decreases (Carr, Robinson, Taylor, & Carlson, 1990; Repp & Karsh, 1990; Rolider & Van Houten, 1990).

The method of strengthening incompatible behaviors is most effective when a desirable behavior that is physically incompatible with the undesirable behavior is reinforced. Sitting in the chair and walking around the classroom are incompatible; the difference is not a matter of degree. When a person is sitting quietly, walking around simply does not exist. Therefore, DRI is most effective in controlling physical responses that involve disruptive hand and feet movements, off-seat behaviors, looking away from the treatment stimulus materials, and so forth. In a group treatment setting, children's physically aggressive behaviors may be effectively controlled with DRI. A child who hits another may be reinforced to draw, write, and hold the book and read. These actions are physically incompatible with hitting.

Most forms of disordered communication are not compatible with forms of appropriate communication. For example, fluency skills, including initiation of soft and gentle phonation after a slight exhalation and prolongation of vowels, are not compatible with abrupt phonatory onset and rapid, stuttered speech. Correct productions of phonemes are incompatible with incorrect productions. However, the difference between some of these correct and incorrect responses may be a matter of degree, not a total incompatibility as in purely physical responses. The manner of phonatory onset or phoneme production, for example, may be more or less acceptable. Still, when correct and incorrect responses are fully discriminated (further apart), they are incompatible. Therefore, in teaching appropriate communicative behaviors, DRI may be effective.

Differential Reinforcement of Alternative Behavior

One reason why children and adults exhibit undesirable behaviors is that they have not learned more useful and socially adaptive alternative behaviors.

When persons do not have more productive behaviors in their repertoire, they tend to produce less productive or even destructive behaviors. Following this logic, researchers have developed the method of **differential reinforcement of alternative behaviors (DRA)**. In this procedure, the clinician reinforces a behavior that is a personally and socially more desirable alternative to an undesirable behavior. In DRA, the clinician targets some specific alternative for reinforcement, whereas in DRO, any desirable behavior suffices, and in DRI, the behavior to be reinforced has to be incompatible with the behavior to be reduced. In DRA, the alternative behavior taught need not be incompatible with the undesirable behavior.

In regular and special classrooms in schools, DRA may be highly useful. A child may behave in an unruly and uncooperative fashion because of lack of social skills. A child who has not learned appropriate play activities may resort to violent or disruptive behaviors on playgrounds. Children who cannot read or write may disrupt other children who quietly read or write. Adolescents without socially acceptable leisure skills may resort to delinquent behaviors. In all these cases, teaching personally and socially useful behaviors tends to reduce the frequency of undesirable behaviors.

Several research studies have shown that developmentally disabled persons who do not have functional communicative skills may resort to unacceptable behaviors (Carr & Durand, 1985; Carr, Robinson, & Palumbo, 1990; Carr, Robinson, Taylor, & Carlson, 1990; Durand & Carr, 1991; Luiselli, 1990; Wacker et al., 1990). Suppose, for example, that in a special educational classroom, a child who lacks communicative skills is asked to assemble a puzzle. The child attempts to comply, but soon finds the task too difficult as none of the pieces seem to fit together. Unable to request help from the teacher, the child resorts to crying, fussing, or other disruptive or inappropriate behaviors. The teacher may interpret this to mean that the child does not want to assemble the puzzle. However, if the same child is taught to say "help me!" when faced with a difficult task, the inappropriate behaviors may not be exhibited.

Several studies have shown that either verbal or nonverbal means of communication, when taught to developmentally disabled persons, can reduce many forms of undesirable behaviors. Sometimes, this approach is also described as **functional equivalence training**. Functional equivalence means that behaviors that are reinforced in the same way or behaviors that have similar causes may be taught as alternatives. For example, the word *water* and the sign in the American Sign Language for the same word are topographically different, but functionally the same. They are produced for the same reason (thirst) and are reinforced by the same object (water). Similarly, a child's crying during treatment sessions may be functionally equivalent to saying to the clinician, "What you are asking me to do is very difficult for me." A nonverbal child's undifferentiated gestures may be reduced by teaching appropriate word responses because the gestures and the words are functionally equivalent alternatives.

Teaching functionally equivalent alternative behaviors is an excellent strategy of reducing undesirable behaviors. In using this method, the clinician must find out the reason for and the consequences that are sought by the undesirable behavior. Then, another behavior that may be produced for the same reason and that may give the client access to the same reinforcer as the undesirable behavior should be taught. For example, if a child in a group session leaves his or her seat to gain attention, the clinician should select a desirable behavior for the child, such as looking into picture books, and should pay much attention to the new target behavior.

A potential problem with DRA is that both the undesirable behavior and the newly acquired functionally equivalent behavior may be exhibited as long as the undesirable behavior is also periodically reinforced. For example, the teacher who finds out the child means "give me help" by his or her fussing behavior, may begin to offer help when the child fusses. This would maintain the unwanted behavior. Therefore, in using DRA, the clinician should stop reinforcing the problem behavior for which an alternative is taught.

Differential Reinforcement of Low Rates of Responding

Some clients exhibit undesirable behaviors at such high frequency that the best strategy might be to reduce their frequency in gradual steps, requiring further reductions in each new step. This method shapes a behavior down, which is the opposite of shaping a desirable behavior up from low frequency to high frequency. This method of gradually reducing the frequency of a problem behavior to a manageable level is called the **differential reinforcement of low rates of responding (DRL)** (Rolider & Van Houten, 1990; Singh et al., 1981).

In one variation of DRL, the clinician sets a criterion of the acceptable level of an unwanted behavior and reinforces the client for not exceeding that criterion. For example, a child who frequently asks inappropriate questions, such as "What is that?" or makes interrupting comments, such as "You know what?" may be reinforced only if the questions or comments are spaced by a fixed interval of time. The clinician might require a minimum interval of 5 minutes between responses. In another variation of DRL, the clinician might set a criterion of a certain number of questions and comments for the entire treatment session. For instance, the clinician might accept three comments or questions and reinforce the child for maintaining that number. In each variation, the acceptable amount of unwanted behavior is lowered in gradual steps.

How the person is reinforced in a DRL is also varied. The clinician may reinforce the client who meets the criterion, but not soon after an unwanted response is made. For instance, when the criterion is two inappropriate behaviors in an entire session, the clinician reinforces the client at the end of the session when the inappropriate behavior is *not* being exhibited. In another variation, the clinician may reinforce responses that fulfill the requirement of a fixed interval between them. In this variation, an unwanted response is reinforced because it was made an appropriate amount of time after the last response was made. It is probably better to avoid reinforcing the undesirable behavior in this manner. It may be better not to reinforce the client soon after an inappropriate response is made.

A potential problem with DRL is that it will reduce but not eliminate an undesirable behavior. However, when the behavior has been substantially reduced, some other procedure, perhaps DRO, may be applied to eliminate it.

Summary of Indirect Methods of Response Reduction

Indirect methods reduce problem behaviors by reinforcing desirable behaviors that replace undesirable behaviors or by reinforcing a reduced frequency of undesirable behaviors. In DRO, any desirable behavior is reinforced; none is specified ahead of time. In DRI, a behavior that is physically incompatible with the undesirable behavior is reinforced. In DRA, an alternative, appropriate behavior is reinforced; the behavior to be reinforced is specified ahead of time; and the alternative behavior often is produced for the same reason and seeks the same effect as the problem behavior. In DRL, a reduced frequency of a troublesome behavior is reinforced.

NEGATIVE SIDE EFFECTS OF AVERSIVE METHODS

The main effects of positive and aversive methods of treatment are, respectively, to increase and to decrease target behaviors. However, both positive and aversive procedures produce certain unplanned side effects. Some of these side effects are positive and others are negative. The clinician should know what side effects his or her procedures produce. The negative side effects should be minimized and positive side effects enhanced. Research has shown that aversive methods may produce one or more of the following negative side effects.

Emotional Reactions

Aversive methods can evoke strong emotional reactions. Most of the intense emotional responses have been noted with highly invasive procedures (electric shock and other stimuli high on aversiveness) used in animal research. However, any aversive stimulus can evoke such negative emotional responses as crying, whining, fear, and tantrum behaviors. Some children may cry when tokens are withdrawn. Occasionally, even a firm verbal "no" can evoke strong emotional reactions in some children.

In speech–language training, clinicians typically give corrective feedback by saying "no" or "wrong" when their clients produce incorrect responses. Studies have generally not reported strong emotional reactions to this type of corrective feedback. In fact, most clients expect the clinician to indicate in some way whether the response was correct. When the clinician fails to give corrective feedback, the client may hesitate because of a lack of specific feedback.

Initial strong emotional reactions to a verbal "no" or token loss may soon subside. But if they do not, the clinician should find another response reduction strategy that may not evoke emotional responses.

Aggression

Some laboratory evidence indicates that strong aversive methods evoke aggressive behaviors. Two types of aggressive behaviors have been described: elicited and operant (Azrin & Holz, 1966; Linscheid & Meinhold, 1990). **Elicited aggression** is directed against any person or object that happens to be around when an aversive stimulus is delivered. It is not directed against the person who delivers the stimulus; hence, it does not seek to eliminate the stimulus. In laboratory experiments, animals receiving shocks have fought with each other or attacked inanimate objects (Van Houten, 1983).

Operant aggression, on the other hand, is directed against the source of the aversive stimulus. Such aggressive acts could lead to a reduction in punishment. For example, children who have been punished may throw objects at parents, who may then stop punishment.

Laboratory research has also shown that aggressive acts are more common when an aversive stimulus is delivered randomly (not contingent on any particular response) and there is no escape or avoidance from the stimulus. When escape is possible, it is more likely than attack (Linscheid & Meinhold, 1990).

Few clinical studies have reported elicited aggression, but, anecdotally, a child may kick the furniture or stamp the feet when told "no." Also, a child, when punished during homework, may throw the pencil on the ground. Similarly, operant aggression also has been reported rarely, but may be observed occasionally. In some treatment sessions, retarded and autistic subjects have tried to bite or scratch therapists administering aversive stimulation (Newsom, Favell, & Rincover, 1983). An appropriately designed and managed response reduction program need not lead to aggressive behaviors, especially when the emphasis is on indirect procedures and positive reinforcement for desirable behaviors.

Escape and Avoidance

In everyday life, a common reaction to aversive stimuli is escape or avoidance. A child who runs away from abusive parents demonstrates escape, and a child who minimizes contact with punitive parents shows avoidance.

Aversive procedures may lead clients to drop out of treatment, in which case they cannot be helped. Both basic and applied research has shown that escape and avoidance behaviors are more likely when an alternative desirable behavior is not reinforced.

Paradoxical Effect

Throughout this chapter, I have noted that, in some cases, procedures known to decrease behaviors may actually increase them. When such a **paradoxical effect** is observed, the behavior reduction procedure used has either not worked or has provided unintended reinforcement for the behavior to be reduced (Azrin & Holz, 1966; Linscheid & Meinhold, 1990).

Several factors cause a paradoxical effect of response reduction procedures. First, very mildly aversive stimuli might reinforce a response. Mild but constant nagging and reprimands may facilitate responses, and mild electric shocks can increase responses. Second, correlated administration of aversive and reinforcing stimuli might increase the response rate. If the delivery of an aversive stimulus is often followed by positive reinforcement, then the aversive stimulus becomes a discriminative stimulus for reinforcement. The result might be a paradoxical increase in response. Third, if the response to be reduced is based on fear or anxiety, the aversive stimulus might reinstate that emotional response, leading to response facilitation. For example, a child's crying behavior might increase under a known response reduction procedure. Fourth, the aversive stimulus may lead to successful escape from the aversive environment. In TO, for example, a child may be sent to his or her room for a specified misbehavior, but this may be reinforcing in the sense that the child escapes the aversive situation, and enters a less aversive personal room. Time-out, in such cases, might increase the response upon which it was made contingent. Fifth, a unique conditioning history of the individual receiving the aversive stimulus may be responsible for the increased response rate. For example, a study showed that children who come from aggressive families are more likely to show increased aggressive behaviors when punished (G. R. Patterson, 1976).

Applied studies have shown that electric shock, TO, overcorrection, and verbal reprimands can increase response rates in some situations. When this happens, the contingency is classified as reinforcing, and the reasons for such paradoxical effects are analyzed. Typically, these reasons are positive reinforcers that become associated with punishment.

Contrast Effect

Contrast effect is another phenomenon of response increase rather than decrease, but it happens when the aversive stimulus is absent. In the paradoxical effect, responses increase even when the aversive stimulus is made contingent on that response. In the contrast effect, however, responses may decrease as long as the aversive stimulus is being presented, but may increase either in the same situation or in a different situation *as long as the aversive stimulus is not being presented.* Suppose that the father of a teenage boy does not allow his son to play music loudly. The boy then does not play music loudly in his father's presence, but as soon as the father leaves home, he blasts his stereo.

Contrast effect has been unequivocally demonstrated in laboratory research. In applied human research, a few studies have indicated that it may occur in some cases. For example, Merbaum (1973) found that self-injurious behaviors decreased when a response reduction procedure was applied in school, but increased when applied at home. The contrast effect has not been systematically studied in the treatment of communicative disorders.

Response Substitution

Sometimes, when one undesirable behavior is decreased, another undesirable behavior may increase. In this case, one response is **substituted** for another. A reduced undesirable response may have been successful in gaining certain reinforcers from others. It is possible that the same reinforcer can be obtained by another undesirable response, which may then increase. For example, an autistic child may have received staff attention by indulging in head banging behavior. When this behavior is reduced by extinction (withdrawal of attention), the child may resort to scratching his or her face to regain attention.

Response substitution has been frequently observed in autistic or profoundly retarded persons with many self-stimulatory or self-injurious behaviors. Although there have been no systematic studies, speech–language clinicians might notice response substitution when certain interfering behaviors are reduced. For example, when a child's excessive hand movements are reduced, disruptive leg movements might increase.

The newly emerged (substituted) undesirable behavior may be reduced similarly to any other undesirable behavior. Extinction, TO, response cost, or one of the differential reinforcement procedures may be useful techniques.

Generalized Suppression

Just as the effect of a reinforcer can spread to other stimulus conditions or responses, the effects of an aversive stimulus can also spread to other situations, persons, or responses. In effect, aversive conditioning may also show stimulus and response generalization. Although stimulus or response generalization of aversive procedures is desirable, as discussed in a later section, generalized suppression is undesirable for two main reasons. First, an aversive procedure that reduces an undesirable behavior may also suppress desirable behaviors. For instance, a child whose hitting behavior has been reduced may not touch other children at all. Second, an aversive procedure intended to reduce a behavior only in one situation may reduce it in all situations. For example, a child who has been told not to talk in church may refuse to talk after returning home.

Fortunately, generalized suppressive effects rarely occur and, when they do, are temporary. Undesirable suppression is more likely when desirable alternative behaviors are not reinforced (Newsom et al., 1983). Like the effect of reinforcement, the effect of aversive procedure has been slow to generalize to untreated settings and responses.

Imitation of Aversive Control

Those who frequently use aversive methods of controlling behaviors set an example, especially for young children. The children, in turn, may be more likely to use aversive means (including aggression) to control other people. These children may not learn positive means. This possibility has been discussed in relation to abusive parents who, as children, may have been excessively punished. There is no strong evidence to support this hypothesis, but it cannot be ruled out.

Research on social learning theory has demonstrated that children do learn aggressive behaviors merely by watching models who exhibit aggression.

In addition, specific aversive procedures may be acquired by children exposed to such procedures. A study by Gelfand and coworkers (1974) showed that children exposed to response cost were likely to use the same procedure with other children.

Imitation of aversive control used in treating communicative disorders has not been studied. It is possible that when the least aversive methods are used and the emphasis is on teaching desirable behaviors through positive reinforcement, imitation of aversive control would not be a problem.

Perpetuation of Aversive Methods

A final concern with the use of aversive methods is that they may perpetuate themselves. Aversive methods affect those who receive as well as those who administer them. A person uses a response reduction procedure precisely because a behavior is aversive to him or her. When a response reduction procedure is successful, an aversive behavior has been terminated. Therefore, the person who used the response reduction procedure is negatively reinforced. The person who has such a history of negative reinforcement may be more likely to use aversive rather than positive reinforcement procedures in controlling other individuals' aversive behaviors.

Perpetuation of aversive methods is socially undesirable. The perpetuation of aversive methods may be checked by making positive reinforcement the predominant method of treatment.

The additional negative effects of aversive procedures described thus far have not posed insurmountable problems in clinical situations. There is much information on the prudent use of response reduction methods, which can minimize chances of undesirable additional effects. In a later section, the most appropriate ways of using response reduction procedures are summarized.

POSITIVE SIDE EFFECTS OF AVERSIVE METHODS

Response reduction procedures may also produce positive (desirable) side effects. There are at least five positive side effects of aversive methods: appropriate generalization, improved social behaviors, positive emotional responding, better attending behaviors, and facilitation of learning (Linscheid & Meinhold, 1990; Newsom et al., 1983).

Appropriate Generalization

Because individual behaviors are members of larger response classes, the elimination or reduction of a single response may affect other responses of the same class. Also, a response reduced in the presence of some stimuli may be automatically reduced in the presence of similar stimuli. When such generalization occurs, reduction of some behaviors leads to reduction of other behaviors without further intervention. Also, undesirable behaviors reduced in the clinical setting may be reduced in nonclinical settings as well.

A certain degree of stimulus and response generalization does take place. However, appropriate generalization does not take place as often as one would wish. As noted earlier, the effects of response reduction procedures are more often discriminated than generalized. However, there are procedures to enhance appropriate generalization. When response reduction procedures are used in different situations and by different clinicians while making an adequate sampling of undesirable behaviors, appropriate generalization may be promoted.

Improved Social Behaviors

When a client's aggressive, uncooperative, and unsociable behaviors are reduced, there may be an increase in socially acceptable behaviors that were not reinforced. Several studies have shown that either during or following aversive treatment, clients become socially more responsive. In clients who are schizophrenic, autistic, and developmentally disabled, reduction of undesirable behaviors has resulted in more cooperation, greater sociability, better interaction with peers and clinical staff, and generally improved behaviors (Newsom et al., 1984).

When not spending much time exhibiting nonproductive behaviors, clients may engage in more productive behaviors that are naturally reinforcing. However, these productive behaviors may be maintained only if they are reinforced.

Improved Emotional Behaviors

An improvement in emotional responding has been reported as a positive side effect of aversive treatment. Again, most of the studies have been done with autistic children whose self-stimulatory or self-injurious behaviors were reduced. As a result, the children have been reported to smile and laugh more often, and to cry and whine less frequently.

Attending Behaviors

Most children who indulge in self-stimulatory and self-injurious behaviors pay little attention to their surroundings. People and events fail to draw their attention. Therefore, it is difficult to teach them adaptive behaviors or academic skills. Some studies have shown that when self-stimulatory and self-injurious behaviors were reduced, the children's attending behaviors and eye contact improved. Subsequent to response reduction, some children began to pay more attention to surrounding events, people, teaching targets, and academic skills training (Newsom et al., 1983).

Facilitation of Learning

Possibly, improved attending behaviors may lead to better learning of specific tasks. Following response reduction, autistic children were better able to imitate various target behaviors. In one study, when an autistic child's oppositional behavior was punished, his speech imitation increased 100% (Newsom et al., 1983). Possibly, suppression of undesirable behaviors removes barriers to learning more appropriate behaviors.

IMPLEMENTING A LEAST AVERSIVE RESPONSE REDUCTION STRATEGY

Most response reduction procedures, as noted earlier, are aversive to the client and the clinician. It is much more pleasant to be able to use only positive reinforcement procedures. When carefully planned and implemented, however, response reduction strategies reduce undesirable behaviors, avoid negative side effects, and enhance positive side effects. Because response reduction procedures are combined with positive reinforcers for desirable behaviors, the overall effectiveness of the treatment program is enhanced as well.

In designing and implementing a response reduction strategy, the clinician should use a hierarchy of options. The first option is to determine whether aversive procedures may be totally avoided; the second option is to use the least aversive methods for as brief a period as necessary; and the third option is to add additional aversive procedures only when necessary. Meanwhile, the clinician must constantly reevaluate the treatment targets and procedures to make sure they are appropriate and effective. Often, the need for using aversive methods is a strong indication that the treatment targets may be inappropriate, the treatment procedures ineffective, or both.

The following suggestions on designing and implementing the least aversive response reduction procedures reflect this hierarchy of options.

Behaviors to Be Reduced Should Be Defined in Operational Terms.

Globally and vaguely defined behaviors are difficult to decrease (or increase). Therefore, the clinician should specify the undesirable behavior in clear, observable terms. For instance, a clinician cannot directly measure or reduce "articulatory incompetence," "language deficiency," "stuttering moments," and "poor voice characteristics." Instead, the clinician should specify what sounds are misarticulated, what language features are misused, and what specific behaviors suggest stuttering or poor voice characteristics.

Behaviors to Be Increased Should Be Defined in Operational Terms.

Response reduction methods should not be used unless there is a clearly defined positive target behavior that will be differentially reinforced. Therefore, the clinician should clearly define the target behaviors that will replace or compete with the undesirable behavior to be reduced.

A Response Reduction Procedure Should Never Be Used Exclusively.

Simply saying "no" to a wrong response when not shaping and reinforcing the correct response is both ineffective and unethical. It has often been said that, although punishment indicates that a behavior is bad, it does not teach a good behavior. Therefore, the clinician should always keep his or her focus on teaching desirable behaviors through positive methods.

If Possible, Undesirable Responses Should Be Prevented.

When undesirable responses are prevented, aversive methods are not needed. If desirable behaviors are shaped in small and carefully planned steps, the undesirable responses may not occur or may occur at such low frequency that they are not a problem. For example, the clinician might shape the correct production of a phoneme in graduated steps instead of simply asking the child to produce it correctly and saying "no" when the child cannot do it. Instead of asking a language delayed child to point to a picture and punishing him or her for not pointing to the correct picture, the clinician might take the child's hand and point to the correct picture and then slowly fade the manual assistance. Prompting a correct response when the client hesitates is also a good strategy of averting a wrong response (hence the aversive stimulus delivery).

An Alternative Behavior that Will Serve the Same Function as the Behavior to Be Reduced Must Be Reinforced (DRA).

An alternative behavior selected for

reinforcement should serve the same function as the behavior to be reduced. For instance, if the undesirable behavior seeks attention, the alternative behavior should be reinforced with attention. To the client, the new, desirable behavior should provide the same advantage the undesirable behavior did. Recall that teaching functional communicative behaviors is often effective in reducing undesirable behaviors in nonverbal or minimally verbal clients.

An Incompatible, Desirable Behavior Should Be Differentially Reinforced (DRI). The clinician must select a desirable behavior that cannot be produced along with the undesirable behavior to be reduced. This desirable behavior then should be systematically reinforced so that it replaces the undesirable behavior.

Any Other Desirable Behavior Should Be Reinforced (DRO). As long as the person omits the undesirable behavior, any of several unspecified desirable behaviors may be reinforced.

A Reduced Rate of Undesirable Behavior May Be Reinforced (DRL). The clinician reinforces the client for exhibiting the undesirable behavior at a lower rate than found in baselines. This method progressively reduces the undesirable behavior.

A High-Probability Undesirable Behavior May Be Used to Reinforce the Low-Probability Desirable Behaviors. Instead of trying to suppress an undesirable behavior, it may be used to reinforce desirable behaviors (Charlop, Kurtz, & Casey, 1990). For example, a child may repeatedly grab the clinician's paper to scribble or draw something. If the clinician were to let the child earn an opportunity to draw on paper by producing a certain number of correct responses, the frequency of desirable behaviors may increase while the interfering paper grabbing behavior may decrease.

Behavioral Momentum May Be Effective. Behavioral momentum is the force of a readily exhibited behavior that promotes the production of an unlikely behavior (Mace et al., 1988). Many children who do not pay attention to the stimulus items or perform required tasks readily perform other tasks that are not treatment targets. For example, a boy who refuses to open his mouth to produce a vowel sound may readily stand up or sit down when asked to. In this case, the clinician may ask the child to stand up and sit down a few times in rapid succession and then suddenly ask the child to open the mouth. The behavior momentum of sitting down and standing up may lead to a sudden production of the target response (mouth opening). In this way, the behavioral momentum decreases the noncompliant behavior.

Treatment Aversiveness Should Be Reduced. For some clients, especially for young children, treatment may be an aversive experience. Treatment may be aversive because, among other reasons, (1) the selected stimuli may lack variety or interest for the child; (2) the selected target behavior may be too difficult for the child; (3) the selected consequences for the target behaviors may not be functioning as reinforcers; (4) the therapy may be scheduled at the end of the day when the child is too tired; (5) the child may be suffering from such chronic conditions as severe allergy; or (6) the therapy may be stagnated at a low and boring level so that there is no movement to varied tasks of increased complexity. Treatment aversiveness may be strong enough for the client that he or she will resort to undesirable behaviors to terminate it. Therefore, the clinician must carefully evaluate the target behaviors and treatment procedures to reduce treatment aversiveness.

In treatment sessions, the clinician should count the number of times positive reinforcers and aversive consequences were delivered to a client. The ratio should always be in favor of reinforcement. There is something wrong with the treatment procedure if the client receives more aversive stimuli than positive reinforcers. Shaping the target behaviors and using functional reinforcers might be helpful.

A Surprising Stimulus May Be Effective in Preventing an Undesirable Response. A suddenly presented stimulus that is unusual, dramatic, and surprising may prevent an undesirable response (Charlop, Burgio, Iwata, & Ivancic, 1988). For example, when the child is about to leave the chair, the clinician may suddenly pull a clown from a bag. This unexpected stimulus may evoke a response of surprise from the child, thus suppressing the imminent off-seat behavior. Loud sounds, colorful pictures, something pulled out of a closet or cupboard, and other surprising stimuli may be effective.

The sudden stimulus presentation should be made before the undesirable behavior is underway. When it looks as though the child is about to cry, leave the chair, or exhibit some undesirable behavior, the clinician should present the surprising stimulus. The clinician who presents a surprising stimulus after the behavior is produced might reinforce that behavior.

Among the Direct Methods, the First Choice Is Extinction Combined With Positive Reinforcement. In this combination, the clinician simply withdraws reinforcers from the behavior to be reduced and heavily reinforces desirable behaviors. In using extinction, the clinician does nothing when an undesirable behavior is produced.

A Continuous Schedule Must Be Used. To make the response reduction contingency effective, it should be applied each time the undesirable behavior is produced. For instance, every instance of off-seat behavior should result in a token loss or time-out.

The Reaction to an Undesirable Behavior Should Be Immediate.
The contingency that reduces an undesirable behavior should be applied immediately. Delayed response weakens the effect. When a wrong response is observed, some clinicians hesitate in saying "no" or "stop." This hesitation and delay in delivering the stimulus is undesirable. Token withdrawal and time-out also should be immediate.

The Clinician Should React to the Earliest Element of a Chain of Response.
Most responses are chains of several different responses. Suppose that a child sitting in a living room decides to swim at the family swimming pool at an inappropriate time. Announcing his or her plan of action, the child might leave the living room, walk toward the bedroom, grab the swimsuit, begin to undress, change into the swimsuit, leave the bedroom, walk toward the patio door, open it, walk toward the swimming pool, and prepare to jump into the pool. This demonstrates that what is normally considered a single integrated act of "going to swim" is actually a chain of responses. Each response in the chain takes the child closer to the terminal response of swimming (which can also be broken down into its component parts). A parent wishing to stop this behavior can intervene at various stages in the sequence. The parent may say "no swimming" as soon as the plan of action was announced, or just before the child is ready to jump into the pool, or anytime in between. The most effective time to say "no" is when the child talks about swimming and begins to leave the living room. Saying "no" immediately before the child is about to jump into the pool is the least effective.

In treatment sessions, it is important that the clinician recognize the sequence of responses that make up a chain of target behaviors so that the first element of the chain can be stopped. In treating a /w/ for /r/ substitution, for example, the clinician may either say "stop" after the child has produced the wrong word "wadio" or say the word as soon as the child begins to round his or her lips for the production of the initial /w/ sound. It is more effective to stop the child as soon as the clinician sees some sign of lip rounding.

In treating stuttering, it is more effective to say "no" or "stop" as soon as the clinician hears the initial repetition of the sound rather than to wait until the person has completed the stuttered word, phrase, or sentence. At times, the client may be stopped even before the stuttered word becomes audible. In some cases, certain articulatory postures or muscular tension precedes the stuttered production of a word. The clinician should stop the client the instant a sign of an abnormal posture or tension is observed.

Chances for Escape Should Be Reduced or Eliminated. When a response is being reduced, as far as possible, there should be no possibility of escape. Under TO, for example, a crying child should not be able to leave the therapy room and go to a parent. When verbal "no" is made contingent on wrong responses, the child should not have a chance to crawl under the table or leave the therapy setting.

Before the clinician resorts to physical means of preventing escape, he or she should reassess the treatment procedure. If the undesirable behavior is due to aversive treatment, the clinician's first responsibility is to reduce this aversiveness.

Reinforcers Should Not Immediately Follow Aversive Stimuli. Aversive stimuli and reinforcing stimuli should not be delivered in close temporal proximity. A clinician who says "no" and immediately smiles and touches the child is committing this mistake. A parent who punishes a child might feel guilty, and immediately hug the child or give something special. In such cases, aversive stimuli lead to positive reinforcers; therefore, aversive stimuli become discriminative stimuli for undesirable responses. Because aversive stimuli in these cases signal reinforcers, a strategy that typically reduces behaviors might increase them. When reinforcement does not follow aversive stimuli, those stimuli will become discriminative of extinction (lack of reinforcement). In essence, aversive stimuli should also be discriminative stimuli for extinction, not for reinforcement.

Reinforcers for Undesirable Behaviors Should Be Eliminated. This is not the same as the discriminative value of aversive stimuli just described. As noted, aversive stimuli become discriminative of reinforcement when reinforcers immediately follow them. However, an undesirable response may be directly reinforced in one situation while it is reduced in other situations and perhaps by other persons. In such cases, response reduction procedures may not be successful.

A response is more easily reduced when extinction (no reinforcement) is combined with another response reduction method. For example, the clinician might use TO or response cost to reduce gestures in a nonverbal child, while reinforcing more appropriate verbal responses. However, if those gestures continue to be reinforced at home and at other places, TO or response cost may be ineffective. Clinicians also might reinforce faulty articulations or stutterings while talking with the client after the session has ended. At home, one parent may reinforce an undesirable behavior while the other tries to reduce it. Such reinforcers must be eliminated or minimized. In the treatment settings, the clinician must insist upon the production of target behaviors from the beginning to the end of interactions, not only during the actual therapy time.

Response Reducing Consequences Must Be Varied. The clinician should not continue to use only one kind of consequence throughout a session. Varied consequences, including different kinds of corrective verbal feedback, TO, response cost, and other procedures, should be used to prevent potential adaptation to the aversive stimulus.

SUMMARY

An important task of the clinician is to decrease certain undesirable behaviors exhibited by clients. Most methods available to reduce behaviors are more or less aversive to the client and even for the clinician. In recent years, less aversive methods of reducing behaviors have been developed.

It is important to assess the maintaining causes of undesirable behaviors before they are treated. Undesirable behaviors may be maintained by positive, negative, or automatic reinforcement.

Behavior reduction procedures may be direct or indirect. In direct methods, a contingency is placed on the behavior to be reduced. In indirect methods, no contingency is placed on the undesirable behavior; instead, a desirable behavior is increased, which has an indirect effect of decreasing the undesirable behavior.

Four direct response reduction methods were described: extinction, stimulus presentation, stimulus withdrawal, and imposition of work. In extinguishing the positively reinforced behaviors, the clinician withdraws reinforcers. Following a possible initial increase, the response rate eventually decreases. In extinguishing negatively reinforced behaviors, the clinician prevents escape. In extinguishing automatically reinforced behaviors, sensory consequences of those behaviors are reduced or eliminated. Extinction must be combined with positive reinforcement for desirable behaviors.

A response that has been reinforced intermittently, with large amounts of reinforcement, over a long period of time, and with no prior history of extinction, is the most difficult to extinguish. Extinction should not be used to reduce aggressive, self-destructive, or highly disruptive behaviors.

Both stimulus presentation and stimulus withdrawal procedures are described as punishment procedures. Technically, punishment is to reduce behaviors by either stimulus presentation or stimulus withdrawal. Because this technical meaning is often confused with the everyday use of "punishment," this term is not preferred in this book.

Corrective feedback is a direct method of reducing responses. Corrective feedback suggests the acceptability of a response. This type of feedback may be verbal, nonverbal, or mechanical.

Withdrawal of the reinforcing stimulus is another direct method of response reduction. A reinforcing stimulus or event is withdrawn immediately after a wrong response is made. Time-out and response cost are the two varieties of stimulus withdrawal. In time-out, a period of nonreinforcement is imposed on an undesirable behavior, which then decreases. In response cost, a tangible reinforcer is withdrawn response contingently. As a result, that response decreases.

Imposition of effort or work contingent on an undesirable behavior is another direct method of response reduction. In overcorrection, a variation of this procedure, a misbehaving person is required to eliminate the effects of misbehavior and practice its counterpart, an appropriate behavior.

Indirect methods of response reduction include the differential reinforcement of other behavior (DRO), the differential reinforcement of incompatible behavior (DRI), the differential reinforcement of alternative behavior (DRA), and the differential reinforcement of low rates of responding (DRL). In the first three, an increase in a desirable behavior indirectly reduces an undesirable behavior; in DRL, a decreased rate of the undesirable behavior is reinforced.

Aversive response reduction methods may have certain undesirable side effects. These include emotional reactions, aggression, escape and avoidance, paradoxical effects, contrast effects, response substitution, generalized suppression, imitation of aversive control, and perpetuation of aversive methods.

Aversive methods also may produce desirable side effects, which include appropriate generalization, improved social behaviors, improved emotional behaviors, attending behaviors, and facilitation of learning.

A carefully planned and implemented program of response reduction strategy is least aversive. In such a strategy, (1) behaviors to be reduced are defined operationally; (2) behaviors to be increased are defined operationally; (3) a response reduction strategy is not used exclusively; (4) if possible, undesirable responses are prevented; (5) an alternative, functionally equivalent behavior is reinforced (DRA); (6) an incompatible, desirable behavior is reinforced (DRI); (7) any other desirable behavior is reinforced (DRO); (8) a reduced rate of the undesirable behavior is reinforced; (9) a high-probability interfering behavior may be used to reinforce the low-probability desirable behavior; (10) behavioral momentum is used; (11) treatment aversiveness is reduced; (12) a surprising stimulus may be presented to prevent an undesirable response; (13) extinction is used; (14) the response reduction contingency is used on a continuous schedule; (15) the reaction to undesirable behavior is immediate; (16) the reaction is to the earliest element of the undesirable behavior; (17) chances of escape are reduced or eliminated; (18) reinforcers do not follow aversive stimuli; (19) reinforcers for undesirable behaviors are eliminated; and (20) varied response reduction strategies are used.

STUDY GUIDE

Answer the following questions in technical language. Check your answers with the text. Rewrite your answers when needed.

1. Describe some undesirable and interfering behaviors of clients.

2. Distinguish between inappropriate and interfering behaviors.

3. Distinguish between aversive and nonaversive events.

4. Define a functional analysis baseline.

5. How are undesirable behaviors reinforced?

6. Give an example of negatively reinforced undesirable behavior.

7. What is automatic reinforcement?

8. What are direct methods of response reduction?

9. Define extinction and give an example.

10. What is an extinction burst?

11. What are the four factors that affect extinction?

12. What is the best way of extinguishing a response? What other contingency would you combine with extinction and how?

13. How is a negatively reinforced behavior extinguished?

14. What are the limitations of extinction?

15. What kinds of behaviors would not be suitable for extinction?

16. Define punishment. Why is this term not preferred in this book?

17. What is corrective feedback? What are its varieties?

18. What are the two varieties of stimulus (reinforcement) withdrawal?

19. Define time-out. What are its varieties?

20. Describe the effective and ineffective uses of time-out.

21. Define response cost and distinguish it from time-out.

22. When is it not possible to use response cost?

23. Describe the effective and ineffective ways of using response cost.

24. Define DRO and give an example. Does it decrease behaviors directly or indirectly?

25. What is DRI? How does it help reduce a behavior?

26. Define DRA and describe how it might be used in reducing behaviors.

27. What is DRL? How is it used? Does it eliminate an undesirable behavior?

28. List, define, and describe all kinds of undesirable effects of punishment that were discussed in the text. Give your own examples.

29. What are the two kinds of aggression described under undesirable side effects of punishment?

30. What are paradoxical effects of aversive stimuli?

31. What is contrast effect?

32. What is imitation of aversive control?

33. How are aversive methods perpetuated?

34. Are there many studies documenting undesirable side effects of punishment in communicative disorders?

35. List, define, and describe all kinds of desirable side effects of aversive methods. Give examples from your own experience.

36. In implementing a least aversive method of response reduction, what steps should be taken?

37. Are response reduction procedures used exclusively? Why or why not?

38. How should an undesirable behavior be prevented?

39. How is a high-probability behavior used to reinforce a low-probability undesirable behavior?

40. What is behavioral momentum? How is it used?

41. What is a potential effect on aversiveness of treatment? How should it be handled?

42. When should a surprising stimulus be presented? Before or after an undesirable behavior?

43. Are aversive stimuli presented continuously or on an intermittent schedule?

44. Should a reinforcer immediately follow an aversive stimulus? Why or why not?

45. Should a single aversive stimulus or a variety be used?

9

Working with Families and Other Persons

- Counseling: Varied concepts and methods
- Outcome-oriented work with families and others
- Peer training
- Working with teachers
- Family members as therapists
- Strategies of working with families and others

Speech–language pathologists receive little professional training in working with family members, peers, friends, colleagues, teachers, employers, and others who are significant in the life of their clients. The need to counsel parents and others and to work with families and others during treatment is widely recognized, but practical training is typically missing. Students are taught mainly how to interview clients to gather information during assessment and provide information after it. Also, there is little controlled research on working with families and others concerned with disordered communication.

Recent emphasis on early assessment of and intervention with infants and toddlers has begun to change this. Professional work with this population invariably requires intensive and sustained work with families. Applied behavior analysts have done significant work in training parents and professionals in managing behavior problems, educational difficulties, deficiencies in self-help skills, and similar problems. Therefore, until a research data base is developed on working with parents and others concerned with communicative disorders, much of what can be said is based on clinical experience and extrapolation from other research fields.

COUNSELING: VARIED CONCEPTS AND METHODS

Counseling and psychotherapy are specialized fields concerned with helping people who have various kinds of emotional, personal, occupational, educational, and social problems. Both medical and nonmedical professionals specialize in counseling and psychotherapy. Among others, psychoanalysts, psychiatrists, clinical psychologists, psychotherapists, personal counselors, family therapists, marriage counselors, social workers, and rehabilitation counselors work with people who have personal problems. Of these specialists, psychoanalysts and psychiatrists are medical professionals who, in addition to psychological methods, may use medical means to control emotional and interpersonal problems. Other professionals rely exclusively on psychological or behavioral means of helping their clients.

A major method used by most counselors and therapists is conversation. They converse with their clients about the problems that need to be solved or reduced. They try to determine what the problem is, what can be done about it, and what may be expected. Both the problems and the solutions are often analyzed at the verbal level. Therapists give information that might help the client take beneficial courses of action. They help the client find solutions through discussion, evaluation, and judgment. The emphasis is on new and more useful or adaptive skills and behaviors, rather than on eliminating some undesirable behaviors. Typically, however, little is done to teach those skills or behaviors. It is expected that the client who realizes what to do to solve or reduce his or her problems will take the necessary steps.

Speech–language pathologists and audiologists also counsel their clients. Both assessment and treatment involve counseling to some extent. All clinicians counsel their clients to provide information about and offer explanations of speech and hearing problems and clinical services. For instance, a clinician who makes an assessment of a client's communicative disorder counsels the client about the assessment results, recommended services, and possible expectations from the services. An audiologist similarly counsels the client after an audiological assessment. Before treatment is started, clinicians counsel their clients about procedures to be used, rationale for using them, and expected results. The client and family members may be counseled on a home treatment program or a maintenance program.

Clinicians may use counseling as the only method of treating a client or in conjunction with other methods. For instance, counseling may be the selected treatment for persons who stutter. The goals of this counseling may be to reduce negative emotions or attitudes, establish realistic expectations of fluency, boost self-confidence, reduce anxiety about speaking situations, and so forth. Similarly, voice clients may be counseled about the damaging effects of vocally abusive behaviors. The clients may be counseled to reduce or eliminate such vocally abusive behaviors as excessive talking, constant throat clearing, or smoking. In such cases, the clinician uses counseling as a treatment procedure or as the only procedure.

Little research has been reported to indicate that merely counseling clients will eliminate or reduce communicative problems. For example, counseling about the effects of vocally abusive behaviors is rarely sufficient to eliminate those behaviors. Stuttering persons who are counseled about their emotional and attitudinal problems may not become fluent speakers. Therefore, clinicians who use counseling usually use it in conjunction with other methods, especially those that rely on teaching certain skills or changing certain behaviors.

It is not my purpose to describe various counseling theories and methods used by counselors, psychologists, and specialists in communicative disorders. Rather, I point out a special kind of work that needs to be done with families and others. This type of work is an extension of treatment from the clinical setting to home and other settings, and is consistent with the philosophy and technology of treatment described in this book.

OUTCOME-ORIENTED WORK WITH FAMILIES AND OTHERS

Clients and their families should be fully informed about the nature of the communicative disorders, the assessment and treatment procedures, alternative services that are available, services offered by other professionals, and so forth. Therefore, all clinicians counsel their clients to offer information of this sort. This type of counseling is not controversial.

Counseling may be controversial when it is used as the method of changing behaviors or teaching new skills. Unless there is controlled and convincing evidence that counseling reduces or eliminates communicative disorders or other behaviors that result in such disorders, counseling may not be used as a method of treatment. For instance, unless research has shown that counseling can reduce or eliminate stuttering or vocally abusive behaviors, there is no justification for using it as a method of treatment.

It is not sufficient to counsel clients only to keep them fully informed about clinical services. Clinicians also should work with clients, their families, and other persons to achieve certain results that often are not achieved by solely working with clients in controlled treatment rooms. This work should have measurable behavioral objectives. An important objective is to effect specific changes in the patterns of interactions involving the client and his or her family, friends, teachers, colleagues, and other persons. However, the methods used to achieve such changes are similar to those used in the treatment room. Therefore, this type of work with families and others associated with clients is different from traditional counseling and psychotherapy.

In Chapter 1, treatment was defined as a rearrangement of communicative relations between a client and his or her typical audience. This definition emphasizes the need to work with people who normally interact with the client. When working closely with these people, clinicians may find that treating communicative disorders takes much more than merely working with clients in a small treatment room. In fact, much work must be done outside the confines of the ubiquitous clinic room.

Working with families and others has two major objectives: training them to teach communicative behaviors and training them to maintain behaviors taught by the clinician. Both are measurable outcomes of working with families and others. In most cases, the clinician establishes the target behaviors. Therefore, family members, peers, and others need not work intensively to establish nonexistent communicative behaviors. Most clients, however, need help beyond the clinic to maintain their newly acquired behaviors. Thus, clinicians must abandon the traditional method of working only with clients and sending at best a progress report home. Because most problems of maintenance are due to a failure in getting significant others involved in treatment, training families and others to maintain behaviors should be implemented in most cases.

In this text, for the sake of brevity, when discussing work with people associated with the client, I use the term *families and others.* The term is used in a generic sense and includes all persons in the client's life. In the case of children, babysitters, day care staff, siblings, school teachers, grandparents, and other caregivers are all potential target people to work with. Friends and playmates of children, often referred to as peers, are an especially important group to train. In the case of adults, spouses, relatives, friends, and colleagues are important. In essence, all those who spend a significant amount of time with the client are potential target persons for training.

Among the many persons with whom the clinician could work, peers, teachers, and family members are the most important. Therefore, the discussion focuses on these three groups. The guidelines on training or working with these groups are generally applicable to other groups, as well.

PEER TRAINING

It is well known that peers strongly influence each other. Sometimes, a child's or an adolescent's behavior may be changed with the help of a peer more efficiently than without such help. Therefore, in teaching communicative behaviors to young clients, clinicians have sought the help of peers.

Because communication is a social activity, children who have communicative problems also have difficulty in social interactions. They often experience social isolation because of their difficulty in communicating with peers. Also, children who have problems communicating need an audience who is especially trained. Peers are the most frequent audience for young speakers. Unless their peers know how to support the communicative attempts that may often be deficient, children with disabilities may give up their attempts. Therefore, successful treatment involves a rearrangement of social roles played by speakers and listeners. Peers, being partners in this activity, also may be effective partners in the treatment process (Paul, 1985).

Although more research is needed, several studies have shown that peers may be effectively trained to play a significant role in supporting communicative behaviors. Peers may be trained to play two kinds of roles: to help establish target communicative behaviors, and to support and maintain communicative behaviors taught by clinicians. In both cases, peers learn a few crucial clinical skills that help establish and maintain target behaviors.

In teaching peers to establish communicative behaviors, the clinician should train them to (1) evoke and model speech and other communicative target behaviors, (2) reinforce the production of communicative behaviors in their peers, and (3) generally provide opportunities for their peers to communicate (Paul, 1985).

In peer training, the peer is the trainee. The child with a communicative disorder who receives treatment is the target child. The clinician teaches both, but the trainee and the target child learn different skills. The trainee learns how to teach communicative behaviors, and the target child learns how to communicate. The clinician shapes the behavior of the trainee, and teaches new communicative skills to the target child through the peer.

In social settings, peers are taught to provide stimuli for speech. They are taught to ask questions and use toys and other naturalistic stimuli to evoke speech. When the target child does not readily respond, the peers are taught to model the target behaviors and prompt their occurrence. The peers selected for such training may have normal communicative skills. These peers are trained to evoke, model, and reinforce communicative behaviors in target children with speech–language problems. This strategy is useful when communicatively handicapped children are mainstreamed. Several research studies have documented the effectiveness of normally speaking peers in teaching language skills to children (Goldstein & Ferrell, 1987; Goldstein & Wickstrom, 1986).

The peers selected for training also may have communicative problems similar to those of the target children under intervention. In this case, the peer needs more advanced communicative skills than the target child. For instance, peers who are developmentally disabled may be trained to model communicative behaviors. Target children, also developmentally disabled, who watch their peers model specific responses may learn them (Goldstein & Mousetis, 1989).

In training peers to help maintain behaviors taught by the clinician, the same procedures as those used to teach the client the target behaviors may be used. The peer training in this case may be less intense than the training needed to establish the behaviors in the first place. Because the target child will already have learned the behaviors, the peer's task will be to evoke or prompt the behaviors and provide appropriate feedback.

The interactions that help teach or sustain communicative behaviors are more naturalistic and more reinforcing to target children. In addition to teaching or maintaining communicative behaviors, peer training also may promote social development in children. The peers who interact with each other are likely to spend more time together, which may lead to the development of additional social skills. Also, the language skills learned through peer or clinician teaching may be expanded further.

WORKING WITH TEACHERS

Historically, specialists in communicative disorders who worked in public schools typically provided services to their students either in small groups or in special classrooms. In recent years, speech–language pathologists, educational audiologists, and educators of the hearing impaired have found that the traditional clinical or special educational activity is limited in effectiveness.

Speech and language skills that promote social communication are essential academic skills. Communicative skills established in restrictive clinical or special classroom settings may not generalize to other settings, including the regular classrooms. Also, to educate children with disabilities in the least restrictive environment, the emphasis in recent years has been on mainstreaming them.

Most children who receive speech and language treatment from itinerant speech–language clinicians are students in regular classrooms. These clinicians work with children twice weekly in small groups. Because of the limited treatment time and high caseload, public school clinicians usually have limited time to work with individual children.

The public school clinician often finds that the communicative skills taught to children are not produced reliably in the regular classroom settings where those skills are most needed. This problem of generalization and maintenance is faced by clinicians in all settings. The limited time that the clinicians have to spend with children makes it especially difficult to implement extensive maintenance programs. In many cases, limited time and high caseload make it difficult to establish all the target behaviors the children need to learn.

A potential solution to these problems is to train regular classroom teachers, other special education specialists, and teacher aids to (1) help maintain clinically taught communicative behaviors in the classrooms and (2) to teach certain communicative skills that may be integrated with academic skills. The methods of training academic personnel are not essentially different from those of training parents and peers. However, a few special considerations apply to the educational setting.

Well-trained educational personnel (regular classroom teachers, special education teachers, and teacher aids) can play an important role in maintaining clinically established communicative behaviors. For instance, in the case of a child who stutters, the teacher might be asked to give a clinically established signal, such as a hand movement, to prompt the child to speak slowly or use other fluency skills. The teacher, after asking a question, might immediately verbally prompt the child to "use the technique." This might increase the chances that the child will use the fluency skills in the classroom. The teacher might also be asked to praise the child for producing fluent utterances, and to stop the child when he or she speaks dysfluently, speaks at a faster rate, or does not manage the airflow properly. The teacher may be asked to provide speaking opportunities for that child so that fluency may be reinforced in the classroom.

Educational personnel also can help a great deal in prompting and promoting maintenance of appropriate voice characteristics in a child receiving voice therapy. The teacher or the aid may be asked to frequently prompt the production of voice with expected characteristics, such as louder, softer, or clearer voice. The teacher might be asked to reinforce the child for producing vocal qualities that are being strengthened by the clinician. The clinician treating a child with hoarseness might ask the teacher to praise the child for talking less or talking softly. Supervisors of playgrounds or cafeterias may be asked to monitor the child's vocal behaviors to control excessive and extremely loud talking.

Educational personnel can play an even more important role in strengthening, expanding, and sustaining oral or sign language skills taught by speech–language pathologists or educators of the deaf. Because these skills are crucial for academic success, language skills taught by the clinicians should be integrated with academic work. If this is done, the clinically established language behaviors may be not only maintained, but also expanded.

When the clinician's time is extremely limited, teachers may be trained to teach certain language structures to children who are language impaired (Campbell, Stremel-Campbell, & Rogers-Warren, 1985; Dyer, Williams, & Luce, 1991; Peck, Killen, & Baumgart, 1989). In this case, the teachers act as primary therapists. The target behaviors selected for the teacher to train should be of immediate academic significance. Therefore, the teachers must play a major role in selecting these target behaviors that are most important for academic success. In consultation with the speech–language pathologist or the educator of the deaf, the teacher must identify communicative skills that must be taught in the classroom and integrated into academic work.

Both the teachers and the specialists in communicative disorders must set aside additional time for training. The teacher training may be accomplished only after the clinician has spent some time analyzing the classroom routines, the typical academic skills required of clients served, the general classroom setting, and the teacher's disposition to getting trained. The resources the teacher has, including aids that might assist in the communication training or maintenance activities, also must be determined.

Initially, the teachers should be given an in-service training session in which general information on communicative disorders and their remediation is offered and discussed. Specific assessment and treatment procedures and the need for maintenance work in the classroom and other school settings should be discussed. Once the teachers and the clinicians agree on the general course of action and mutual support, formal training of teachers involving specific children should be attempted.

In teaching speech and language skills, the clinician and the teacher together should develop an Individualized Education Plan (IEP) for each child. The clinician and the teacher should select client-specific, academically useful, and socially relevant target behaviors for children under consideration. The teacher should agree that the skills taught are important and are easily integrated into academic activities. Some research suggests that having the teachers and other staff participate in the selection of treatment targets and the general treatment strategy is effective (Peck et al., 1989).

The teachers should be asked to suggest ways of teaching or facilitating the target behaviors in the classrooms. How these behaviors must be integrated into academic work should also be the teacher's decision. The clinician may offer suggestions to improve the strategy suggested by the teacher.

The teacher then should observe the clinician as he or she teaches specific target behaviors to selected children. If time is a problem, the teacher may directly observe the clinician for brief periods of time and then watch videotaped treatment sessions in full. The clinician should clearly define for the teacher the target behaviors and show how the consequences must be programmed. Suggestions on using stimulus materials, including modeling, prompting, and manual guidance, should be offered. The teacher should also know how the target behavior productions are documented. The teacher must use the more naturalistic training methods that create opportunities to use speech and language skills in the classroom.

The teacher should then conduct brief treatment sessions in the presence of the clinician, who will give feedback on the teacher's performance. The teacher should be able to use the evoking, modeling, and reinforcing procedures. The teacher also should be able to record the occurrences of target behaviors on recording sheets. When the teacher becomes proficient in the selected treatment procedure, he or she may be encouraged to use it in the regular classroom and other situations.

The clinician should periodically observe the teacher's work to monitor the progress and the accuracy with which the teacher implements the program. Teacher's recording sheets, audiotape recordings, or videotapes may be used to evaluate the teacher's work.

Whether they train the target behaviors or help maintain clinically established behaviors, teachers are an indispensable resource for the public school clinician. Enlisting their cooperation is a significant part of the school clinician's job.

FAMILY MEMBERS AS THERAPISTS

Most parents whose children receive speech and language treatment should be trained to support and maintain clinically established behaviors. However, some parents may have to be trained to be their children's primary therapists. The methods of promoting maintenance were described in Chapter 7. Therefore, in this chapter, the emphasis is on training family members and others to establish behaviors. It was also pointed out in Chapter 7 that methods of maintaining behaviors are no different from establishing them. Therefore, those who learn to establish behaviors will be better able to maintain them.

Families in many rural areas may not have access to speech, language, hearing, and aural rehabilitation services. Such families may be able to make only periodic visits to a distant clinic. This schedule will not permit the clinician to implement a regular treatment program. As an alternative to professionally implemented treatment, the clinician may develop a home treatment program to be implemented by parents.

In a home treatment program, parents act as therapists. They hold formal, regular treatment sessions at home. Although similar methods are used, there is a difference between home treatment sessions held by parents and others and sessions held to promote maintenance of clinically established behaviors. Under a maintenance program, parents and others help sustain behaviors the clinician establishes. Under a home treatment program, parents and others establish target behaviors and then take steps to sustain them. Therefore, parents and others who implement a home treatment program are the primary therapists.

Home treatment programs are useful when intensive early intervention is needed. For instance, infants, toddlers, and children who are language delayed, hearing impaired, mentally retarded, neurologically handicapped, and autistic need early and prolonged intervention. Depending on the degree of impairment, these children may need daily work on communicative skills. In such cases, training parents to act as therapists at home may be the only or the most effective alternative.

In other cases, home treatment may be adjunct to professional treatment. Clients who need intensive and prolonged treatment may receive professional treatment once or twice a week and more frequent treatment at home. In such cases, home treatment supplements and parallels professional treatment. Families who conduct supplemental home treatment may frequently consult with the professional so that the clinician can provide immediate and consistent feedback to the family members on their performance. The family members may also observe the professional treatment, which helps ensure that they augment what the clinician does. Therefore, adjunct family treatment may be more effective than stand-alone family treatment.

Another class of clients, adults included, may need home treatment. Some families travel to out-of-state clinics to consult with speech–language pathologists who offer unique treatment programs. After the client has received treatment for a short duration, the significant others may continue treatment at home. To do this, they need to be trained in the implementation of the treatment procedure.

Several controlled research studies have shown that parent training can be effective in promoting language behaviors in children. In addition, behavioral research has shown that developmentally disabled mothers may be taught various parenting skills, including language stimulation in their children. For instance, developmentally disabled (mentally retarded) mothers were taught to express greater physical affection to their children, imitate their children's vocalizations, and praise their children for producing target behaviors. The results were that when the mothers learned these skills, the children's vocalizations increased (Feldman, Case, Rincover, Towns, & Betel, 1989; Feldman et al., 1986).

Parents of autistic children may also be trained to enhance language in their children by evoking, modeling, and reinforcing target responses in naturalistic play situations (Laski, Charlop, & Schreibman, 1988). Parents (and their children) may be initially trained in the clinic. Subsequently, the training sessions may be held at home. Such parent training tends to enhance generalization and maintenance of target communicative behaviors because the child learns those behaviors in the natural setting where it is expected to be maintained.

General Guidelines on Developing Home Treatment Programs

In training the parents to implement treatment programs at home, the clinician should take several steps. First, the clinician should thoroughly evaluate the client's communicative behaviors. In assessing infants and young children, the clinician must evaluate their general development, as well as associated disabilities, including mental retardation, hearing impairment, genetic syndromes, and other conditions that might predispose them to later speech–language problems.

Early speech–language behaviors, including babbling, cooing, and single-word utterances, should be assessed. If the client is multiply handicapped, most likely a team of specialists will evaluate all aspects of development and functioning. A psychologist, for example, may evaluate the client's intellectual status, motor development, attention to environmental stimuli, and social responsiveness. Medical specialists may evaluate physical and neurological functioning. An audiologist may assess hearing. The team's findings and recommendations will determine the nature of home intervention.

Second, the speech–language pathologist should treat the client during a trial period to develop a program the parents might implement at home. Because treatment procedures may be client specific, a period of trial treatment is necessary to make sure that the recommended treatment will be effective. Parents should never be asked to implement a program that has not been tried with their child. All home treatment programs must be client specific, tested, and found to be effective.

Third, the clinician should train the parents and other family members in the implementation of the home treatment program. The clinician should use the trial treatment to train parents in recognizing target behaviors, treatment techniques, and record-keeping procedures. The parents should be trained to model, prompt, and reinforce target behaviors. They also should be trained in stopping the undesirable behaviors at the earliest possible time.

To begin with, the parents should watch the clinician implement the treatment procedure for their child. Later, the parents should implement the procedures while the clinician watches them. Whereas treatment involves modification of client behaviors, parent training involves modification of parent behaviors. The parents who thus acquire new skills will, in turn, modify their child's behavior.

A significant part of parent training is to teach them the methods of record keeping. The parents should record target behavior productions and their use of the techniques. The clinician should give them prepared forms on which to record the frequency of target behaviors produced at home and in other natural settings. The parents may be asked to audio record or, if practical, video record sample sessions. The parents should submit all forms of recorded information to the clinician.

After the parents are trained in the implementation of a home treatment program that works, they should receive a written description of the program. If practical, some key features of the program may be videotaped and given to the parents. For instance, in treating stuttering children, the clinician may videotape the use of airflow, prolonged speech, and other target behaviors. How to reinforce and sustain these behaviors also may be demonstrated on the tape. As time passes, parents and other family members may forget specific aspects of treatment programs; therefore, it is useful to have a visual record of the program for them to periodically review to make sure that they follow the clinician's procedure.

Fourth, the clinician and the parents should stay in touch during the period of home treatment implementation. The clinician should evaluate the effectiveness of home treatment programs by examining data supplied by parents on how the procedure is implemented at home and on how the client is progressing. If practical, the clinician may periodically visit the home and observe the parent's implementation of the program. A more practical method of monitoring the parents' work is to make frequent phone calls and exchange written information.

In many cases, it may be necessary to retrain the parents after a period of trial treatment at home. Also, brief retraining sessions may be needed when the client is ready to move on to a more complex level of training.

The clinician should schedule periodic assessment of the child at his or her office. If the home treatment data and the clinic assessment data indicate that the client is not making satisfactory progress, professional treatment at a clinical facility must be recommended.

A more detailed discussion of development of home treatment programs is outside the scope of this chapter. Before training family members and others to implement a home treatment program, the clinician should refer to other sources devoted to this topic (Girolametto, 1988; McCormick & Schiefelbusch, 1990; McDonald & Gillette, 1986; Odom & Karnes, 1988; Rossetti, 1986, 1990).

STRATEGIES OF WORKING WITH FAMILIES AND OTHERS

Training families and others either to be the primary therapists or to implement maintenance procedures poses many challenges, some of which are discussed below. Because implementation of clinical programs in homes requires rearranging the lives of many persons, it is a difficult enterprise. It also is difficult because most specialists in communicative disorders have not done anything like what it requires to implement such programs. There are frequent unexpected problems that require a change in strategy. The following sections highlight a few major problems and offer some suggestions for handling them.

Scheduling Problems

Scheduling is a major problem in working with families and others. In some clinical settings, it is relatively easy to schedule persons associated with clients for observation of treatment sessions and for training them in methods of response maintenance. For instance, clinicians working in university speech–hearing clinics, private clinics, and hospitals are better able to establish frequent contacts with families and others than clinicians working in public schools. It is easy to schedule parents for maintenance work when they bring children for clinical services. Spouses, siblings, parents, or grandparents are likely to accompany clients who attend university and private clinics. In public schools, children who receive services for communicative disorders are at the school for the day. Therefore, it is more difficult to have family members attend treatment sessions held in public schools because they are not accompanying the child to an established appointment.

The public school clinician will have to send frequent reminders to family members to attend training sessions. In progress reports sent home, the clinician should emphasize that the treatment is not complete without parent training and that the responses the child has learned may not be maintained unless the family members work with the child at home. It must be made clear to family members that if they do not receive training in response maintenance, the child's dismissal from treatment will be premature regardless of how long the clinician continues treatment. Whether continued treatment of a child may be made contingent on family participation is a question that the school districts may eventually have to consider.

In all settings, the family members should be scheduled initially for observation of treatment sessions. They should be scheduled to observe entire sessions, not only portions of them. Eventually, the family members should be scheduled for training sessions in which they learn to recognize, reinforce, and record the production of target behaviors at home and in other nonclinical settings.

Emotional Involvement of Parents

A significant problem in training parents to manage their children's communicative behaviors at home is their emotional involvement. Each family member will have developed some unique reactions to the client's communicative problem. Most reactions are likely to be colored emotionally, and most need to be changed.

The clinician should encourage family members to prompt the correct behavior or stop the incorrect behavior in its earliest stage. The family members who do this may not appreciate the tone in which this must be done. Many tend to react emotionally when the client produces incorrect responses. Instead of giving a subtle hint to stop the behavior or saying the word "stop" in a neutral tone, they may give an emotional and even angry lecture. Instead of simply saying "slow down" in a friendly and nonpunitive tone, the parent may shout, "Pay attention to your speech now! You are going at a hundred miles an hour!"

That the clinician asks the family members to be especially discrete in front of others may have no initial effect. In front of guests, the mother may tell her stuttering son, "Did you forget what your therapist told you? Talk slowly, for God's sake!" Then, she may turn toward her astonished or embarrassed guests and say, "If he slows his speech, he has no trouble at all!" The humiliated son may ask his mother to keep quiet the next time he stutters in front of others.

Many parents and siblings find it difficult to give objective, prompt, and subtle signals. Some think that they must make the message clear via an emotionally laden, punitive, and boisterous response to the client. Others continue to respond the way they have, only more frequently because the clinician has given them some responsibility. Instead of prompting the correct response when an incorrect response is imminent, they make negative or hurtful comments after the incorrect response has been made. The family members may save their verbal praise for correct behavior for another time, or, when they do express praise, it may be half-hearted.

Some clients who receive such reactions from their family members may report them to the clinician. Others may not. It is the clinician's job to ensure that the responses of the family are appropriate. The clinician should periodically check how the client is taking the family's attempts at monitoring target behaviors. The clinician should ask for tape-recorded evidence of response monitoring at home. Whenever opportunities arise, the clinician should carefully observe how the family members and the client react to each other. The clinician should talk to family members when it is evident that their reactions may have been inappropriate. Again, the clinician should illustrate how not to prompt, reduce, or increase behaviors. Objective response monitoring should be modeled for them.

A parent who is a speech–language pathologist may paradoxically find it especially difficult to teach or monitor his or her child's troubled communicative behaviors. There is little research on how speech–language pathologists handle communicative disorders in their children, but limited experience with such parents suggests that their professional training may or may not help in dealing with the problems. Most do not wish to treat their children; it is probably better that they do not. Sometimes, a professional parent's emotional responses to the child's speech or language problem may be stronger than those of persons without training in speech–language pathology. More systematic information is needed on this group of parents.

The Client's Acceptance of the Family's Newfound Role

If the family members have difficulty changing their long-standing reactions to the client's speech, the client also may have difficulty accepting the family members' new role as therapists. Although very few will admit it, most clients are reluctant to accept the role of the therapist from his or her family. Even very young children may object to their mothers telling them what to do, as I once found out. As instructed, a mother asked her 3-year-old son who stuttered to slow down his speech at home. The boy promptly told her, "You are not Dr. Hegde."

Teenagers are especially reluctant to accept prompts and signals from family members, and some adults resent their spouses' new therapeutic role. When the wife reminds her stuttering husband to slow down his speech, he may say "Okay, okay," but not change his rate at all. Most clients wish that treatment could be limited entirely to the clinician's office. When clinicians suggest to clients that their friends, bosses, colleagues, and family members should get involved, some clients are dismayed that the experts cannot do it alone.

In working with clients and their families, the clinician must be convincing and persuasive. While being sympathetic to their initial reluctance, the clinician should also be persistent. To a parent who typically drops off a child and disappears until the end of the treatment session, the clinician should say, "I want you to join us today so you know what we are doing." Sometimes the clinician should be firm and allow little choice; at other times, family members' willingness to participate may have to be won over a few sessions of discussion and persuasion. A few parents find it emotionally difficult to watch treatment involving their loved one. These parents find it hard to participate in treatment.

The clinician should explain to the client the importance of the family's role in helping response learning or maintenance at home. The client's unwillingness to involve friends or colleagues must be discussed. The client should understand that friends and colleagues are usually happy to help. The clinician may give examples of reluctant clients who eventually brought their friends and family into treatment sessions and felt pleased about the results. The clinician should bring up the topic often, discuss it briefly, and thus let the client know that he or she is serious about it.

Dealing with Excuses

When the clinician requests taped conversations from home, evidence of response monitoring, and records of brief and informal therapy conducted at home, some clients and families may give endless excuses for not bringing the records. In such cases, it is likely that not only the audiotape is missing. Probably, response monitoring at home has also been missing. Parents or clients who complete their assignments at home are usually eager to bring evidence. They often borrow a tape recorder if they do not have one. Generally, those who do not bring the records have done nothing worth reporting.

The clinician should not accept excuses. Politely, the clinician should suggest a firm solution to a seeming hurdle for holding a 10-minute conversation to monitor the client's target behaviors. If the family has no tape recorder, the clinician should loan one right away; if this is not possible, the family members may be asked to borrow one from a friend or colleague. If the family claims to be too busy, the clinician should talk about the family's daily schedule for the next few days and gently but firmly select a time slot before the next session and suggest that they tape the speech then. If possible, the clinician may call the family a day or two before the next session to remind them to bring the recorded tape.

Some family members produce results only when the clinician gives them a form to complete. For example, if the clinician wants parents to chart episodes of loud talk their child exhibits at home, a recording sheet with dates and observational time slots already typed on it may prompt them to make observations and record the results.

If a client says he or she could not reach the colleague who is expected to observe treatment, the clinician should ask for the person's phone number. The clinician should offer to call the person and request help. If the client's excuse is, "I have no objection to bringing my boss, but I don't think she will like it," then the clinician should offer to discuss the matter with the boss. The clinician should take the responsibility to contact other persons once the client agrees to their involvement but does not follow through. Under no circumstance, however, should a clinician discuss a client's problem with someone without the client's approval. Doing so is unethical because it violates client confidentiality.

If possible, the clinician should visit the client's home and demonstrate what the family members need to do. The clinician should hold informal training sessions to show how to monitor the target behaviors in the family room and at the dining table. This often helps both the reluctant parties—the family and the client.

Talking with Families and Others

Working with the significant others involves more than teaching them to evoke and consequate target behaviors. In addition to dealing with the problems described thus far, the clinician should answer the questions the family members have about the client's communicative disorder and what they should do about it. The family members are likely to ask questions such as the following: What caused the disorder? How should we react to the client? What should we do and not do? What personal, educational, and occupational problems might the client face? How can we help solve those problems? What is the treatment, and how long is it going to last? How can we find resources to pay for treatment? In answering these and other questions, the clinician should know what to say and how to say it.

Whether at the initial interview when the case history is taken or during the several subsequent conversations held with the family and the client, the clinician should be able to talk to them on any issue or question that affects clinical services offered to the client. The following sections give some guidelines on what the clinician can say to the clients and their families and how to say it.

Give Accurate Information

The clinician is likely to have answers to many commonly asked questions. Occasionally, however, the clinician may not have an answer to an unusual or complex question. When not sure of an answer, the clinician should simply say so and state that he or she will find an answer to the question.

The clinician should never give inaccurate information. It is unethical to bluff with jargon and smoke people out with incomprehensible technicalities. Often asked questions include: What caused the problem? Why does my son stutter? Why can't this child of mine speak when I have two others who talk fine? Why can't my child make an *es*? To answer these questions, the clinician needs scientific information; however, the scientific information may not support a clear-cut answer that points out a cause in a given case.

The clinician can tell the client and family that it is difficult to say what caused the disorder in a particular client. The knowledge of disorders applies to groups of people, not to individuals. For example, there are many potential causes of cleft palate, language delay in children, stuttering, and other problems, but determining the exact cause in a given client is not easy. In talking with stuttering adults and their families, the clinician may say, "We know many potential causes of stuttering. For example, genetic predisposition, environmental stress, faulty learning or conditioning, instability in the nervous system, and many other factors can contribute to the development of stuttering. Typically, several such factors come together to produce stuttering in an individual. Some or all of these factors may have contributed to stuttering in your case. Other, unknown factors also may have contributed. It is difficult to pinpoint causes in individual cases." The clinician then can point out that stuttering is treatable, even though the specific cause cannot be determined. A similar answer is appropriate for many disorders of communication. Although the cause of an articulation disorder or delayed language may be unknown, a clinician can remediate the problem. For most people, this reassurance is more important than some speculative causation of a disorder.

The clinician may be tempted to say that certain conditions associated with a communicative disorder are the causes of those disorders. The clinician should avoid this temptation. Even if a child is retarded and has a language delay, has cerebral palsy and is communicatively handicapped, or has autism and speech–language problems, the clinician should not reinforce the popular notion that mental retardation, cerebral palsy, or autism is the cause of the communicative disorders. Those conditions and communicative disorders coexist. It is difficult to establish a cause–effect relation among factors or events that cannot be separated.

Talk in Probabilistic Terms

The clinician should answer parents' questions about treatment in probabilistic terms, and avoid definitive terms. The clinician should use conditional answers for questions relative to treatment outcome; rate of progress; eventual maintenance; educational, occupational, and personal consequences of the communicative disorder; and the effects of treatment on some of these consequences.

The outcome of treatment depends on many factors, most of which are not under the clinician's control. These factors include the client's motivation, punctuality, and uninterrupted attendance at treatment sessions; cooperation of family members; the client's rate of learning; and the presence or absence of other complicating or handicapping conditions. Therefore, the clinician should tell clients and their families that the outcome depends on many factors, and should describe some of these factors. The clinician might say what most clients are likely to achieve with a specified treatment program, not what the particular client shall attain. It should be noted that the Code of Ethics of the American Speech–Language–Hearing Association (ASHA Council on Professional Ethics, 1991) prohibits the clinician from guaranteeing treatment outcome.

Talk in Simple Terms

The clinician should use simple words and everyday examples. When technical terms are necessary, their meaning should be explained in everyday language. The following are some examples:

For statements like these	*Use statements like these*
• I will teach a few phonemes to your child.	• I will teach a few speech sounds to your child.
• I will teach some language structures and grammatical morphemes.	• I will teach words such as *in, on,* and *under.* They are called prepositions.
• I will try to enhance your child's linguistic competence.	• I will teach words and sentences.
• Your son can't close his velopharyngeal port.	• Your child has trouble shutting off the nasal passage at the back of his throat.
• Your child has syllable interjections.	• Your child says "um" a lot.
• Your dysfluency rate is high.	• You repeat words, repeat parts of words, and prolong sounds. We call these behaviors dysfluencies (or stutterings).
• Please reinforce your daughter at home for her target behaviors.	• Praise your daughter when she says the *es* sound correctly.

For each of the examples given, the clinician may have to give further explanations and additional examples.

Although simple and accurate explanations are fine, misleading oversimplifications of complex matters are not. If simplicity or accuracy has to be sacrificed, it should be simplicity. However, the clinician should realize that an inability to simplify something often is due to limited information. When the clinician knows more about a phenomenon, he or she can simplify and still be accurate.

Do Not Talk Down

Although it is good to avoid the use of jargon and complex language, it is not good to talk down to clients and their families. From the case history and the initial conversation with the client and family, the clinician can judge their educational level and general sophistication. Based on this judgment, the clinician should tailor his or her language to suit the listeners.

The type and the level of education of clients and their families may create an exception to the general rule that the clinician should avoid technical terms and talk in simple language. For instance, if the father of a language delayed child is an English teacher or linguistics professor, the clinician need not struggle to explain prepositions or other linguistic aspects of language in everyday language. If the mother of a child with velopharyngeal insufficiency is a physician, it is appropriate to use technical terms.

In conclusion, much research needs to be done on the development and effectiveness of home treatment programs. Families and others vary widely in how fast and efficiently they can learn to teach and monitor communicative behaviors. Research should identify the most effective and economical ways of training family members. Research also should find methods of documenting the precision with which parents implement treatment programs at home. How to document the client's progress or lack of progress in a home treatment program is also a matter for further research.

SUMMARY

Counseling and psychotherapy are specialized fields concerned with helping people who have emotional, personal, occupational, and social problems. Many different professions are involved in counseling and psychotherapy. Specialists in communicative disorders also counsel their clients.

In providing services, all speech–language pathologists and audiologists give information to clients and families about assessment results, available treatment programs, expected outcome, and the role of the family. This is counseling.

Counseling also may be used as a method of changing behaviors or solving problems. A counselor or psychotherapist does this in dealing with emotional and social problems. However, in communicative disorders, there is not much research supporting the exclusive use of counseling as a method of treating speech, language, voice, fluency, and hearing problems.

The clinician should counsel clients and families about available services and their effects. The clinician's work with families and others should have measurable outcomes.

Clinicians working in public schools should train teachers to support and sustain clinically established behaviors in their classrooms. Teachers also may be trained to help establish communicative behaviors, especially language skills.

Research has shown that peers may be trained to evoke, model, and reinforce various kinds of communicative and other behaviors. Peer training may be used either to establish the target behaviors or to maintain target behaviors taught by the clinician. Parents also may be trained to establish target behaviors, to maintain already established behaviors, or both.

Home treatment programs should be attempted only after the clinician has treated a client during a trial period to make sure that the recommended procedure works. During this treatment, the parents are trained in the implementation of the procedure. The clinician should consistently monitor parents' work at home. If the home program is not successful, the client should receive professional training.

A strategy of working with families and others should overcome several problems. First, the clinician should offer a flexible schedule to meet and work with families and others. Second, the clinician should consider the emotional involvement of parents and others, and train them in giving objective and subtle prompts, hints, and response consequences that might evoke and sustain responses. Third, the client may not accept the family's role of home therapists. This needs work with both clients and their families. Fourth, the clinician will have to find effective ways of dealing with excuses. Fifth, the clinician should give accurate information, talk in probabilistic terms, use simple terms, but should not talk down.

STUDY GUIDE

1. Define counseling and psychotherapy.

2. List the various professionals who counsel people.

3. What is a major method of counseling people?

4. Distinguish between giving information and using counseling as a means of changing behaviors.

5. Can counseling, used exclusively, teach new communicative behaviors?

6. What is outcome-oriented work with families and others?

7. Are treatment methods useful in working with families and others? Why or why not?

8. Who needs home treatment programs?

9. What are the two major objectives in training others?

10. Point out the importance of training teachers.

11. What kinds of training can the teachers receive from the clinician?

12. Can teachers help establish target communicative behaviors?

13. Describe how a teacher can work with a child who stutters to help maintain fluency.

14. What kinds of language targets should the teacher be encouraged to select for training?

15. How does a clinician monitor a teacher's work in establishing language skills?

16. Why is it good to train peers?

17. Why should a clinician evaluate a trial treatment before recommending it to the family?

18. When should a clinician recommend professional help for a client who has been receiving home treatment?

19. What major problems must be considered in working with families and others?

20. Describe how parents' emotional involvement may be a problem in working with them. How can these problems be overcome?

21. What steps can a clinician take to convince the client to accept help from family members?

22. How can a clinician deal with excuses given by family members and others for not following through with suggestions?

23. What guidelines should the clinician follow in talking with families and others?

24. What is meant by "talk in probabilistic terms"?

25. Distinguish between "talk in simple terms" and "do not talk down."

26. To whom can the clinician talk in technical language?

10

Treatment Program II: How to Write, Modify, and Implement Programs

- How to write treatment programs

- An outline of a general treatment program

- How to modify treatment programs

- Sequences of training

- Concluding remarks

In Chapter 5, a basic treatment program was described. In the subsequent chapters, other aspects of the program were described. The techniques described to this point should make it possible for a clinician to establish certain target behaviors and get them generalized to and maintained in everyday situations. In this final chapter, some advanced features of the program are described. Also, the information presented in all the previous chapters is integrated into a single treatment perspective. The main focus of this chapter is on writing comprehensive treatment programs for individual clients. The related issue of how to modify a written program in light of clinical data is described, as well as follow-up and booster treatment procedures.

HOW TO WRITE TREATMENT PROGRAMS

Careful planning is necessary before treatment can be started. There are two approaches to treatment planning: writing lesson plans and preparing a comprehensive treatment program. The more traditional approach involves writing **lesson plans** that briefly describe short-term treatment objectives and procedures. The plans are at best sketchy, only hinting at what may be done during the current week or two weeks. Often, they merely list activities for single sessions. Not being comprehensive, lesson plans do not provide a total picture of the treatment planned for the client. Often, the clinician who writes lesson plans may not have a long-range plan or perspective. This piecemeal approach to treatment planning is not a desirable strategy.

An alternative to writing lesson plans is to prepare a comprehensive **treatment program** for the client at the outset. The treatment program should include (1) the target behaviors that need to be trained; (2) a tentative sequence in which they will be trained; (3) complete treatment and probe procedures; (4) a maintenance program; (5) various criteria that will suggest movement throughout the training stages and sequences; and (6) record keeping, follow-up, and booster treatment procedures.

Writing a comprehensive treatment program requires additional planning time before initiating treatment. However, this time is well spent because the clinician does not have to think of target behaviors and treatment procedures on a daily or weekly basis. Such planning might minimize some clinician anxiety due to uncertainties about what to do this week or next week. The written program can be easily modified as suggested by the ongoing performance data.

What follows is an outline of a treatment program. Much of the information needed to develop a training program has been presented in the previous chapters, including selection and definition of target behaviors, tentative training sequence, treatment and probe procedures, maintenance program, criteria of movement throughout the treatment and probe sequences, record-keeping procedures, and follow-up and booster treatment. Therefore, these aspects of the program are not elaborated in this outline. The outline is intended as a checklist of areas that should be covered in a comprehensive treatment plan. It contains definitions of key terms and brief descriptions of most of the procedures that should be specified in a treatment program.

The treatment program is written in a narrative form, much like an assessment report. With the format presented here, it should be possible to write comprehensive treatment programs for a variety of clients exhibiting different kinds of communicative disorders.

AN OUTLINE OF A GENERAL TREATMENT PROGRAM

Assess the Client's Communicative Behaviors

When a client applies for clinical services, thoroughly assess that client's speech and language behaviors. **Assessment** is measurement of the client's relevant behaviors.

Take a case history.

Take reliable and valid speech and language samples. Whenever possible, take samples from the client's natural environment. Repeated samples help establish reliability.

Briefly assess the client's general and speech-related motor behaviors. Make a more detailed assessment if there is evidence of neuromotor involvement, and then refer the client to a neurologist.

Screen the client's hearing; refer him or her to an audiologist when warranted.

If you administer standardized tests, select those that directly sample observable speech and language behaviors instead of unobservable psychological, neurological, or cognitive processes presumed to underlie those behaviors. Keep in perspective the limitations of standardized tests, and treat all test results as tentative.

Develop and use client-specific measurement procedures. Do not hesitate to replace standardized tests with such procedures along with carefully planned baselines.

Analyze the assessment data: length of typical utterance (the statistical mode); longest and shortest utterances; mean length of utterances; missing grammatic features based on obligatory contexts; frequency with which various grammatic, semantic, and pragmatic structures are used by the client; number and frequency of response classes produced; types of sentences used and not used; types and amounts of dysfluencies and associated motor behaviors; articulation of speech sounds at different levels of response complexity; voice characteristics and deviations; and number of manual signs, symbolic behaviors, or other nonverbal behaviors produced.

Make sure the summarized client behaviors are objective and measurable. Avoid inferred and unmeasurable processes and subjective statements not backed up by objective data.

Select Target Behaviors for Training

After the assessment, select target behaviors for the client. **Target behaviors** are empirical response classes that, when taught or modified, reduce or eliminate the disorder under consideration.

Select short- and long-term target behaviors. The short-term target behaviors can be arbitrarily defined as those that can be trained in 2 to 3 months, whereas the long-term targets include most of the communicative behaviors that a given client needs to learn. Maintenance of communicative behaviors in the natural environment is the final, long-term objective.

Consider the following issues: What are communicative behaviors? What behaviors are to be trained? Consider the normative versus the client-specific strategies: norms and normative sequences; relevancy, usefulness, and maintenance considerations; empirically based response classes; responses that are modifiable; and so on.

Consider the best sequence of training: Should the target behaviors be trained in their normative sequence if known, or should the order depend upon clinical evidence?

Establish the Baselines of Target Behaviors

Once the target behaviors are selected, the next step is to establish the baselines of those behaviors. **Baselines** are reliable response measures in the absence of the planned treatment variables. Because of the limitations of the traditional assessment data, baselines are critical in establishing clinician accountability and treatment effectiveness.

Prepare the stimulus materials for evoking responses during baseline trials or periods. In many cases, the same stimuli can be used to train and probe.

Write sentences, phrases, and words that will serve as target behaviors. Write specific questions designed to evoke the target responses.

Establish baselines of conversational speech.

Establish baselines in all relevant response modes (modeled, evoked, and conversational speech; oral reading).

When necessary, use the discrete-trial procedure. A **trial** is a sequence of events that involves presenting a stimulus, asking a question, modeling a response when planned, waiting for a response (few seconds), recording the response, and moving or removing the stimulus. The sequence is then repeated with an intertrial interval of 3 to 4 seconds. Use a two-trial (evoked and modeled) procedure.

During the baseline sessions, reinforce the client noncontingently.

Design a recording sheet on which every response is recorded as either correct, incorrect, or absent, using separate symbols. Record baseline, training, and probe sessions on separate recording sheets.

Whenever possible, obtain measures of communicative behaviors tape-recorded in the client's home and other extraclinical situations.

Calculate the percentages of correct and incorrect productions of target responses.

Design a Flexible Therapeutic Environment

A **therapeutic environment** is a somewhat controlled and isolated situation in which the treatment variables are applied to initially establish the target behaviors.

The initial therapeutic setup is a controlled environment in which the stimuli and opportunities for the target behaviors are provided at full strength, whereas those for undesirable behaviors are minimized or eliminated.

The setup should be flexible, however, so that, during the latter stages of training, generalization can be enhanced and maintenance programs implemented by fading the difference between the treatment and the natural settings.

Plan and Write a Comprehensive Treatment Program

A **treatment program** specifies what the client will be required to do, what the clinician will do, and how the two will interact. Ideally, the program is written after baselines are established and before treatment is started. Sometimes this may not be possible, as the clinician may wish to informally experiment with a few procedures in the first few sessions. The program should be written as soon as possible.

Give **identification data** (name, address, etc.). Summarize background information, assessment data, and the purposes of treatment.

Describe the **target behaviors** in measurable terms. Define both the correct and the incorrect responses.

Describe the **training procedures**. Specify how the target behaviors will be evoked and modeled on training trials. Describe stimulus presentation, evoking questions, modeling of the correct response, time allowed to respond, and recording procedure.

Suggest the **reinforcing and response reducing consequences** that may initially be used. Specify the types of reinforcing stimuli and response reduction procedures to be used when incorrect responses are given. Plan to use conditioned generalized reinforcers and differential reinforcement procedures to increase behaviors that will indirectly reduce undesirable behaviors.

Suggest the **schedules** on which the consequences will be delivered. Initially, the reinforcers are delivered on a continuous schedule. When the target behaviors show some significant increases (roughly a 50% increase above the baseline), an intermittent schedule is used. Starting with a fixed ratio 2 schedule, the ratio is stretched gradually.

Specify when modeling will be discontinued and evoked trials started. When the discrete-trials procedure is used, training starts with modeled trials, but when the client is able to imitate reliably, evoked trials are introduced. In many cases, **five consecutively correct imitated responses** may be sufficient to discontinue modeling.

Suggest when modeling will be reinstated. **Modeling is reinstated** when the client gives wrong responses on two consecutive evoked trials presented soon after the termination of modeling. Subsequently, the clinician can be more flexible: up to five incorrect responses may be accepted.

Describe when the evoked trials will be reinstated. **Evoked trials are reinstated** every time the client gives five consecutively correct imitated responses.

Specify the training criteria. Training criteria can differ depending upon the level of training and response topography. When discrete trials are used, the **training criterion** is usually a specified number of correct responses on a set of trials. Typically, 90% correct response rate, based on at least 20 trials, is a criterion used in the initial stages of training. When discrete sentences or phrases are trained, 10 consecutively correct responses on a given sentence or phrase may be the initial criterion. In the treatment of fluency and voice, 98% accuracy may be appropriate at all levels of treatment.

Describe when probes may be held. A **probe** is a procedure designed to assess generalization or maintenance of clinically trained behaviors. Probes may be administered at the completion of a training stage. When target responses are trained to a criterion at the level of single words, a probe may be administered to see if the behaviors generalize. Successive probes can be administered when target behaviors attain the training criterion at the level of phrases, sentences, or conversational speech. In the treatment of language disorders, probes may be administered after having trained four to six stimulus items.

Specify the probe criterion. The **probe criterion** is usually 90% correct response rate on probe items. In the case of persons who stutter, 98% fluency may be required.

Describe the types of probes and when they will be used. **Intermixed** probes are used in the early stages, and **pure probes** in the final stages. Responses given to the probe items are not reinforced.

Suggest the steps to be taken when the client does not meet a probe criterion. Any time a probe criterion is not met, training is **reinstated**. The response topography or level that did not meet the probe criterion is trained again.

Describe the dismissal criterion. **Clients are dismissed** when they meet the final dismissal criterion. This is also a probe criterion. The client may be dismissed from the continuous treatment program when responses meet at least a 90% probe criterion in conversational speech at home and possibly in other nonclinical situations.

Describe the response maintenance procedure. **Responses are maintained** when people in the client's life prompt and reinforce the target behaviors. Describe how maintenance will be promoted by training other people in contingency management.

Suggest a schedule and procedure of follow-up. **Follow-up** consists of periodic measurement of trained behaviors to assess their maintenance. Follow-up assessment is done initially at monthly (or 3-month) intervals and later at biannual and annual intervals.

Describe booster treatment. Given some time following the client's dismissal from the original treatment, **booster treatment** strengthens the target behaviors. Any time a follow-up measure shows a decline in the rate of target behaviors, booster treatment should be given.

A comprehensive treatment program written according to the guidelines summarized here will make it possible to move smoothly from one level of training to the other. If the client's performance data warrant it, the written program is modified.

Implement the Treatment Program

Careful management of behavioral contingencies is the most important aspect of implementing treatment programs. The clinician manages two types of contingencies: those that will increase some responses, and those that will decrease others. Certain contingencies are applied to the desirable target behaviors, and certain other contingencies are applied to undesirable target behaviors.

Apply the Selected Contingencies to Desirable Target Behaviors

1. Select potential reinforcers from the client's natural environment.

2. Give instructions to the client; describe the target behaviors.

3. Model the correct responses until imitative responses are produced reliably.

4. Shape the desired response whenever necessary. Do not allow the intermediate responses to stabilize. Raise the criterion of reinforcement gradually, resulting in the terminal response.

5. Prompt the responses to prevent the occurrence of incorrect responses.

6. Use manual guidance if responses are not readily imitated.

7. Fade the stimulus control in gradual steps.

8. Reinforce responses immediately. When you use primary reinforcers, also use social reinforcers.

9. Withdraw the primary reinforcer eventually. Try to maintain responses on social and conditioned generalized reinforcers.

10. Shift to an intermittent schedule of reinforcement.

11. Whenever possible, use generalized conditioned reinforcers. Backup tokens with a variety of reinforcers.

12. Reinforce progressively more complex responses.

Apply the Selected Contingencies to Undesirable Behaviors

1. Select the response reducing consequences.

2. Whenever possible, identify reinforcers that may be maintaining those responses.

3. Withhold the reinforcers for inappropriate behaviors (extinction).

4. Whenever possible, remove opportunities for emitting inappropriate behaviors.

5. Give corrective feedback ("no," "wrong," "not correct," etc.) promptly and response contingently.

6. When appropriate, use response cost or time-out. When using the response cost procedure, withdraw reinforcers response contingently. When using time-out, say "stop," avoid eye contact, and freeze your position for a few seconds.

7. Use one of the differential reinforcement procedures to increase any other desirable behavior, an alternative behavior, or an incompatible behavior. Shape the undesirable behavior down by reinforcing a progressively lower rate.

8. Use a high-probability interfering behavior to reinforce a low-probability target behavior.

9. Use behavioral momentum.

10. Eliminate negative reinforcement for undesirable behaviors by making treatment less aversive and more positive.

11. Use a surprising stimulus to prevent an undesirable response.

12. Present the response reduction consequence on a continuous schedule.

13. Do not allow escape.

14. Apply the response reducing consequence at the very first sign of the behavior to be reduced.

15. Minimize the use and the duration of response reduction procedures. Let the client experience more positive consequences than aversive consequences.

16. Watch for possible undesirable additional effects of response reduction procedures.

Implement a Maintenance Program

Almost all clients need a maintenance program. The target behaviors trained in clinical situations may show some amount of generalization to natural environments. This generalization must be measured. However, generalized target behaviors may not be maintained over time; therefore, a maintenance program must be implemented.

1. Select responses that are useful to the client.
2. Use the probe procedure throughout the training period to monitor generalization.
3. Train responses in relation to a variety of stimuli.
4. Use conditioned generalized reinforcers.
5. Use intermittent schedules of reinforcement.
6. Have observers, parents, friends, and siblings attend training sessions.
7. Hold treatment sessions in natural settings during the latter stages of training.
8. Train the production of target responses in conversational speech.
9. Teach the client self-monitoring skills.
10. Teach the client to prime others for reinforcement.
11. Reinforce generalized responses.
12. Train parents, teachers, siblings, and others to manage the treatment contingencies at home, school, and other places.
13. Train parents and others in creating opportunities for emitting target responses.
14. Train parents in recording speech–language samples that you can use to assess generalization and maintenance.
15. Give an adequate amount of treatment.
16. Arrange for booster treatment.

Keep Continuous Objective Records

Target behaviors must be measured continuously. The traditional pretests and posttests are inadequate. Continuous objective records help establish clinician accountability.

1. Before you begin to baserate, design a recording sheet and a measurement procedure.

2. Measure the frequency of desirable and undesirable responses and record them separately.

3. Record baseline, training, and probe data on separate sheets.

4. Obtain response rates in extraclinical situations.

5. Specify the measured behaviors in absolute numbers and percentages.

6. Avoid subjective statements that are not supported by objective measures.

7. Record the occurrence of desirable and undesirable target behaviors in each session.

8. Summarize measurement-based observations at the end of each session.

9. Measure target behaviors in natural settings.

10. Obtain the measures of target behaviors produced at home.

Follow Up the Client

Follow-up is a procedure designed to assess response maintenance in the natural environment and across time. Responses are measured in the absence of treatment variables.

1. Before dismissing the client, assess generalization and maintenance of all the trained responses in as many situations and contexts as possible.

2. Schedule initial follow-up sessions in 3- to 6-month intervals and subsequently on an annual basis.

3. Use the conversational probe procedure to assess response maintenance.

4. Whenever possible, take the follow-up measures in nonclinical situations involving people not associated with treatment.

Arrange for Booster Treatment

Many clients can benefit from **booster treatment** after they have been dismissed from the program. A few booster sessions can strengthen responses to a great extent and thus promote maintenance.

1. Whenever a follow-up measure shows a decline in the response rate, conduct booster treatment sessions. Typically, the original treatment procedure is used.

2. Newer and more effective procedures, if they are available at the time of booster treatment, should be used.

3. Subsequent to booster treatment sessions, follow-up sessions should be as frequent as they were to begin with.

The above outline can be modified as deemed necessary. It lists components of treatment programs that are common to most disorders. Additional or modified procedures needed to suit individual disorders or clients may be easily incorporated.

HOW TO MODIFY TREATMENT PROGRAMS

A written treatment program is useful because the clinician can organize treatment according to the planned sequence. However, a treatment program is not a set of rules that must be followed regardless of client performance. A written program is a tentative plan of action, but what exactly the clinician does throughout the sessions depends mostly upon the client performance. The program may be executed the way it was written, or client responses may dictate changes. Very often, treatment programs need to be modified because of changing patterns of client behaviors. Every clinician ought to know when and how to modify planned treatment procedures.

Treatment programs are modified because of several client-specific reasons. Although these reasons vary across individuals, a few common reasons may be identified. The distinction between treatment principles and procedures is helpful in considering potential modifications of a treatment program. Some suggestions for program modifications follow. Each suggestion is based upon a reason that would necessitate a change.

Principles Do Not Change; Procedures Do

Frequently, a program needs modification because a procedure is not working with a given client. In such cases, the clinician should analyze the reasons for failure and make necessary changes. It is important to note that changes are almost always made in procedures, not in principles. The principles of response contingency, positive and negative reinforcement, extinction, response reduction, discrimination, generalization, and environmental control (maintenance) are not modified by uncontrolled clinical activity.

What fails is a treatment procedure, not the principle behind it. Because each principle can generate different treatment procedures, it is possible to modify ineffective procedures within the framework of those principles. Usually, a more effective procedure can be derived from the same principle. The clinician may replace ineffective stimuli with more effective stimuli or discard consequences that do not work in favor of those that do.

Selected Consequences May Not Be Effective

Probably the most common problem encountered in treatment programs is that the selected response consequences do not work. The clinician may select a seemingly wonderful reinforcer, but it may not increase the rate of the target response when presented contingently. The clinician might present tokens, but they may be ineffective. Undesirable target behaviors may not decrease when consequated with verbal "no." In situations such as these, some clinicians say that reinforcement or corrective feedback (punishment) did not work. What happened was that selected response consequences did not act as reinforcers or punishers, and it is no reflection on the principle of reinforcement or punishment. The modification in this case is simple: Change the particular consequence.

Before a selected consequence is abandoned, however, the clinician must make sure that it was used correctly. Were the consequences delivered response contingently? If the training stage was initial, were they used continuously? If tokens were used, were they backed up by another kind of reinforcer? A common mistake is to present plastic chips and assume that they are reinforcers. If there were no mistakes in the use of the selected consequences, then the clinician must select new consequences. In the case of tokens, different backups must be found. If such verbal stimuli as "good" and "excellent" have not been effective, perhaps primary reinforcers or a well backed-up token system will be effective. If corrective feedback did not reduce wrong or undesirable responses, then perhaps time-out or response cost might.

The clinician should always define response consequences empirically. An event is a reinforcer only when it increases a response rate. An event is a punisher only when it decreases a response rate. Within this philosophy, one cannot complain about "ineffective" reinforcers or punishers, which is a contradiction in terms. One can only talk about not having found a reinforcer or punisher, which means that the clinician should search for the consequences that will have the desired effect on behaviors.

Individual Histories Necessitate Changes

Treatment programs that cannot be modified to suit individual behavioral histories are not very useful to clinicians. In fact, the most important need to modify a treatment program is an individual client's unique history. The history of individual clients renders certain consequences effective. As noted in earlier chapters, a child who is nonverbal, for example, may not react to verbal praise in the same way a highly verbal client might.

It is well known that what is reinforcing to one client may not be reinforcing to another. Also, for the same client, what is reinforcing at one time may not be reinforcing at other times. Punishing events may also vary accordingly. Some clients generalize relatively easily, whereas others do not. The reasons for such differences are not well understood, but it is well known that multiple procedures are needed to achieve the same goals in different clients and at different times in the same client.

Antecedents of Responses May Require Changes

Antecedents of target behaviors are a significant part of treatment contingencies. Defective antecedents may fail to evoke responses. For example, pictorial and other stimulus materials selected for training may be ambiguous or poor representations of real stimulus events. Persons with adequate verbal skills may correctly name poorly drawn pictures, whereas those with limited language skills may not.

Questions may not be direct enough to evoke answers from the client. In training the regular past tense inflection, for example, the clinician may have to first state what is happening in the picture and then ask what happened yesterday (e.g., "Today the man is painting; yesterday he did the same. What did he do yesterday?"). While training the present progressive, the clinician may not be able to evoke the *ing* by simply telling the client to "Tell something about the picture." The question may have to be more specific, such as "What is the boy doing?" Writing questions for evoking grammatic features and sentence forms requires some thought.

In some forms of stuttering treatment, the clinician initially evokes single words or short phrases. This strategy may also be needed in the treatment of voice disorders. How to ask questions that restrict answers to one or two words also needs some prior planning.

When treatment is shifted from one stage to the next, discriminative stimulus control may be lost. For example, a response that has come under the control of a modeling stimulus may be adversely affected when modeling is discontinued. Whenever loss of discriminative stimulus control seems to be the problem, the stimulus must be faded in gradual steps. If all *ing* responses were trained with the verbal antecedent "What is the boy doing?" then other antecedents may fail to evoke that response.

Response Topographies May Have to Be Changed

Another reason for modifying treatment programs is the changing nature of response properties. Verbal behavior consists of complex chains, the elements of which are continuously variable. As noted in earlier chapters, target behaviors can be trained at various levels of response complexity. Clients may fail to learn because a wrong response topography was selected for training. In such cases, there may be nothing wrong with the contingencies used by the clinician.

The clinician who began training a certain phoneme at the phrase level might find that the correct responses are too infrequent to keep the positive:aversive consequence ratio in favor of positive consequences. Then, the response topography must be changed. The assumption is that the initial topography selected for training was not appropriate for the client. Perhaps the client needed training at the level of single words.

In training grammatic features, a clinician might initially select a sentence form, but the client may not show systematic increases in that behavior. Assuming that other procedures were correctly used, the clinician at this point might consider training the feature in the context of single words or two-word phrases.

Topographic considerations are important in the treatment of fluency disorders. The treatment technique can be applied initially at the level of isolated words. If the treatment is started at the level of continuous speech, the client may not sustain such target behaviors as reduced rate or soft initiation of phonation.

Treatment of voice disorders can pose similar problems. For example, the client may not be able to sustain the desirable pitch at the level of sentences, but may be able to do so when asked to produce single words or short phrases.

Some clients can learn certain target responses more easily than others. A guideline the clinician can use is the differential baserates of selected target behaviors. If the correct production of plural morpheme /s/ was baserated at 0%, and the present progressive *ing* at 37%, then *ing* may be trained first. Possibly, because of the higher initial baseline, the *ing* is learned faster than the plural /s/. Clinical experience suggests that a response already produced to some extent is easier to train than a response not being produced at all.

Two or more behaviors that have similar baselines may be more or less difficult to learn. When a target behavior does not seem to increase under the training contingency, one must proceed to another target. It is difficult to determine when the clinician should stop the training efforts on a given target, but it should not be done too prematurely. The clinician should always remember that most target behaviors must be shaped. A complex response topography can be simplified by breaking that response into smaller targets that are shaped in successive stages. Before dropping a particular target from training, one must make sure that the shaping procedure was tried. After dropping a target, the clinician must return to that difficult target behavior at a later time.

Most programs, no matter how carefully written, require some modifications during implementation. In modifying treatment programs, the most important criterion to follow is the client's rate of responses. If desirable responses do not increase, and undesirable responses do not decrease, then something is wrong: Perhaps the consequences were not functional; stronger reinforcers were needed; the selected stimulus materials were not relevant; the response selected for training was not appropriate; the response was appropriate, but a shaping procedure was not used effectively; or the clinician may not have found an initial response that exists in the client's repertoire. In modifying a program, such possibilities must be considered.

SEQUENCES OF TRAINING

In Chapter 5, a basic sequence of treatment was described. The description specified an initial sequence of training, probe, and progression across different target behaviors. In addition to describing what the client and the clinician will be doing, a treatment program describes *movement*. Both the client and the clinician move across different parameters. It means that "what to do next" is an important question for the program writer.

In this section, a few major factors that determine particular sequences of treatment are considered. Treatment must be sequenced because of (1) response topographies, (2) response modes, (3) multiple targets, (4) generalization and maintenance, and (5) shifts in contingencies.

Sequenced Response Topographies

Final target behaviors are often complex and chained. Most clients are unable to learn them in total. Therefore, the final target behavior is usually taught in small steps. The clinician first identifies what the client can do that is in some way related to the final target behavior. By making this occur more reliably, the clinician moves to the next response, which may be slightly more complex. In this way, the final target may be achieved. This technique is the well-known shaping procedure. In essence, the most basic reason for sequencing treatment is that the clinician must first teach simpler components of complex responses and then integrate the total response.

Generally, the more difficult the task for a given client, the smaller the response topography at which the training is initiated. For example, when training is started at the level of syllables, it must move through the stages of words, phrases, sentences, and conversational speech. At each stage, the client's responses must meet certain training and probe criteria. For instance, when the correct production of the target phoneme in syllables reaches 90% correct across 20 consecutive trials, the clinician might shift training to the word level. A 90% correct response rate at the word level might suggest that the training be shifted to the phrase level, and so on.

Based upon response topographies, language training is similarly sequenced. A basic vocabulary training program, for example, might involve certain simple words. However, each word response may have to be broken into smaller responses, such as the production of syllables. The syllables are then "put together" to form the word. Once a few words are taught, the clinician might move on to teaching phrases consisting of those words. Phrases may then be expanded into sentences. Essentially, training moves from simpler to more complex response classes involving varied response topographies. Similar sequences may be used to teach nonverbal languages or communication systems, including the American Sign Language. Most academic skills are also taught in sequenced steps.

In treating stuttering, the typical starting point is single words or short phrases. Target behaviors, such as rate reduction through syllable prolongation, inhalation and slight exhalation before phonation, gentle onset of phonation, and soft articulatory contacts, are practiced and reinforced at the level of single words or short phrases. When these skills are stabilized at this level, the training may be shifted to expanded utterances. Eventually, the target behaviors are practiced in conversational speech.

In treating voice disorders, the sequences are similar to those used in stuttering treatment. Whether it is the modification of vocal pitch, intensity, tremors, or other vocal qualities, the treatment is started at a level of response topography that the client can handle with some degree of success. The client may be asked to reduce tremors while saying simple words, or even while vocalizing a syllable. If the tremors are successfully controlled at this level, the training may be shifted to words or phrases, and finally to the level of conversational speech, where the response topography is allowed to vary. Success at each stage, defined operationally, means that the client is ready for the next stage of higher response complexity.

Sequenced Response Modes

Different modes of responses create a need for sequencing training, because the target behaviors can be taught more easily in some modes than in others. The mode in which treatment is started may not be the terminal mode for that response. Therefore, the clinician often starts with one mode and finishes with another.

The most frequently used initial mode is imitative. The clinician models the correct response and the client tries to duplicate it. Success leads to reinforcement. When the target behavior is imitated reliably by the client, the modeling stimulus is faded. If additional discriminative stimuli are required, prompts are used. These are also faded. Then, the training is shifted to a nonimitative response mode (evoked speech).

In some cases, oral reading may be an initial response mode. While treating adult stutterers, it is often easier to train the target responses in oral reading than in conversational speech. Oral reading frees the stutterer from the speech formulation task. The client can then concentrate on how to produce speech (using slow rate, gentle onset, etc.). Also, topographical expansion, such as movement from the one-word to the two-word level, is easier in oral reading. Once the skills are practiced in the oral reading mode, the client must shift to the conversational speech mode. Thus, the sequence in this case might be oral reading and conversational speech, with topographically based sequences within each of these modes of responses.

Sequenced Multiple Targets

In earlier chapters, it was noted that most clients have multiple responses missing in their repertoires. Especially in the case of articulation and language disorders, multiple targets are the rule. Occasionally, a client might need training on a single phoneme, but such cases are few. When multiple behaviors need to be trained, they must be sequenced.

In Chapter 5, the essential sequence involving multiple responses was described. When the first target behavior has reached an initial probe criterion, the clinician might select the next behavior for training. While the second behavior is being trained, the first behavior may be moved to the next topographic level. For instance, if the first behavior has reached the probe criterion at the single-word level, it may be moved to the phrase level of training. The training on the second behavior is then initiated at the word level. In this manner, additional behaviors are newly brought under the training contingency while already trained behaviors keep advancing through sequences based upon response topography, mode, or other factors.

Theoretically, it is possible to train multiple targets in a single session at the same or different levels of response topography. In the beginning, however, it may be preferable to train only one behavior, or a few. In the subsequent phases of treatment, multiple responses may be trained, each at a different topographic level. For example, the first grammatic feature selected for training may be at the level of conversational speech mode while the second behavior is being trained at the controlled sentence level, the third behavior is at the phrase level of training, and so on. How many target behaviors can be simultaneously handled in a single session depends upon the client's sustained response rates and the length of sessions.

Training- and Maintenance-Based Sequences

Another factor that necessitates sequencing is the training–generalization–maintenance aspect of all treatment programs. Target behaviors are first trained to a certain probe criterion. A behavior trained at the highest topographic level and in the conversational speech mode may generalize to natural settings. However, after completing the initial training, a maintenance procedure must be implemented. Observers, parents, or siblings may be brought into the treatment sessions. The treatment setting may be changed. Informal treatment sessions may be held at the client's home, school, or occupational setting. The parents may be trained to administer probes and the treatment contingencies at home. All of these activities must be sequenced.

Some aspects of generalization and maintenance may be considered at the outset of the treatment program. Selecting target behaviors that are likely to be produced and reinforced in the natural environment is an example. Most other aspects of generalization and maintenance are implemented only after a certain amount of training has been completed. Shifting training from a controlled to a more natural setting, for example, may not be productive if done at the earliest stage of treatment. Furthermore, some parents may find it hard to reinforce a target that is still being shaped by the clinician. Therefore, these aspects of maintenance are better implemented at a later time, after responses have been shaped and can be reinforced by parents.

Sequenced Shifts in Contingencies

The final factor that dictates a sequence arises from the need to manage contingencies differently at different stages of treatment. In the beginning of treatment, the reinforcers are presented on a continuous schedule because this can speed up learning. However, to strengthen already learned responses, reinforcers must be given on an intermittent schedule during the latter stages of treatment.

Any time an intermittent schedule is introduced, or a shift is made to a larger schedule, the response rate might drop. Whenever this happens, the clinician should reinstate continuous reinforcement. The intermittent schedule introduced for the first time must not require a large number of responses or great intervals between reinforcers. When properly sequenced, contingency shifts can help maintain responses in natural environments.

CONCLUDING REMARKS

I hope that the 10 chapters of this book can provide speech–language pathologists with some conceptual and methodologic bases of clinical intervention. In conclusion, it may be appropriate to summarize the philosophic assumptions of this book.

First, a strong scientific basis is needed for a clinical profession, such as that concerned with communicative disorders. Unless clinical practice is based on the concepts and methods of science, it is unlikely to gain public recognition as a profession and as a scientific discipline. In fact, unless the field is first recognized as a scientific discipline, it may not gain much recognition as a clinical profession. Throughout the book, emphasis has been on the view that experimental evidence should support clinical practice. There is an urgent need to expand clinical–experimental research activities in communicative disorders, and I hope that increasing numbers of clinicians will be inclined to gather experimental evidence as a part of their clinical services.

Second, science and clinical activities are more similar than different because they share common goals and procedures. Scientists and practitioners alike seek to analyze and control phenomena of their interests.

Third, as clinical scientists, specialists in communicative disorders must base treatment procedures on experimental evidence and not on speculative reasoning. Although this should go without saying, it needs to be said. Also, clinical practice cannot be based on mere observational data, such as developmental trends. Clinical procedures must be experimentally tested under controlled clinical conditions.

Fourth, treatment programs must be client specific. A clinical science is needed that looks at individual client's real behaviors and not statistical averages based on group performances. The requirements of law and science both dictate that clinicians develop a philosophy of practice that treats individual behaviors as the ultimate test of the efficacy of treatment techniques. All treatment techniques should be modifiable in light of client-specific data.

Fifth, there are principles of treatment that apply across disorders of communication. From these principles, it is possible to derive procedures to treat individual clients and specific disorders.

Sixth, there is a treatment paradigm that fulfills these and other philosophical and methodological requirements. Throughout this book, that paradigm, which describes environmental events and the client and clinical actions in terms of a contingency, has been enumerated. Treatment in communicative disorders involves a contingent relation between environmental events, client responses, and clinician actions. It is a relation between speakers and their listeners. A successful clinician rearranges this communicative relation to effect objectively measured changes in the behaviors of clients and the people surrounding them. The goal of treatment is to generate a new pattern of functional communication between clients and people associated with them.

SUMMARY

In planning treatment for specific clients, one can either write the traditional lesson plans or write comprehensive treatment programs. The latter is preferred because it gives a better treatment perspective.

The written treatment program should include target behaviors, treatment sequences, treatment and probe procedures, maintenance program, various criteria of "movement," and procedures for record keeping, follow-up, and booster treatment.

The treatment program that can be applied across disorders includes the following steps: (1) assessment of the client's communicative behaviors, (2) selection of target behaviors, (3) establishing the baselines, (4) designing a flexible therapeutic environment, (5) planning and writing a comprehensive treatment program, (6) implementing the treatment program, (7) planning and implementing a maintenance program, (8) keeping continuous objective records, (9) follow-up of the client, and (10) arranging booster treatment.

Most treatment programs need to be modified in light of the client response data. However, it is the treatment procedures that are changed, not the principles. The reasons for program modification include the following: (1) ineffective consequences, (2) unique individual histories, (3) inadequate stimulus control, and (4) inappropriate response topographies.

Most treatment programs have to be sequenced for the following reasons: (1) varied response topographies, (2) different response modes, (3) multiple targets, (4) training and maintenance considerations, and (5) contingency shifts.

The specialists in communicative disorders have a treatment paradigm that fulfills the legal, social, and scientific demands that are made upon the profession. Additional research within this conceptually and methodologically integrated model can be expected to help refine treatment procedures and extend their generality.

STUDY GUIDE

Answer the following questions in technical language. Check your answers with the text. Rewrite your answers when needed.

1. What are the two approaches to treatment planning?

2. Which one of those approaches was not recommended?

3. Why should a clinician write a comprehensive treatment program at the very beginning?

4. What are the six major elements of a comprehensive treatment program?

5. List the 10 steps given in the outline of a general treatment program. Describe each step briefly.

6. What is assessment as defined in this chapter?

7. What is a therapeutic environment?

8. Why should a therapeutic environment be flexible?

9. What major questions should a treatment program answer?

10. What items are involved in applying selected contingencies to the desirable target behaviors?

11. What items are involved in applying selected contingencies to undesirable behaviors?

12. List at least 10 elements of a maintenance program.

13. How can a clinician measure and record target behaviors?

14. What is a follow-up?

15. Should a clinician reinforce during follow-up measurement?

16. How often should a clinician schedule follow-up sessions?

17. What is booster treatment?

18. When is booster treatment necessary?

19. How is booster treatment given?

20. What are the five reasons that might necessitate program modifications?

21. What are the five reasons for sequencing training?

22. What are the clinical and philosophic assumptions of this book?

Glossary

ABA design—A single-subject research design in which target behaviors are first baserated (A), taught (B), and then reduced (A) to show that the teaching was effective.

ABAB design—A single-subject research design in which target behaviors are first baserated (A), taught (B), reduced (A), and then taught again (B) to show that the teaching was effective.

ABAB reversal design—A single-subject design in which a desirable behavior is baserated (A), taught (B), reduced by teaching its counterpart (A), and then taught again (B) to show that the teaching was effective.

ABAB withdrawal design—A single-subject design in which a desirable behavior is baserated (A), taught (B), reduced by eliminating teaching (A), and then taught again (B) to show that the teaching was effective.

Antecedents—Events that occur before responses; stimuli.

Assessment—A set of clinical procedures with which information is obtained on a client's existing and nonexisting communicative behaviors, communicative problems, and potential factors associated with these problems; the information is evaluated to understand and treat the problems. Also defined as measurement of client's behaviors.

Audience generalization—Production of unreinforced responses in the presence of persons not involved in training.

Automatic reinforcers—Sensory consequences of responses that reinforce those responses.

Aversive stimuli—Events that people work hard to avoid or move away from.

Avoidance—A behavior that prevents the occurrence of an aversive event and hence gets reinforced.

Avoidance conditioning—Teaching behaviors that terminate, reduce, or avoid aversive events.

Backup reinforcers—Events, objects, and opportunities that become available to clients who earn tokens in treatment sessions.

Baselines—Rates of responses in the absence of planned intervention.

Behavioral momentum—Rapidly evoking a high-probability response and immediately commanding a low-probability response to reduce noncompliance.

Booster treatment—Treatment given any time after the client was dismissed from the original treatment to maintain responses.

Client-specific strategy—A method of selecting target behaviors that are relevant and useful for the individual client.

Conditioned generalized reinforcers—Tokens, money, and other reinforcers that are effective in a wide range of conditions.

Conditioned reinforcers—Events that reinforce behaviors because of past learning experiences. The same as *secondary reinforcers.*

Concurrent stimulus–response generalization—Production of new and unreinforced responses in relation to new stimuli. The most complex form of generalization.

Constituent definitions—Dictionary definitions of terms with no reference to how what is defined is measured. See also *operational definitions.*

Contingency—An interdependent relation between events or factors. See *environmental contingency* and *genetic/neurophysiological contingency.*

Contingency priming—Seeking reinforcers for one's own behaviors.

Continuous reinforcement—A schedule in which all responses are reinforced.

Contrast effect—Increased rate of a response in a situation where the aversive stimulus that decreases it is absent.

Control group—The group that does not receive treatment and hence shows no change.

Controlled evidence—Data that show that a particular treatment, not some other factor, was responsible for the positive changes in the client's behavior.

Corrective feedback—Response-contingent presentation of a stimulus that evaluates the response as unacceptable and has the effect of decreasing the response.

Criteria—Rules to make various clinical judgments, including when to model, when to stop modeling, and when a behavior is trained. *Criteria* is plural; *criterion* is singular.

Dependent variables—Effects studied by scientists; behaviors taught to clients and pupils. See also *independent variables.*

Deteriorating baselines—Baselines of a worsening problem; desirable behaviors that are lower each time they are measured.

Determinism—A philosophical position that nothing happens without a cause.

Diagnosis—In medicine, detection of causes of diseases or disorders. In communicative disorders, description and assessment of disorders.

Differential reinforcement—The method of establishing discrimination by reinforcing a response in the presence of one stimulus and not reinforcing the same response in the presence of another stimulus.

Differential reinforcement of alternative behaviors (DRA)—Reinforcing a specified desirable behavior that serves the same function as the one to be reduced.

Differential reinforcement of incompatible behaviors (DRI)—Reinforcing a behavior that is not compatible with a behavior targeted for reduction.

Differential reinforcement of low rates of responding (DRL)—Reinforcing a progressively lower frequency of an undesirable behavior to shape it down.

Differential reinforcement of other behaviors (DRO)—Reinforcing many unspecified behaviors while not reinforcing a specified response targeted for reduction.

Direct methods of response reduction—Reducing behaviors by placing a contingency on them. See also *indirect methods of response reduction.*

Discrete trials—Opportunities for producing responses that are clearly separated in time.

Discrimination—A behavioral process of establishing different responses to different stimuli.

Effectiveness (of treatment)—Assurance that treatment, not some other factor, was responsible for the positive changes documented in a client under treatment.

Elicited aggression—Aggressive behavior directed against any object or person when an aversive stimulus is delivered.

Empirical validity—Credibility or truthfulness of statements based on research data.

Empiricism—A philosophical position that statements must be supported by observational or experimental evidence.

Environmental contingency—Interdependent relation between stimuli, responses, and consequences faced by the responses.

Escape—A behavior that reduces or terminates an aversive event and hence increases in frequency. See also *avoidance.*

Escape extinction—Blocking an escape response to prevent negative reinforcement for it.

Evoked trial—A structured opportunity to produce a response when the clinician does not model.

Exclusion time-out—Response-contingent exclusion of a person from a reinforcing environment; the typical effect is response reduction.

Exemplar—A response that illustrates a target behavior.

Experiment—A controlled condition in which an independent variable is manipulated to produce changes in a dependent variable.

Experimental group—The group that receives treatment and hence shows changes. See also *control group*.

Explanation—A statement that fully describes an event and points out its causes.

Extinction—The procedure of terminating reinforcers for responses to be reduced.

Extinction burst—An initial and temporary increase in responses when reinforcers are withdrawn.

Factorial stimulus generalization—Production of unreinforced responses given in relation to new stimuli, settings, audience, and so forth; the most complex form of stimulus generalization.

Fading—A method of reducing the controlling power of a stimulus while still maintaining the response.

Fixed interval schedule—An intermittent schedule of reinforcement in which an invariable time duration separates opportunities to earn reinforcers.

Fixed ratio schedule—An intermittent schedule of reinforcement in which a certain number of responses are required to earn a reinforcer.

Follow-up—Probe or assessment of response maintenance subsequent to dismissal from treatment.

Functional equivalence training—Reinforcing desirable behaviors that serve the same function as the undesirable behaviors.

Generality (of treatment)—The applicability of a treatment procedure in a wide range of situations involving other clients and clinicians.

Generalization—A declining rate of unreinforced response in the presence of untrained stimuli.

Genetic/neurophysiological contingency—Relation between genetic and neurophysiological variables that determine or influence physical and behavioral characteristics.

Gradient of generalization—Progressively decreasing response rate as a stimulus is varied on a given dimension, resulting in a curve that approximates the bell-shaped curve.

Group design strategy—Methods in which treatment effects are demonstrated by treating individuals in one group and not treating individuals in another group.

High probability behaviors—Frequently exhibited behaviors that reinforce less frequently exhibited behaviors.

IEPs—Individualized Education Programs for children with disabilities or special needs.

IFSPs—Individualized Family Service Plans developed for infants and toddlers and their family members.

Imitation—Learning in which responses take the same form as their stimuli; modeling provides the stimuli.

Imitation of aversive control—Use of aversive methods to control others by persons who were subjected to aversive control themselves.

Imposition of effort—Response-contingent imposition of work that decreases the response.

Improvement—Documented positive changes in a client's behavior under treatment; no guarantee that the treatment was effective.

Incompatible behaviors—Behaviors that cannot be produced simultaneously.

Independent variables—Causes scientists investigate; treatment methods clinicians use. See also *dependent variables*.

Indirect methods of response reduction—Reducing certain behaviors by increasing other behaviors; indirect because no contingency is placed on behaviors to be decreased.

Informative feedback—Information on the performance levels that reinforce behaviors.

Initial response—The first, simplified component of a target response used in shaping.

Instructions—Verbal stimuli that gain control over other persons' actions.

Interfering behaviors—Behaviors that interrupt the treatment process.

Intermediate response—Responses other than the initial and final responses used in shaping.

Intermittent reinforcement—Reinforcing only some responses or responses produced with some delay between reinforcers.

Intermixed probes—Procedures of assessing generalized production by alternating trained and untrained stimulus items.

Intraverbal generalization—Stimulus and response generalization with forms of verbal behaviors.

Isolation time-out—Response-contingent removal of a person from a reinforcing environment and placing him or her in a nonreinforcing environment; the typical effect is the reduction of that response.

Logical validity—Consistency of statements that do not violate rules of logic.

Maintenance strategy—Extension of treatment to natural settings.

Manual guidance—Physical guidance provided to shape a response.

Matching—A method in which individuals of similar characteristics are placed in the experimental and control groups.

Mode (of responses)—Manner or method of a response; imitation, oral reading, and conversational speech are different modes.

Modeled trial—An opportunity to imitate a response when the clinician models it.

Modeling—The clinician's production of the target response the client is expected to learn; used to teach imitation.

Multiple baseline design—A set of single-subject designs in which the effects of a treatment are demonstrated by showing that untreated baselines did not change and that only the treated baselines did.

Multiple baseline across behaviors design—A single-subject design in which several behaviors are sequentially taught to show that only treated behavior changed and hence the treatment was effective.

Multiple baseline across settings design—A single-subject design in which a behavior is sequentially taught in different settings to show that the behavior changed only in a treated setting and hence the treatment was effective.

Multiple baseline across subjects design—A single-subject research design in which several subjects are taught behaviors sequentially to show that only treated subjects changed and hence the treatment was effective.

Multiple causation—The concept that most events, including communicative behaviors and their disorders, have several causes.

Negative reinforcers—Aversive events that are removed, reduced, postponed, or prevented; responses that do these increase in frequency.

Nonexclusion time-out—Response-contingent arrangement of a brief duration of time in which all interaction is terminated; the typical effect is response reduction.

Normative strategy—A method of selecting target behaviors for clients based on age-based norms.

Norms—Averaged (mean) performance of a typical group of persons on a selected test or measure.

Objectivity—Agreement among different clinicians and scientists who observe or measure the same event.

Omission training—Reinforcing a person for not exhibiting a certain behavior; the same as DRO.

Operant aggression—Aggressive behavior directed against the source of an aversive stimulus.

Operational definitions—Scientific definitions that describe how what is defined is measured.

Overcorrection—A procedure of reducing behaviors by requiring the person to eliminate the effects of his or her misbehavior and practice its counterpart, a desirable behavior.

Paradigm (of treatment)—An overall philosophy or viewpoint of treatment.

Paradoxical effects—Increase in response rates when a known response reduction procedure is used.

Partial modeling—Withdrawing modeling in gradual steps.

Peer training—Training peers of clients to evoke and reinforce target behaviors in natural settings.

Perpetuation of aversive methods—Continued use of aversive methods because of negative reinforcement.

Physical setting generalization—Production of unreinforced responses in a setting not used in training.

Physical stimulus generalization—Production of unreinforced responses in the presence of untrained stimuli because of their similarity to trained stimuli.

Population—A large, defined group with certain characteristics identified for the purposes of a study. See also *sample*.

Positive practice—Required and unreinforced practice of a desirable behavior following restitution for an undesirable behavior.

Positive reinforcers—Events that, when presented immediately after a response is made, increase the future probability of that response.

Postreinforcement pause—A period of no responding after receiving a reinforcer.

Posttests—Measures of behaviors established after completing an experimental teaching program. See also *pretests*.

Pretests—Measures of behaviors established before starting an experimental teaching program. See also *posttests*.

Primary reinforcers—Unconditioned reinforcers whose effects do not depend upon past learning.

Principles (of treatment)—Empirical rules from which treatment procedures are derived.

Probes—Procedures to assess generalized production of responses. See also *intermixed probes* and *pure probes*.

Procedures (of treatment)—Technical operations the clinician performs to effect changes in the client behaviors; behaviors of clinicians.

Program (of treatment)—An overall description of target behaviors, treatment variables, measurement procedures, generalization measures, maintenance strategies, follow-up, and so forth.

Prompts—Special stimuli that increase the probability of a response; prompts may be verbal or nonverbal.

Punishment—Procedures of reducing a behavior by response-contingent presentation or withdrawal of stimuli.

Pure probes—Procedures for assessing generalized production with only untrained stimulus items.

Random assignment—A method of assigning randomly selected subjects to either the experimental or the control group without bias.

Random procedure—A method of selecting subjects from a large population without bias; each subject in the population has the same chance of being selected.

Ratio strain—Reduction in response rate due to a sudden thinning of reinforcement.

Reinforce—Strengthen, increase.

Reinforcement—A method of selecting and strengthening behaviors of individuals by arranging consequences under specific stimulus conditions.

Reinforcement withdrawal—Taking away reinforcers to decrease a response.

Reinforcers—Events that follow behaviors and thereby increase the future probability of those behaviors. See also *positive* and *negative reinforcers.*

Reliability—Consistency with which the same event is repeatedly measured.

Replication—Conducting repeated research to show that a given procedure works with different clients, in different settings, and for different clinicians.

Response class—A group of responses created by the same or similar contingencies; functionally, but not necessarily structurally, similar responses.

Response cost—Response-contingent withdrawal of reinforcers that decreases those responses.

Response generalization—Production of unreinforced new (untrained) responses.

Response mode generalization—Production of unreinforced responses in a mode not involved in training.

Response substitution—Increase in a different undesirable behavior when one is reduced.

Restitution—An element of overcorrection in which the person eliminates the effects of his or her misbehavior and then improves the situation.

Sample—A smaller number of individuals selected from a larger population. See also *population.*

Satiation—Temporary termination of a drive or need because it has been satisfied.

Schedules of reinforcement—Different patterns of reinforcement that generate different patterns of responses.

Science—A certain philosophy of nature and events, a particular disposition exhibited by scientists, and a set of methods used in investigating events.

Secondary reinforcers—Conditioned reinforcers whose effects depend upon past learning.

Self-control—A behavior that monitors other behaviors of the same person.

Shaping—A method of teaching nonexistent responses that are not even imitated. The responses are simplified and taught in an ascending sequence. Also known as *successive approximations.*

Significant others—People who are important in the lives of clients.

Single-subject strategy—Methods of demonstrating treatment effects by showing contrasts between conditions of no treatment, treatment, withdrawal of treatment, and other control procedures when all subjects are treated. See also *group design strategy.*

Social reinforcers—A variety of conditioned reinforcers, which include verbal praise.

Stimulus generalization—Production of a newly learned response to stimuli not used in training. See also *response generalization.*

Targets—Behaviors a client is taught.

Terminal response—The final response targeted in shaping.

Time-out—A response-contingent period of nonreinforcement; the typical effect is reduced rate of that response.

Tokens—Objects that are earned during treatment and exchanged later for back-up reinforcers.

Topography—The form or shape of behaviors; how behaviors sound, feel, or appear.

Treatment—In communicative disorders, the management of contingent relations between antecedents, responses, and consequences; a rearrangement of communicative relationships between a speaker and his or her listener.

Treatment variables—Technical operations performed by the clinician to create, increase, or decrease behaviors.

Trial—A structured opportunity to produce a response.

Validity—The degree to which a measuring instrument measures what it purports to measure.

Variable interval schedule—An intermittent reinforcement schedule in which the time duration between reinforcers is varied around an average.

Variable ratio schedule—An intermittent reinforcement schedule in which the number of responses needed to earn a reinforcer is varied around an average.

Verbal stimulus generalization—Production of unreinforced responses when untrained verbal stimuli are presented.

References

Angelo, D. H., & Goldstein, H. (1990). Effects of a pragmatic teaching strategy for requesting information by communication board users. *Journal of Speech and Hearing Disorders, 55,* 231–243.

American Speech–Language–Hearing Association Congressional Relations Division, Government Affairs Department. (1989). *Current federal legislative regulatory issues: Issues of interest to speech–language pathologists and persons with communication disorders.* Rockville Pike, MD: American Speech–Language–Hearing Association.

American Speech–Language–Hearing Association Council on Professional Ethics. (1991). Code of ethics of the American Speech–Language–Hearing Association. *ASHA, 33,* 103–104.

American Speech–Language–Hearing Association Government Affairs Review. (1990). *Reauthorization of EHA discretionary programs.* Rockville Pike, MD: American Speech–Language–Hearing Association.

Arena, J. (1978). *How to write an I.E.P.* Novato, CA: Academic Therapy.

Azrin, N. H., & Holz, W. C. (1966). Punishment. In W. K. Honig (Ed.), *Operant behavior: Areas of research and application* (pp. 380–447). New York: Appleton-Century-Crofts.

Bachrach, A. J. (1969). *Psychological research: An introduction.* New York: Random House.

Bailey, J. S., Timbers, G. D., Phillips, E. L., & Wolf, M. M. (1971). Modification of articulation errors of predelinquents by their peers. *Journal of Applied Behavior Analysis, 4,* 266–281.

Baker, R. D., & Ryan, B. P. (1971). *Programmed conditioning for articulation.* Monterey, CA: Monterey Learning Systems.

Barlow, D. H., Hayes, S. C., & Nelson, R. O. (1984). *The scientist practitioner.* New York: Pergamon.

Barlow, D. H., & Hersen, M. (1984). *Single case experimental designs: Strategies for studying behavior change.* New York: Pergamon.

Barrera, R. D., & Sulzer-Azaroff, B. (1983). An alternating treatment comparison of oral and total communication training programs with echolalic autistic children. *Journal of Applied Behavior Analysis, 16,* 379–394.

Barton, E. S., & Osborne, J. G. (1978). The development of classroom sharing by a teacher using positive practice. *Behavior Modification, 2,* 231–250.

Bennett, C. W. (1974). Articulation training in two hearing impaired girls. *Journal of Applied Behavior Analysis, 7,* 439–445.

Berg, W. K., & Wacker, D. P. (1989). Evaluation of tactile prompts with a student who is deaf, blind, and mentally retarded. *Journal of Applied Behavior Analysis, 22,* 93–99.

Bernthal, J. E., & Bankson, N. W. (1988). *Articulation and phonological disorders.* Englewood Cliffs, NJ: Prentice-Hall.

Blake, P., & Moss, T. (1967). The development of socialization skills in an electively mute child. *Behavior Research and Therapy, 5,* 349–356.

Bourgeois, M. (1990). Caregiver training, generalization, and maintenance of communicative behaviors in patients with Alzheimer's disease. In L. B. Olswang, C. K. Thompson, S. F. Warren, & N. J. Minghetti (Eds.), *Treatment efficacy research in communication disorders* (pp. 203–213). Washington, DC: American Speech–Language–Hearing Foundation.

Brantner, J. P., & Doherty, M. A. (1983). A review of timeout: A conceptual and methodological analysis. In S. Axelrod & J. Apsche (Eds.), *The effects of punishment on human behavior* (pp. 87–132). New York: Academic Press.

Brown, R. (1973). *A first language: The early stages.* Cambridge, MS: Harvard University Press.

Campbell, C. R., Stremel-Campbell, K., & Rogers-Warren, A. K. (1985). Programming teacher support for functional language. In S. F. Warren & A. K. Rogers-Warren (Eds.), *Teaching functional language* (pp. 311–339). Austin, TX: PRO-ED.

Capelli, R. (1985). *An experimental analysis of morphologic acquisition.* Unpublished master's thesis, California State University, Fresno.

Carr, E. G. (1979). Teaching autistic children to use sign language: Some research issues. *Journal of Autism and Developmental Disorders, 9,* 345–359.

Carr, E. G. (1982). *How to teach sign language to developmentally disabled children.* Lawrence, KS: H&H Enterprises.

Carr, E. G., Binkoff, J. A., Kologinsky, E., & Eddy, M. (1978). Acquisition of sign language by autistic children: I. Expressive labeling. *Journal of Applied Behavior Analysis, 11,* 489–501.

Carr, E. G., & Durand, V. M. (1985). Reducing behavior through functional communication training. *Journal of Applied Behavior Analysis, 18,* 111–126.

Carr, E. G., & Kologinsky, E. (1983). Acquisition of sign language by autistic children: II. Spontaneity and generalization effects. *Journal of Applied Behavior Analysis, 16,* 297–314.

Carr, E. G., Robinson, S., & Palumbo, L. W. (1990). The wrong issues: Aversive versus nonaversive treatment. The right issue: Functional versus nonfunctional treatment. In A. C. Repp & N. N. Singh (Eds.), *Perspectives on the use of aversive and nonaversive interventions for persons with developmental disabilities* (pp. 362–379). Sycamore, IL: Sycamore.

Carr, E. G., Robinson, S., Taylor, J. C., & Carlson, J. (1990). *Positive approaches to the treatment of severe behavior problems in persons with developmental disabilities: A review and analysis of reinforcement and stimulus-based procedures.* Seattle: The Association for Persons with Severe Handicaps.

Charlop, M. H., Burgio, L. D., Iwata, B. A., & Ivancic, M. T. (1988). Stimulus variation as a means of enhancing punishment effects. *Journal of Applied Behavior Analysis, 21*, 89–95.

Charlop, M. H., Kurtz, P. F., & Casey, F. G. (1990). Using aberrant behaviors as reinforcers for autistic children. *Journal of Applied Behavior Analysis, 23*, 163–181.

Charlop, M. H., & Milstein, J. P. (1989). Teaching autistic children conversational speech using video modeling. *Journal of Applied Behavior Analysis, 22*, 275–285.

Chomsky, N. (1957). *Syntactic structures.* Hague: Mouton.

Chomsky, N. (1965). *Aspects of the theory of syntax.* Cambridge, MS: MIT Press.

Clark, S., Remington, B., & Light, P. (1988). The role of referential speech in sign learning by mentally retarded children: A comparison of total communication and sign-alone training. *Journal of Applied Behavior Analysis, 21*, 419–428.

Cole, K. N., & Dale, P. (1986). Direct language instruction and indirect language instruction with language delayed preschool children. *Journal of Speech & Hearing Research, 29*, 206–217.

Connell, P. (1987). An effect of modeling and imitation teaching procedures on children with and without specific language impairment. *Journal of Speech and Hearing Research, 30*, 105–113.

Connell, P., & McReynolds, L. V. (1981). An experimental analysis of children's generalization during lexical learning: Comprehension or production. *Applied Psycholinguistics, 2*, 309–332.

Costello, J. M. (1975). The establishment of fluency with timeout procedures: Three case studies. *Journal of Speech and Hearing Disorders, 40*, 216–231.

Costello, J. M., & Onstine, J. M. (1976). The modification of multiple articulation errors based on distinctive feature theory. *Journal of Speech and Hearing Disorders, 46*, 199–215.

De Cesari, R. (1985). *Experimental training of grammatic morphemes: Effects on the order of acquisition.* Unpublished master's thesis, California State University, Fresno.

Doyle, P. J., Goldstein, H., & Bourgeois, M. S. (1987). Experimental analysis of syntax training in Broca's aphasia: A generalization and social validation study. *Journal of Speech and Hearing Disorders, 52*, 143–155.

Doyle, P. J., Goldstein, H., Bourgeois, M. S., & Oleyar, K. (1990). Facilitating generalized requesting behavior in Broca's aphasia: An experimental analysis of a generalization training procedure. In L. B. Olswang, C. K. Thompson, S. F. Warren, & N. J. Minghetti (Eds.), *Treatment efficacy research in communication disorders* (pp. 189–202). Washington, DC: American Speech–Language–Hearing Foundation.

Drabman, R. S., Hammer, D., & Rosenbaum, M. S. (1979). Assessing generalization in behavior modification with children: The generalization map. *Behavioral Assessment, 1*, 203–204.

Duker, P. C., & Morsink, H. (1984). Acquisition and cross-setting generalization of manual signs with severely retarded individuals. *Journal of Applied Behavior Analysis, 17*, 93–103.

Durand, V. M., & Carr, E. G. (1991). Functional communication training to reduce challenging behavior: Maintenance and application in new settings. *Journal of Applied Behavior Analysis, 24*, 251–264.

Dyer, K., Williams, L., & Luce, L. C. (1991). Training teachers to use naturalistic communication strategies in classrooms for students with autism and other severe handicaps. *Language, Speech, and Hearing Services in Schools, 22,* 313–323.

Elbert, M., Dinnsen, D. A., Swartzlander, P., & Chin, S. B. (1990). Generalization to conversational speech. *Journal of Speech and Hearing Disorders, 55,* 694–699.

Elbert, M., & McReynolds, L. V. (1975). Transfer of /r/ across contexts. *Journal of Speech and Hearing Disorders, 40,* 380–387.

Emerick, L. L., & Haynes, W. O. (1986). *Diagnosis and evaluation in speech pathology* (3rd ed.). Englewood Cliffs, NJ: Prentice-Hall.

Ezell, H. K., & Goldstein, H. (1989). Effects of imitation on language comprehension and transfer to production in children with mental retardation. *Journal of Speech and Hearing Disorders, 54,* 49–56.

Faw, G. D., Reid, D. H., Schepis, M. M., Fitzgerald, J. R., & Welty, P. A. (1981). Involving institutional staff in the development and maintenance of sign language skills with profoundly retarded persons. *Journal of Applied Behavior Analysis, 14,* 411–423.

Feldman, M. A., Case, L., Rincover, A., Towns, F., & Betel, J. (1989). Parent Education Project III: Increasing affection and responsivity in developmentally handicapped mothers: Component analysis, generalization, and effects on child language. *Journal of Applied Behavior Analysis, 22,* 211–222.

Feldman, M. A., Towns, F., Betel, J., Case, L., Rincover, A., & Rubino, C. A. (1986). Parent Education Project II: Increasing stimulating interactions of developmentally handicapped mothers. *Journal of Applied Behavior Analysis, 19,* 23–37.

Ferster, C. B., Culbertson, S., & Boren, M. C. P. (1975). *Behavior principles* (2nd ed.). Englewood Cliffs, NJ: Prentice-Hall.

Ferster, C. B., & Skinner, B. F. (1957). *Schedules of reinforcement.* New York: Appleton-Century-Crofts.

Fitch, J. L. (1973). Voice and articulation. In B. B. Lahey (Ed.), *The modification of language behavior* (pp. 130–177). Springfield, IL: Charles C. Thomas.

Flanagan, B., Goldiamond, I., & Azrin, N. H. (1958). Operant stuttering: The control of stuttering behavior through response-contingent consequences. *Journal of the Experimental Analysis of Behavior, 1,* 173–177.

Fleece, L., Gross, A, O'Brien, T., Kistner, J., Rothblum, E., & Drabman, R. (1981). Elevation of voice volume in young developmentally delayed children via an operant shaping procedure. *Journal of Applied Behavior Analysis, 14,* 351–355.

Foxx, R. M., & Bechtel, D. R. (1983). Overcorrection: A review and analysis. In S. Axelrod & J. Apsche (Eds.), *The effects of punishment on human behavior* (pp. 133–220). New York: Academic Press.

Foxx, R. M., Faw, G. D., McMorrow, M. J., Kyle, M. S., & Bittle, R. G. (1988). Replacing maladaptive speech with verbal labeling responses: An analysis of generalized responding. *Journal of Applied Behavior Analysis, 21,* 411–417.

Foxx, R. M., & Jones, J. R. (1978). A remediation program for increasing the spelling achievement of elementary and junior high school students. *Behavior Modification, 2,* 211–230.

Garcia, E., & DeHaven, E. (1974). Use of operant techniques in the establishment and generalization of language: A review and analysis. *American Journal of Mental Deficiency, 79,* 169–178.

Gelfand, D. M., Hartmann, D. P., Lamb, A. K., Smith, C. L., Mahan, M. A., & Paul, S. C. (1974). The effects of adult models and described alternatives on children's choice of behavior management techniques. *Child Development, 45,* 585–593.

Georges, J., Bellaire, K. J., & Thompson, C. K. (1990). Acquisition and generalization of gestures and communication board use in aphasia. In L. B. Olswang, C. K. Thompson, S. F. Warren, & N. J. Minghetti (Eds.), *Treatment efficacy research in communication disorders* (p. 246). Washington, DC: American Speech–Language–Hearing Foundation.

Gierut, J. (1989). Maximal opposition approach to phonological treatment. *Journal of Speech and Hearing Disorders, 54,* 9–19.

Gierut, J. (1990). A functional analysis of phonological contrast treatments. In L. B. Olswang, C. K. Thompson, S. F. Warren, & N. J. Minghetti (Eds.), *Treatment efficacy research in communication disorders* (p. 252). Washington, DC: American Speech–Language–Hearing Foundation.

Girolametto, L. E. (1988). Improving the social–conversational skills of developmentally delayed children: An intervention study. *Journal of Speech and Hearing Disorders, 53,* 156–167.

Gleason, J. B. (1989). *The development of language.* Columbus, OH: Merrill.

Goldstein, H., & Ferrell, D. R. (1987). Augmenting communicative interaction between handicapped and nonhandicapped preschool children. *Journal of Speech and Hearing Disorders, 52,* 200–211.

Goldstein, H., & Mousetis, L. (1989). Generalized language learning by children with severe mental retardation: Effects of peers' expressive modeling. *Journal of Applied Behavior Analysis, 22,* 245–259.

Goldstein, H., & Wickstrom, S. (1986). Peer intervention effects on communicative interaction among handicapped and nonhandicapped preschoolers. *Journal of Applied Behavior Analysis, 19,* 209–214.

Gray, B., & Ryan, B. (1971). *Programmed conditioning for language: Program book.* Monterey, CA: Monterey Learning Systems.

Gray, B., & Ryan, B. (1973). *A language program for the nonlanguage child.* Champaign, IL: The Research Press.

Guess, D. (1969). A functional analysis of receptive language and productive speech. *Journal of Applied Behavior Analysis, 2,* 55–64.

Guess, D., & Baer, D. M. (1973). Some experimental analyses of linguistic development in institutionalized retarded children. In B. B. Lahey (Ed.), *The modification of language behavior* (pp. 3–60). Springfield, IL: Charles C. Thomas.

Guess, D., Sailor, W., Rutherford, G., & Baer, D. M. (1968). An experimental analysis of linguistic development: The productive use of the plural morpheme. *Journal of Applied Behavior Analysis, 1,* 225–235.

Halvorson, J. (1971). The effect on stuttering frequency of pairing punishment (response cost) with reinforcement. *Journal of Speech and Hearing Research, 14,* 356–364.

Harris, S. L., Handleman, J. S., & Alessandri, M. (1990). Teaching youth with autism to offer assistance. *Journal of Applied Behavior Analysis, 23,* 297-305.

Hart, B. M. (1985). Naturalistic language training techniques. In S. F. Warren & A. K. Rogers-Warren (Eds.), *Teaching functional language* (pp. 63–88). Austin, TX: PRO-ED.

Hegde, M. N. (1980). An experimental–clinical analysis of grammatical and behavioral distinctions between verbal auxiliary and copula. *Journal of Speech and Hearing Research, 23,* 864–877.

Hegde, M. N. (1985). Treatment of fluency disorders: State of the art. In J. M. Costello (Ed.), *Speech disorders in adults: Recent advances* (pp. 155–188). Austin, TX: PRO-ED.

Hegde, M. N. (1987). *Clinical research in communicative disorders: Principles and strategies.* Austin, TX: PRO-ED.

Hegde, M. N. (1988). Principles of management and remediation. In N. J. Lass, L. V. McReynolds, J. L. Northern, & D. F. Yoder (Eds.), *Handbook of speech–language pathology* (pp. 377–394). Toronto: Decker.

Hegde, M. N., & Gierut, J. (1979). The operant training and generalization of pronouns and a verb form in a language delayed child. *Journal of Communication Disorders, 12,* 23–34.

Hegde, M. N., & Heidt, S. (1990). The independent and interactive effects of rate reduction and airflow in stuttering treatment. In L. B. Olswang, C. K. Thompson, S. F. Warren, & N. J. Minghetti (Eds.), *Treatment efficacy research in communication disorders* (pp. 125–138). Washington, DC: American Speech–Language–Hearing Foundation.

Hegde, M. N., & McConn, J. (1981). Language training: Some data on response classes and generalization to an occupational setting. *Journal of Speech and Hearing Disorders, 46,* 353–358.

Hegde, M. N., Noll, M. J., & Pecora, R. (1979). A study of some factors affecting generalization of language training. *Journal of Speech and Hearing Disorders, 44,* 301–320.

Hegde, M. N., & Parson, D. (1990). The relative effects of Type I and Type II punishment on stuttering. In L. B. Olswang, C. K. Thompson, S. F. Warren, & N. J. Minghetti (Eds.), *Treatment efficacy research in communication disorders* (p. 251). Washington, DC: American Speech–Language–Hearing Foundation.

Holland, J. C., & Skinner, B. F. (1961). *The analysis of behavior.* New York: McGraw-Hill.

Hurlbut, B. I., Iwata, B. A., & Green, J. D. (1982). Nonvocal language acquisition in adolescents with severe physical disabilities: Blissymbol versus iconic stimulus formats. *Journal of Applied Behavior Analysis, 15,* 241–258.

Ingham, R. J. (1984). *Stuttering and behavior therapy: Current status and experimental foundations.* Austin, TX: PRO-ED.

Iwata, B. A. (1987). Negative reinforcement in applied behavior analysis: An emerging technology. *Journal of Applied Behavior Analysis, 20,* 361–387.

Iwata, B. A., Pace, G. M., Cowdery, G. E., Kalsher, M. J., & Cataldo, M. F. (1990). Experimental analysis and extinction of self-injurious escape behavior. *Journal of Applied Behavior Analysis, 23,* 11–27.

Iwata, B. A., Vollmer, T. R., & Zarcone, J. H. (1990). The experimental (functional) analysis of behavior disorders: Methodology, applications, and limitations. In A. C. Repp & N. N. Singh (Eds.), *Perspectives on the use of aversive and nonaversive interventions for persons with developmental disabilities* (pp. 301–330). Sycamore, IL: Sycamore.

Jackson, D. A., & Wallace, R. F. (1974). The modification and generalization of voice loudness in a fifteen-year-old retarded girl. *Journal of Applied Behavior Analysis, 7,* 461–471.

James, J. E. (1981). Behavioral self-control of stuttering using time-out from speaking. *Journal of Applied Behavior Analysis, 14,* 25–37.

Jung, J. H. (1989). *Genetic syndromes in communication disorders.* Austin, TX: PRO-ED.

Kalish, H. I. (1981). *From behavioral science to behavior modification*. New York: McGraw-Hill.

Kazdin, A. E. (1984). *Behavior modification in applied settings* (3rd ed.) Homewood, IL: The Dorsey Press.

Keller, M., & Bucher, B. (1979). Transfer between receptive and productive language in developmentally disabled children. *Journal of Applied Behavior Analysis, 12*, 311.

Koegel, R. L., Koegel, L. K., & Ingham, J. C. (1986). Programming rapid generalization of correct articulation through self-monitoring procedures. *Journal of Speech and Hearing Disorders, 51*, 24–32.

Koegel, R. L., Koegel, L. K., Voy, K. V., & Ingham, J. C. (1988). Within-clinic versus outside-of-clinic self-monitoring of articulation to promote generalization. *Journal of Speech and Hearing Disorders, 53*, 392–399.

Koegel, R., & Rincover, A. (1977). Research on the difference between generalization and maintenance in extra-therapy responding. *Journal of Applied Behavior Analysis, 10*, 1–12.

Lane, H. L. (1964). Differential reinforcement of vocal duration. *Journal of the Experimental Analysis of Behavior, 7*, 107–115.

Laski, K. E., Charlop, M. H., & Schreibman, L. (1988). Training parents to use the natural language paradigm to increase their autistic children's speech. *Journal of Applied Behavior Analysis, 21*, 391–400.

Lenneberg, E. H. (1967). *Biological foundations of language*. New York: Wiley.

Lerner, J., Dawson, D., & Horvath, L. (1980). *Cases in learning and behavior problems: A guide to individualized education programs*. Boston: Houghton Mifflin.

Linscheid, T. R., & Meinhold, P. (1990). The controversy over aversives: Basic operant research and the side effects of punishment. In A. C. Repp & N. N. Singh (Eds.), *Perspectives on the use of aversive and nonaversive interventions for persons with developmental disabilities* (pp. 435–450). Sycamore, IL: Sycamore.

Lovaas, I. O. (1966). A program for the establishment of speech in psychotic children. In J. K. Wing (Ed.), *Early childhood autism*. London: Pergamon.

Luiselli, J. K. (1990). Recent developments in nonaversive treatment: A review of rationale, methods and recommendations. In A. C. Repp & N. N. Singh (Eds.), *Perspectives on the use of aversive and nonaversive interventions for persons with developmental disabilities* (pp. 73–86). Sycamore, IL: Sycamore.

Mace, C. F., Hock, M., Lalli, J. S., West, B. J., Belfiore, P., Pinter, E., & Brown, D. K. (1988). Behavioral momentum in the treatment of noncompliance. *Journal of Applied Behavior Analysis, 21*, 123–141.

Martin, R. R., & Haroldson, S. K. (1988). An experimental increase in stuttering frequency. *Journal of Speech and Hearing Research, 31*, 272–274.

Martin, R. R., Kuhl, P., & Haroldson, S. K. (1972). An experimental treatment with two preschool children. *Journal of Speech and Hearing Research, 15*, 743–752.

Matson, J. L., & DiLorenzo, T. M. (1984). *Punishment and its alternatives*. New York: Springer.

Matson, J. L., Esveldt-Dawson, K., & O'Donnell, D. (1979). Overcorrection, modeling and reinforcement procedures for reinstating speech in a mute boy. *Child Behavior Therapy, 1*, 363–371.

Matson, J. L., Sevin, J. A., Fridley D., & Love, S. R. (1990). Increasing spontaneous language in three autistic children. *Journal of Applied Behavior Analysis, 23,* 227–234.

McCormick, L., & Schiefelbusch, R. L. (1990). *Early language intervention: An introduction* (2nd ed.). Columbus, OH: Merrill.

McDonald, J. D., & Blott, J. P. (1974). Environmental language intervention: The rationale for diagnostic training strategy through rules, context, and generalization. *Journal of Speech and Hearing Disorders, 39,* 244–256.

McDonald, J. D., & Gillette, Y. (1986). Communicating with persons with severe handicaps: Roles of parents and professionals. *Journal of the Association for the Severely Handicapped, 11*(4), 225–265.

McNeil, D. (1970). *The acquisition of language.* New York: Harper & Row.

McReynolds, L. V. (Ed.). (1974). *Developing systematic procedures for training children's language.* Rockville, MD: American Speech–Language–Hearing Association, ASHA Monographs no. 18.

McReynolds, L. V., & Elbert, M. F. (1981). Generalization of correct articulation in clusters. *Applied Psycholinguistics, 2,* 119–132.

McReynolds, L. V., & Engmann, D. L. (1974). An experimental analysis of the relationship between subject noun and object noun phrases. In L. V. McReynolds (Ed.), *Developing systematic procedures for training children's language* (ASHA Monograph no. 18, pp. 30–46). Rockville, MD: American Speech–Language–Hearing Association.

McReynolds, L. V., & Kearns, K. P. (1983). *Single-subject experimental designs in communicative disorders.* Baltimore: University Park Press.

Merbaum, M. (1973). The modification of self-destructive behavior by a mother–therapist using aversive stimulation. *Behavior Therapy, 4,* 442–447.

Moore, J. C., & Holbrook, A. (1971). The operant manipulation of vocal pitch in normal speakers. *Journal of Speech and Hearing Research, 14,* 283–290.

Mowrer, D. E. (1977). *Methods of modifying speech behaviors.* Columbus, OH: Merrill.

Nelson, K. E. (1977). Facilitating children's syntax acquisition. *Developmental Psychology, 13,* 101–107.

Newsom, C., Favell, J. E., & Rincover, A. (1983). Side effects of punishment. In S. Axelrod & J. Apsche (Eds.), *The effects of punishment on human behavior* (pp. 285–316). New York: Academic Press.

Odom, S. L., & Karnes, M. B. (Eds.). (1988). *Early intervention for infants and children with handicaps.* Baltimore: Brooks.

Onslow, M., Costa, L., & Rue, S. (1990). Direct early intervention with stuttering: Some preliminary data. *Journal of Speech and Hearing Disorders, 55,* 405–416.

Owens, R. E. (1988). *Language development: An introduction.* Columbus, OH: Merrill.

Patterson, G. R. (1976). The aggressive child: Victim and architect of a coersive system. In E. J. Mash, L. J. Hamerlynck, & L. C. Handy (Eds.), *Behavior modification and families* (pp. 267–316). New York: Brunner/Mazel.

Patterson, R. L., Teigen, J. R., Liberman, R. P., & Austin, N. K. (1975). Increasing speech intensity of chronic patients ("mumblers") by shaping techniques. *The Journal of Nervous and Mental Diseases, 160,* 182–187.

Paul, L. (1985). Programming peer support for functional language. In S. F. Warren & A. K. Rogers-Warren (Eds.), *Teaching functional language* (pp. 290–307). Austin, TX: PRO-ED.

Pazulinec, R., Meyerrose, M., & Sajwaj, T. (1983). Punishment via response cost. In

S. Axelrod & J. Apsche (Eds.), *The effects of punishment on human behavior* (pp. 71–86). New York: Academic Press.

Peck, C. A., Killen, C. C., & Baumgart, D. (1989). Increasing implementation of special education instruction in mainstream preschools: Direct and generalized effects of nondirective consultation. *Journal of Applied Behavior Analysis, 22,* 197–210.

Peterson, H. A., & Marquardt, T. M. (1990). *Appraisal and diagnosis of speech and language disorders* (2nd ed.). Englewood Cliffs, NJ: Prentice-Hall.

Prins, D., & Hubbard, C. P. (1988). Response contingent stimuli and stuttering: Issues and implications. *Journal of Speech and Hearing Research, 31,* 696–709.

Pyles, D. A. M., & Bailey, J. S. (1990). Diagnosing severe behavior problems. In A. C. Repp & N. N. Singh (Eds.), *Perspectives on the use of aversive and nonaversive interventions for persons with developmental disabilities* (pp. 381–402). Sycamore, IL: Sycamore.

Remington, B., & Clark, S. (1983). Acquisition of expressive signing by autistic children: An evaluation of the relative effects of simultaneous communication and sign-alone training. *Journal of Applied Behavior Analysis, 16,* 315–328.

Repp, A. C., & Karsh, K. G. (1990). A taxonomic approach to the nonaversive treatment of maladaptive behavior of persons with developmental disabilities. In A. C. Repp & N. N. Singh (Eds.), *Perspectives on the use of aversive and nonaversive interventions for persons with developmental disabilities* (pp. 332–347). Sycamore, IL: Sycamore.

Repp, A. C., & Singh, N. N. (Eds.). (1990). *Perspectives on the use of aversive and nonaversive interventions for persons with developmental disabilities.* Sycamore, IL: Sycamore.

Rheingold, H. L., Gewirtz, J. L., & Ross, H. Q. (1959). Social conditioning of vocalizations in the infant. *Journal of Comparative and Physiological Psychology, 52,* 65–72.

Rolider, A., & Van Houten, R. (1990). The role of reinforcement in reducing inappropriate behavior: Some myths and misconceptions. In A. C. Repp & N. N. Singh (Eds.), *Perspectives on the use of aversive and nonaversive interventions for persons with developmental disabilities* (pp. 119–127). Sycamore, IL: Sycamore.

Roll, D. R. (1973). Modification of nasal resonance in cleft-palate children by informative feedback. *Journal of Applied Behavior Analysis, 6,* 397–403.

Rossetti, M. (1986). *High-risk infants: Identification, assessment, and intervention.* Austin, TX: PRO-ED.

Rossetti, M. (1990). *Infant–toddler assessment: An interdisciplinary approach.* Austin: TX: PRO-ED.

Ryan, B. P. (1974). *Programmed therapy for stuttering in children and adults.* Springfield, IL: Charles C. Thomas.

Sailor, W., Guess, D., Rutherford, G., & Baer, D. M. (1968). Control of tantrum behavior by operant techniques during experimental verbal training. *Journal of Applied Behavior Analysis, 1,* 237–243.

Schumaker, J., & Sherman, J. A. (1970). Training generative verb usage by imitation and reinforcement procedures. *Journal of Applied Behavior Analysis, 3,* 273-287.

Schumaker, J., & Sherman, J. A. (1978). Parents as intervention agents. In R. L. Schiefelbusch (Ed.), *Language intervention strategies* (pp. 237–326). Baltimore: University Park Press.

REFERENCES

Schwartz, M. L., & Hawkins, R. P. (1970). Application of delayed reinforcement procedures to the behavior of an elementary school child. *Journal of Applied Behavior Analysis, 3,* 85–96.

Scott, R. R., Himadi, W., & Keane, T. (1983). A review of generalization in social skills training: Suggestions for future research. In M. Hersen, R. M. Eisler, & P. M. Miller (Eds.), *Progress in behavior modification* (Vol. 15, pp. 114–172). New York: Academic Press.

Shames, G. H., & Florence, C. L. (1980). *Stutter-free speech: A goal for therapy.* Columbus, OH: Merrill

Shipley, K. G., & Banis, C. (1981). *Teaching morphology developmentally.* Tucson, AZ: Communication Skill Builders.

Singh, N. N., Dawson, M. J., & Manning, P. (1981). Effects of spaced responding DRL on the stereotyped behavior of profoundly retarded persons. *Journal of Applied Behavior Analysis, 14,* 521–526.

Skinner, B. F. (1953). *Science and human behavior.* New York: Macmillan.

Skinner, B. F. (1957). *Verbal behavior.* New York: Appleton-Century-Crofts.

Skinner, B. F. (1969). *Contingencies of reinforcement: A theoretical analysis.* New York: Appleton-Century-Crofts.

Skinner, B. F. (1974). *About behaviorism.* New York: Vintage Books.

Skinner, B. F. (1989). *Recent issues in the analysis of behavior.* Columbus, OH: Merrill.

Skinner, B. F. (1990). Can psychology be a science of mind? *American Psychologist, 45,* 1206–1210.

Stoel-Gammon, C., & Dunn, C. (1985). *Normal and disordered phonology in children.* Austin, TX: PRO-ED.

Stokes, T. M., & Baer, D. M. (1977). An implicit technology of generalization. *Journal of Applied Behavior Analysis, 10,* 349–367.

Thompson, C. K., & McReynolds, L. V. (1986). *Wh* interrogative production in agrammatic aphasia: An experimental analysis of auditory–visual stimulation and direct-production treatment. *Journal of Speech and Hearing Research, 29,* 193–206.

Till, J. A., & Yoye, A. (1988). Acoustic phonetic effects of two types of verbal feedback in dysarthric subjects. *Journal of Speech and Hearing Disorders, 53,* 449–458.

Todd, G. A., & Palmer, B. (1968). Social reinforcement of infant babbling. *Child Development, 39,* 591–596.

Van Houten, R. (1983). Punishment: From the animal laboratory to the applied setting. In S. Axelrod & J. Apsche (Eds.), *The effects of punishment on human behavior* (pp. 13–44). New York: Academic Press.

Wacker, D. P., Steege, M. V., Northrup, J., Sasso, G., Berg, W., Reimers, T., Cooper, L., Cigrand, K., & Donn, L. (1990). A component analysis of functional communication training across three topographies of severe behavior problems. *Journal of Applied Behavior Analysis, 23,* 417–429.

Wacker, D. P., Wiggins, B., Fowler, M., & Berg, W. K. (1988). Training students with profound or multiple handicaps to make requests via microswitches. *Journal of Applied Behavior Analysis, 21,* 331–344.

Wambaugh, J. L., & Thompson, C. K. (1989). Training and generalization of agrammatic aphasic adults' *Wh*–interrogative productions. *Journal of Speech and Hearing Disorders, 54,* 509–529.

Warren, S. F., & Bambara, L. M. (1989). An experimental analysis of milieu language intervention: Teaching the action-object form. *Journal of Speech & Hearing Disorders, 54,* 448–461.

Warren, S. F., & Kaiser, A. P. (1986). Incidental language teaching: A critical review. *Journal of Speech & Hearing Disorders, 51,* 291–299.

Weisberg, P. (1961). Social and nonsocial conditioning of infant vocalizations. *Child Development, 34,* 377–388.

Weismer, S. E., & Murray-Branch, J. (1989). Modeling versus modeling plus evoked production training: A comparison of two language intervention methods. *Journal of Speech & Hearing Disorders, 54,* 269–281.

Welch, S. (1981). Teaching generative grammar to mentally retarded children: A review and analysis of a decade of behavioral research. *Mental Retardation, 19,* 277–284.

Whitney, J. L., & Goldstein, H. (1990). Using self-monitoring to reduce disfluencies in connected speech of speakers with minimal aphasia. In L. B. Olswang, C. K. Thompson, S. F. Warren, & N. J. Minghetti (Eds.), *Treatment efficacy research in communication disorders* (p. 246). Washington, DC: American Speech–Language–Hearing Foundation.

Williams, G. C., & McReynolds, L. V. (1975). The relationship between discrimination and articulation training in children with misarticulation. *Journal of Speech and Hearing Research, 18,* 401–412.

Winokur, S. (1976). *A primer of verbal behavior: An operant view.* Englewood Cliffs, NJ: Prentice-Hall.

Author Index

Subject Index

317